Lung Cancer and Imaging

IPEM–IOP Series in Physics and Engineering in Medicine and Biology

About the Series

The Series in Physics and Engineering in Medicine and Biology will allow IPEM to enhance its mission to 'advance physics and engineering applied to medicine and biology for the public good'.

Focusing on key areas including, but not limited to:

- clinical engineering
- diagnostic radiology
- informatics and computing
- magnetic resonance imaging
- nuclear medicine
- physiological measurement
- radiation protection
- radiotherapy
- rehabilitation engineering
- ultrasound and non-ionizing radiation.

A number of IPEM–IOP titles are published as part of the EUTEMPE Network Series for Medical Physics Experts.

Lung Cancer and Imaging

Edited by
Ayman El-Baz
University of Louisville, KY, USA

Jasjit S Suri
AtheroPoint, CA, USA

IOP Publishing, Bristol, UK

ISBN 978-0-7503-2540-0 (ebook)
ISBN 978-0-7503-2538-7 (print)
ISBN 978-0-7503-2541-7 (myPrint)
ISBN 978-0-7503-2539-4 (mobi)

DOI 10.1088/978-0-7503-2540-0

Version: 20191201

IOP ebooks

British Library Cataloguing-in-Publication Data: A catalogue record for this book is available from the British Library.

Published by IOP Publishing, wholly owned by The Institute of Physics, London

IOP Publishing, Temple Circus, Temple Way, Bristol, BS1 6HG, UK

US Office: IOP Publishing, Inc., 190 North Independence Mall West, Suite 601, Philadelphia, PA 19106, USA

With love and affection to my mother and father, whose loving spirit sustains me still.

—Ayman El-Baz

To my late loving parents, immediate family, and children.

—Jasjit S Suri

Contents

Preface

This book covers the state-of-the-art automated non-invasive approaches for the early detection of lung cancer. Lung cancer is the second most common cancer in men and women all over the world, after prostate cancer in men and after breast cancer in women. Moreover, it is considered the leading cause of cancer-related death among both genders in the USA, as the number of people who die each year of lung cancer is greater than the number of people who die of breast and prostate cancers combined. Early detection of lung cancer increases the chances of patient survival, which increases the motivation to develop accurate and fast diagnostic tools to detect lung cancer earlier.

Although resection of pulmonary nodules is the ideal and a reliable method of diagnosis, there is a crucial need for developing a non-invasive diagnostic tool to eliminate the risks associated with this surgical procedure. There are several imaging modalities that could be used to non-invasively diagnose pulmonary nodules, e.g. chest radiography (x-ray) and computed tomography (CT) scans, which will be discussed in the book. Among the topics discussed in the book are lung nodule classification approaches using 3D convolutional neural networks (3D-CNNs) and capsule networks (CapsNets). Lung cancer epidemiology, biomarkers, radiomics, and photodynamic diagnosis are also explained. Moreover, this book presents studies involving synergetic therapy, exhaled aerosol fingerprints, ground-glass opacity (GGO) nodules, and electromagnetic imaging.

In summary, the main aim of this book is to help advance scientific research within the broad field of early detection of lung cancer. The book focuses on major trends and challenges in this area, and presents work aimed at identifying new techniques and their use in biomedical analysis.

Ayman El-Baz
Jasjit S Suri

Acknowledgements

The completion of this book would not have been possible without the participation and assistance of so many people whose names may not all be enumerated. Their contributions are sincerely appreciated and gratefully acknowledged. However, the editors would like to express their deep appreciation and indebtedness in particular to Dr Ali H Mahmoud and Kamal Hammouda for their endless support.

Ayman El-Baz
Jasjit S Suri

Editor Biographies

Ayman El-Baz

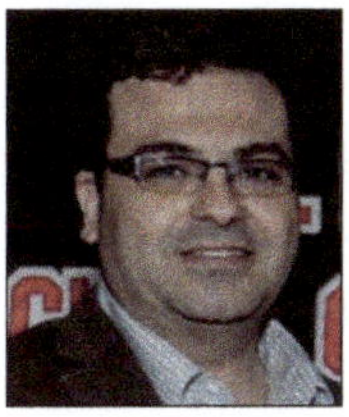

Ayman El-Baz is a Professor, University Scholar, and Chair of the Bioengineering Department at the University of Louisville, USA Dr El-Baz earned his BSc and MSc degrees in electrical engineering in 1997 and 2001, respectively. He earned his PhD in electrical engineering from the University of Louisville in 2006. In 2009, Dr El-Baz was named a Coulter Fellow for his contributions to the field of biomedical translational research. Dr El-Baz has 17 years of hands-on experience in the fields of bio-imaging modeling and non-invasive computer-assisted diagnosis systems. He has authored or co-authored more than 500 technical articles (141 journals, 25 books, 78 book chapters, 225 refereed-conference papers, 171 abstracts, and 30 US patents and disclosures).

Jasjit S Suri

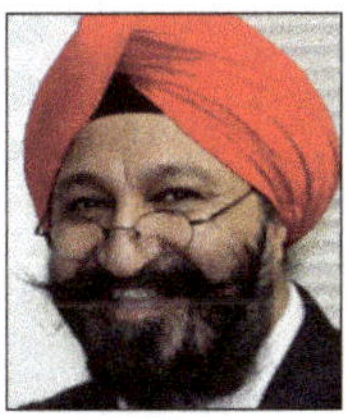

Jasjit S Suri is an innovator, scientist, visionary, industrialist, and an internationally known world leader in biomedical engineering. Dr Suri has spent over 25 years in the field of biomedical engineering/devices and management. He received his PhD from the University of Washington, Seattle and his Business Management Sciences degree from Weatherhead, Case Western Reserve University, Cleveland, OH. Dr Suri was awarded the President's Gold medal in 1980 and made a Fellow of the American Institute of Medical and Biological Engineering for his outstanding contributions. In 2018, he was awarded the Marquis Life Time Achievement Award for his outstanding contributions and dedication to medical imaging and its management.

Contributors

Heidi Abrahamse
Laser Research Centre, Faculty of Health Sciences, University of Johannesburg, Doornfontein, South Africa

Hadil Abu Khalifeh
Chemical Engineering Department, Abu Dhabi University, Abu Dhabi, UAE

Anine Crous
Laser Research Centre, Faculty of Health Sciences, University of Johannesburg, Doornfontein, South Africa

Filippo Del Grande
Clinica di Radiologia EOC, Istituto di Imaging della Svizzera Italiana (IIMSI), Lugano, Switzerland

Adel Elmaghraby
Computer Engineering and Computer Science Department, University of Louisville, KY, USA

Naveen Garg
University of Texas MD Anderson Cancer Center, Houston, TX, USA

Mohammed Ghazal
Department of Electrical and Computer Engineering, Abu Dhabi University, Abu Dhabi, UAE

Kazuhiko Hamamoto
Tokai University, School of Information and Telecommunication Engineering, Tokai University, Tokyo, Japan

Iqra
Microbiology and Biotechnology Research Lab, Fatima Jinnah Women University, Rawalpindi, Pakistan

Wentong Li
Department of Pathology, Weifang Medical University, Weifang, Shandong, China
Shandong Engineering Research Center for Smart Materials and Regenerative Medicine, Weifang, Shandong, China

Chung-Ming Lo
Graduate Institute of Library, Information and Archival Studies, National Chengchi University, Taipei City, Taiwan

Ali Mahmoud
BioImaging Laboratory, Bioengineering Department, University of Louisville, KY, USA

Saima Shakil Malik
Microbiology and Biotechnology Research Lab, Fatima Jinnah Women University, Rawalpindi, Pakistan

Nosheen Masood
Microbiology and Biotechnology Research Lab, Fatima Jinnah Women University, Rawalpindi, Pakistan

Aryan Mobiny
Department of Electrical and Computer Engineering, University of Houston, TX, USA

Supratik Moulik
Triradiate Industries, Sugar Land, TX, USA

Hien V Nguyen
Department of Electrical and Computer Engineering, University of Houston, Houston, TX, USA

May Phu Paing
Faculty of Engineering, King Mongkut's Institute of Technology Ladkrabang, Bangkok, Thailand

Francesco Petrella
Department of Thoracic Surgery, IEO European Institute of Oncology IRCCS, Milan, Italy

Chuchart Pintavirooj
Faculty of Engineering, King Mongkut's Institute of Technology Ladkrabang, Bangkok, Thailand

Stefania Rizzo
Clinica di Radiologia EOC, Istituto di Imaging della Svizzera Italiana (IIMSI), Lugano, Switzerland

Ahmed Shaffie
BioImaging Laboratory, Bioengineering Department, University of Louisville, KY, USA

Xiuhua April Si
Department of Aerospace, Industrial, and Mechanical Engineering, California Baptist University, Riverside, CA, USA

Ahmed Soliman
BioImaging Laboratory, Bioengineering Department, University of Louisville, KY, USA

Fatma Taher
College of Technological Innovation, Zayed University, Dubai, UAE

Meng-Hua Tao
Department of Biostatistics and Epidemiology, University of North Texas Health Science Center, Fort Worth, TX, USA

Supan Tungjitkusolmun
Faculty of Engineering, King Mongkut's Institute of Technology Ladkrabang, Bangkok, Thailand

Lulu Wang
Shenzhen Technology University, Pingshan District, Shenzhen Guangdong, China

Carol C Wu
University of Texas MD Anderson Cancer Center, Houston, TX, USA

Jinxiang Xi
Biomedical Engineering, University of Massachusetts, Lowell, MA, USA

Hongli Yu
College of Pharmacy, Weifang Medical University, Weifang, Shandong, China
Shandong Engineering Research Center for Smart Materials and Regenerative Medicine, Weifang, Shandong, China

Weifen Zhang
College of Pharmacy, Weifang Medical University, Weifang, Shandong, China
Shandong Engineering Research Center for Smart Materials and Regenerative Medicine, Weifang, Shandong, China

IOP Publishing

Lung Cancer and Imaging

Ayman El-Baz and Jasjit S Suri

Chapter 1

Early diagnosis system for lung nodules based on the integration of a higher-order MGRF appearance feature model and 3D-CNN

Ahmed Shaffie, Ahmed Soliman, Ali Mahmoud, Hadil Abu Khalifeh, Fatma Taher, Mohammed Ghazal, Adel Elmaghraby and Ayman El-Baz

Lung cancer is a leading cause of death by cancer for both men and women worldwide, which is why creating systems for early diagnosis with machine learning algorithms and nominal user intervention is of huge importance. In this chapter, a new system for lung nodule diagnosis, using features extracted from one computed tomography (CT) scan, is presented. To obtain an accurate diagnosis of the detected lung nodules, the proposed framework integrates the following two groups of features: (i) appearance features that are modeled using a higher-order Markov–Gibbs random field (MGRF) model that has the ability to describe the spatial inhomogeneities inside the lung nodule and (ii) local features that are extracted using 3D convolutional neural networks (3D-CNN) because of their ability to exploit the spatial correlation of input data in an efficient way. The novelty of this chapter is accurately modeling the appearance of the detected lung nodules using a newly developed seventh-order MGRF model that has the ability to model the existing spatial inhomogeneities for both small and large detected lung nodules, in addition to the integration with the extracted local features from 3D-CNN. Finally, a deep autoencoder (AE) classifier is fed by the above two feature groups to distinguish between malignant and benign nodules. To evaluate the proposed framework, we used the publicly available data from the Lung Image Database Consortium (LIDC). We used a total of 727 nodules that were collected from 467 patients. The proposed system's diagnostic accuracy, sensitivity, and specificity were 92.90%, 91.39%, and 94.04% respectively. The proposed framework demonstrated its promise as a valuable tool for lung cancer detection, evidenced by its higher accuracy.

1.1 Introduction

Lung cancer is the main cause of cancer-related mortality not only in the United States but all over the world. Its rate is increasing, despite the extraordinary evolution of imaging devices and hospital care, because it is usually diagnosed at the late stages. Lung cancer is the second most common cancer in men and women, after prostate cancer in men and after breast cancer in women. Moreover, it is considered the leading cause of cancer-related death among both genders in the USA, as the number of people who die each year of lung cancer is greater than the number of people who die of breast and prostate cancers combined [1]. The number of patients suffering from lung cancer has recently increased significantly all over the world, which increases the motivation to develop accurate and fast diagnostic tools to detect lung cancer earlier in order to increase the patient survival rate. Lung nodules are the first indication to start diagnosing lung cancer. Lung nodules can be benign (normal subjects) or malignant (cancerous subjects). Figure 1.1 shows some samples of benign and malignant lung nodules.

Histological examination through biopsies is considered the gold standard for the final diagnosis of pulmonary nodules as malignant or benign. Even though the resection of pulmonary nodules is the ideal and most reliable method of diagnosis, there is a crucial need to develop non-invasive diagnostic tools to eliminate the risks associated with this surgical procedure.

In general, several imaging modalities are used to diagnose pulmonary nodules, such as chest radiography (x-ray), magnetic resonance imaging (MRI), positron emission tomography (PET), and computed tomography (CT) scans. Some researchers prefer to use MRI to avoid exposing the patient to ionizing radiation, which can have very bad effects and has the potential to increase lifetime cancer risk [2]. Diffusion weighted MRI (DW-MRI) has been reported as being used for lung cancer diagnosis, as it can be used to qualitatively check high b-value images and apparent diffusion coefficient (ADC) maps, in addition to quantitatively generating the mean and median tumor ADCs [3]. However, CT and PET scans are the most widely used modalities for diagnosis and staging of lung cancer. A CT scan is more

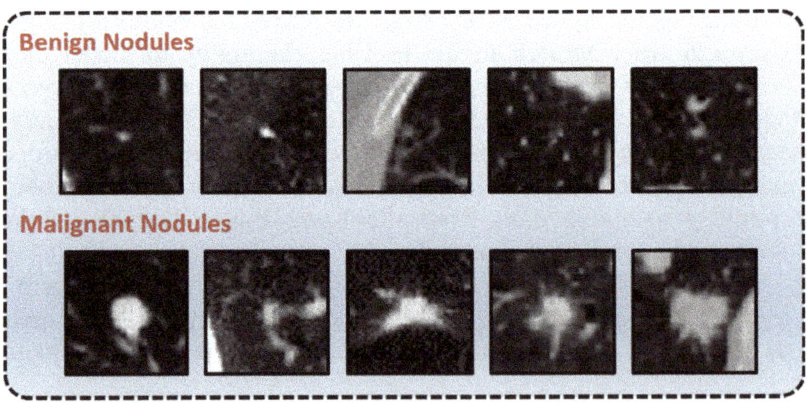

Figure 1.1. Sample 2D axial projection for benign (top row) and malignant (bottom row) lung nodules.

likely to show lung tumors than other modalities because of its high resolution and clear contrast compared to the other modalities. It can also show the size, shape, and accurate position of any lung tumor. We will focus on and utilize CT scans in our study as this is considered a routine procedure for patients who have lung cancer, in addition to its ability to provide high resolution pulmonary anatomical details.

Recently, a lot of researchers have tried to develop computer aided diagnostic (CAD) systems to classify the detected lung nodules to detect lung cancer earlier. Sun *et al* [4] studied the feasibility of using deep learning algorithms for benign/malignant classification on the Lung Image Database Consortium (LIDC) dataset. Radiologists provided marks that they used to segment the nodules on each CT slice. After rotating and down-sampling, they collected 174 412 samples with 52-by-52 pixels each and the corresponding ground truth. They designed and implemented three deep learning algorithms called the deep belief networks (DBNs), convolutional neural network (CNN), and stacked denoising autoencoder (SDAE). They compared the performance of deep learning algorithms to traditional computer aided diagnostic (CADx) systems by designing a scheme with 28 image features and a support vector machine (SVM). The accuracies of CNN, SDAE, and DBNs were 0.7976, 0.7929, and 0.8119, respectively; the accuracy of their designed traditional CADx was 0.7940, which was lower than DBNs and CNN. Shen *et al* [5] studied the problem of classification of lung nodules as benign or malignant using CT images. They focused on modeling raw nodule patches without any prior definition of nodule morphology. They proposed a hierarchical learning framework based on multi-scale convolutional neural networks (MCNNs), to capture nodule heterogeneity by extracting discriminative features from alternatingly stacked layers. Their framework used multi-scale nodule patches to learn a set of known features simultaneously by concatenating response neuron activations obtained at the last layer from each input scale. They evaluated the proposed method on CT images from the LIDC dataset, which provides nodule annotations as being benign or malignant. Likhitka *et al* [6] proposed a framework modeled in four steps: image enhancement, segmentation, feature extraction, and classification. For lung nodule diagnosis, they used the nodule size, nodule spine values, structure, and volume as input features for the SVM classifier to distinguish between benign and malignant nodules. An unsupervised spectral clustering algorithm has been studied by Weia *et al* [7] to classify benign and malignant nodules. They constructed a new Laplacian matrix in their algorithm using local kernel regression models (LKRM) and incorporating a regularization term, which can deal with the out-of-sample problem. To verify the accuracy of their algorithm, they assembled a ground truth dataset from the LIDC dataset including 375 malignant and 371 benign lung nodules. Another study by Nishio *et al* [8] analyzed 73 lung nodules from 60 sets of CT images. They performed contrast-enhanced CT in 46 CT examinations. They used images from the LUNGx Challenge, which does not have the ground truth of the nodules; this is why radiologists constructed a surrogate ground truth. Their method was based on novel patch-based feature extraction using principal component analysis, pooling operations, and image convolution. They compared their method to three other systems for the extraction of nodule features: histogram of CT density, three-dimensional random local binary pattern, and local binary pattern on three orthogonal planes. They analyzed the probabilistic outputs of the systems and surrogate ground truth using the receiver operating characteristic (ROC) curve and area under the curve (AUC). Given the ground truth, the AUCs were as follows: histogram of CT density, 0.640; three-dimensional random local binary pattern, 0.725; and local binary pattern on three orthogonal planes, 0.688 and their method, 0.837. A set of handcrafted features has been used by Wang *et al* [9] to reduce the false positive rate and deep feature fusion for non-medical training. Their results show that the deep fusion feature can achieve sensitivity and specificity of 69.3% and 96.2% at 1.19 false positives per image compared to public datasets. Dhara *et al* [10] focused on the classification of benign and malignant nodules using an SVM-based CAD system. Nodules were segmented using a semi-automated technique, which needed only a seed point from the user. They computed shape-based, margin-based, and texture-based features to represent the nodules. They determined a set of relevant features as a second step for an efficient representation of nodules in the feature space. They validated their classification method on 891 nodules of the LIDC dataset. They evaluated the performance of the classification using the AUC. They obtained AUCs of 0.9505, 0.8822, and 0.8488, respectively, for three different configurations of datasets. Song *et al* [11] developed three types of deep neural networks (e.g. CNN, DNN, and SAE) for lung cancer calcification. They used those networks on the CT image classification task with some modification for the benign and malignant lung nodules. They evaluated those networks on the LIDC dataset. The experimental results showed that the CNN network reached the best performance with an accuracy of 84.15%, specificity of 84.32%, and sensitivity of 83.96%. Shewaye *et al* [12] proposed an automated system to diagnose benign or malignant nodules in CT images. The experimental results were illustrated using a combination of histogram and geometric lung nodule image features and different linear and nonlinear discriminant classifiers. They experimentally validated their proposed approach on the LIDC dataset. The classification results were 93% correctly classified as benign and 82% correctly classified as malignant of the test data. A fusion framework between PET and CT features has been proposed by Guo *et al* [13]. They applied SVM to train a vector of CT texture features and PET heterogeneity features to improve the diagnosis and staging of lung cancer. In their study they included 32 subjects with lung nodules (19 M, 13 F, age 70 ± 9 yr) who underwent PET/CT scans.

The existing methods for the classification of lung nodules have the following limitations: (i) some methods depend on the Hounsfield unit (HU) values as the appearance descriptor without taking any spatial interaction into consideration; (ii) most of the reported accuracy is low compared to the clinically accepted threshold; and (iii) some of the methods just depend on raw data and disregard the morphological information. The proposed framework overcomes the previously mentioned limitations through the integration of a novel appearance feature using a seventh-order Markov–Gibbs random field (MGRF) that takes into account 3D spatial interaction between the nodule's voxels and local features extracted from the segmented lung nodule using 3D-CNN, with the deep autoencoder to achieve high classification accuracy.

1.2 Methods

The proposed framework presents a new automated non-invasive clinical diagnostic system for the early detection of lung cancer by classification of the detected lung nodule as benign or malignant. It integrates appearance features and local information derived from a single computed tomography (CT) scan to significantly improve the accuracy, sensitivity, and specificity of early lung cancer diagnosis (figure 1.2). In the computed tomography markers method, two types of features are integrated (appearance and local features). The appearance feature is modeled using an MGRF model that is used to relate the joint probability of the nodule appearance and the energy of repeated patterns in the 3D scans in order to describe the spatial inhomogeneities in the lung nodule. The new higher seventh-order MGRF model is developed in order to have the ability to model the existing spatial inhomogeneities for both small and large detected pulmonary nodules. Local features are extracted from the segmented nodules using 3D-CNN to describe the pulmonary nodule local information. Details of the framework's main components are given below.

1.2.1 Appearance features using MGRF energy

The Hounsfield values' spatial distribution differs from benign nodules to malignant ones: the smoother the homogeneityof the nodule is, the more likely it is to be benign. Describing the visual appearance features using the MGRF model will distinguish between benign and malignant nodules showing highly distinctive features (see figure 1.3). To describe the texture appearance of pulmonary nodules, Gibbs energy values are calculated using the seventh-order MGRF model to distinguish between benign and malignant nodules, because the Gibbs energy values show the interaction between the voxels and their neighbors [14] (see figure 1.4). Let $\mathbb{Q} = \{0, \ldots, Q-1\}$ denote a finite set of signals (HU values) in the lung CT scan, $s: \mathbb{R}^3 \rightarrow \mathbb{Q}$, with signals $\mathbf{s} = [s(r): r = (x, y, z) \in \mathbb{R}^3]$. The interaction graph,

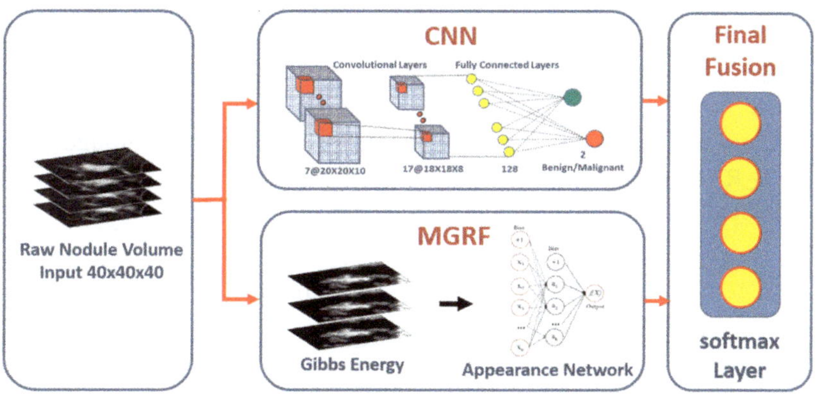

Figure 1.2. Lung nodule classification framework.

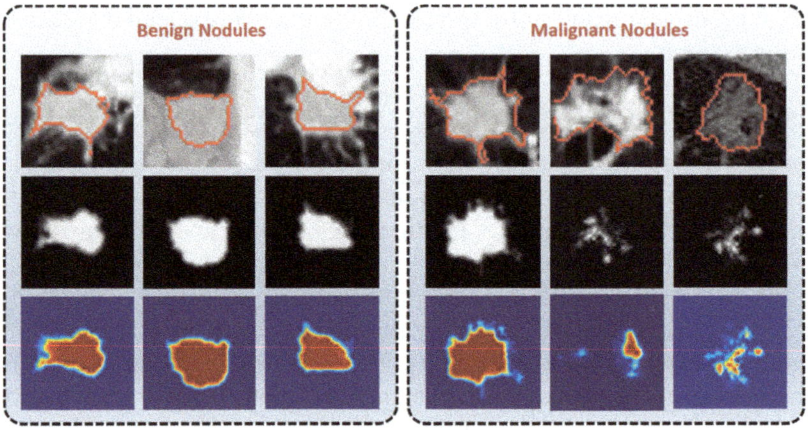

Figure 1.3. 2D axial projection for three benign and three malignant lung nodules (top row), along their calculated Gibbs energy (middle row), and their colormap visualization of the Gibbs energy (bottom row).

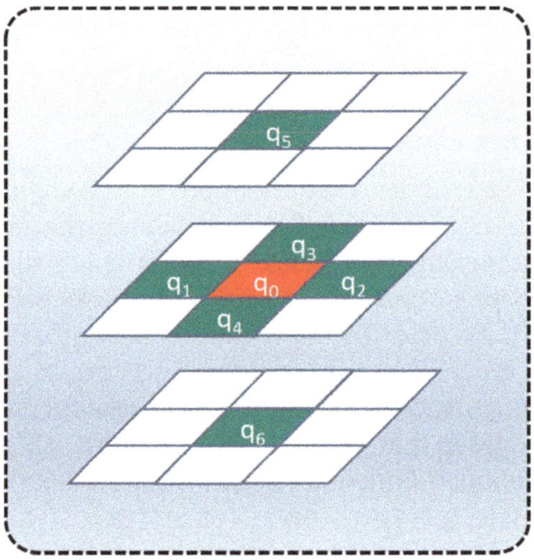

Figure 1.4. The seventh-order clique. Signals q_0, q_1,…, q_6 are at the central pixel and its six central-symmetric neighbors are at the radial distance r. Note that the selection of the neighborhood geometry takes into account the nodules sphericity.

$\Gamma = (\mathbb{R}^3, \mathbb{E})$, quantifies the signal probabilistic dependences in the images with nodes at voxels, $r \in \mathbb{R}^3$, that are connected with edges $(r, r') \in \mathbb{E} \subseteq \mathbb{R}^3 \times \mathbb{R}^3$. An MGRF of images is defined by a Gibbs probability distribution (GPD)

$$\boldsymbol{\Upsilon} = \left[\Upsilon(\mathbf{s}):\ \mathbf{s} \in \mathbb{Q}^{|\mathbb{R}|};\ \sum_{\mathbf{s}\in\mathbb{Q}^{|\mathbb{R}|}} \Upsilon(\mathbf{s}) = 1 \right] \tag{1.1}$$

factored over a set $\mathbb{C}$ of cliques in Γ supporting non-constant factors, logarithms of which are Gibbs potentials [15]. To make modeling more efficient at describing the visual appearance of different nodules in the lung CT scans, the seventh-order MGRF models the voxel's partial ordinal interaction within a radius r rather than modeling the pairwise interaction as in the second-order MGRF.

Let a translation-invariant seventh-order interaction structure on $\mathbb{R}$ be represented by A, $A \geqslant 1$, families, $\mathbb{C}_a$; $a = 1, \ldots, A$, of seventh-order cliques, $\mathbf{c}_{a:r} \in \mathbb{C}_a$, of the same shape and size. Every clique is associated with a certain voxel (origin), $r = (x, y, z) \in \mathbb{R}^3$, supporting the same (7)-variate scalar potential function, $V_a: \mathbb{Q}^7 \rightarrow (-\infty, \infty)$.

The Gibbs probability distribution for this contrast/offset-, and translation-invariant MGRF is

$$\Upsilon_7(\mathbf{s}) = \frac{1}{Z}\phi(\mathbf{s})\exp\left(-E_7(\mathbf{s})\right), \tag{1.2}$$

where $E_{7:a}(\mathbf{s}) = \sum_{\mathbf{c}_{a:r} \in \mathbb{C}_a} V_{7:a}(g(r')\colon r' \in \mathbf{c}_{a:r})$ and $E_7(\mathbf{s}) = \sum_{a=1}^{A} E_{7:a}(\mathbf{s})$ denote the Gibbs energy for each individual and all the clique families, respectively, Z is a normalization factor, while $\phi(\mathbf{s})$ is a core distribution. The calculated Gibbs energy, $E_7(\mathbf{s})$, will be used to discriminate between benign and malignant tissues and gives an indication of malignancy. While a high potential of malignancy is indicated by lower energy, a high potential to be benign is indicated by higher energy. To calculate $E_7(\mathbf{s})$, the Gibbs potentials for the seventh-order model are calculated using the maximum likelihood estimates (MLE) by generalizing the analytical approximation in [16, 17]:

$$V_{7:a}(\xi) = \frac{F_{7:a:\mathrm{core}}(\xi) - F_{7:a}(\xi|\mathbf{s}^\circ)}{F_{7:a:\mathrm{core}}(\xi)(1 - F_{7:a:\mathrm{core}}(\xi))}, \tag{1.3}$$

where $a = 1, \ldots, A$; $\xi \in \vartheta_7$, $\mathbf{s}^\circ$ denotes the training malignant nodule images, ξ denotes a numerical code of a particular seventh-order relation between the seven signals on the clique, ϑ_7 is a set of these codes for all seventh-order signal co-occurrences, $F_{7:a}(\mathbf{s}^\circ)$ is an empirical marginal probability of the relation ξ, $\xi \in \vartheta_7$, over the seventh-order clique family $\mathbb{C}_{7:a}$ for $\mathbf{s}^\circ$, and $F_{7:a:\mathrm{core}}(\xi)$ is the core probability distribution.

The proposed seventh-order MGRF appearance model is summarized in algorithm 1.

Algorithm 1. Learning the seventh-order MGRF appearance model.

1. Given training malignant nodules $\mathbf{g}^\circ$, find the empirical nodule ($l = 1$) and background ($l = 0$) probability distributions, $\mathbf{F}_{l:7:r}(\mathbf{g}^\circ) = [F_{l:7:r}(\beta|\mathbf{g}^\circ)\colon \beta \in \mathbb{B}]$ of the local binary pattern (LBP)-based descriptors for different clique sizes $r \in \{1, \ldots, r_{\max}\}$ where the top size $r_{\max} = 10$ in our experiments below.
2. Compute the empirical distributions $\mathbf{F}_{7:r:\mathrm{core}} = [F_{7:r:\mathrm{core}}(\beta)\colon \beta \in \mathbb{B}]$ of the same descriptors for the core independent random field (IRF) $\psi(\mathbf{g})$, e.g. for an image, sampled from the core.
3. Compute the approximate MLE of the potentials:

$$V_{l:7:r}(\beta) = \frac{F_{7:r:\text{core}}(\beta) - F_{l:7:r}(\beta|\mathbf{g}^{\circ})}{F_{7:r:\text{core}}(\beta) \cdot (1 - F_{7:r:\text{core}}(\beta))}.$$

4. Compute partial Gibbs energies of the descriptors for equal and all other clique-wise signals over the training image for the clique sizes $r = 1, 2, \ldots, 10$ to choose the size ρ_l, making both energies the closest one to another.

1.2.2 Local feature extraction using a 3D-CNN

A 3D-CNN has the ability to exploit the spatial correlation of input data in an efficient way. The motive for adding a CNN is to try to exploit and add the local features to the proposed framework through the automatic extraction of the most discriminative statistical features from raw data. The used 3D-CNN architecture consists of four layers (two convolutional layers, one fully connected layer, and one classification layer). The input to the first convolution layer is the lung nodules as 3D gray scale volumes of size $40 \times 40 \times 40$. A kernel of size $5 \times 5 \times 5$ is used in this layer with a stride of 2. The final output of this layer is seven feature maps (FMs) of size $20 \times 20 \times 10$. The input for the second convolution layer is the output FMs of the first convolution layer. A kernel of size $5 \times 5 \times 3$ is used in this layer with a stride of 1. The output of this layer is 17 FMs of size $18 \times 18 \times 1$. In order to prevent over-fitting we used a drop ratio of 0.8 to enhance the quality of the classification on the test data which have not been seen before in the training data. The final fully connected layers combine the detected features from the raw CT volume to be ready for the classification process. Its input feature map size is 128, which are finally classified as benign or malignant.

1.2.3 Nodule classification using autoencoders

Our CADx system utilizes a feed-forward deep neural network to classify the pulmonary nodules as malignant or benign. The implemented deep neural network comprises a two-stage structure of a stacked autoencoder (AE).

The first stage consists of autoencoder-based classifiers for the appearance and 3D-CNN to extract the local features, which are used to give an initial estimation for the probabilities of the classification, which are augmented together to be considered as the input for the second stage autoencoder to give the final estimation of the classification probabilities (see figure 1.1 for more details).

The autoencoder is employed in order to diminish the dimensionality of the input data (1000 histogram bins for the Gibbs energy image in the network of the appearance) with multi-layered neural networks to obtain the most discriminating features by greedy unsupervised pre-training.

After the AE layers, a softmax output layer is stacked in order to refine the classification by reducing the total loss for the training labeled input.

For each AE, let $W = \{W_j^e, W_i^d : j = 1, \ldots, s; i = 1, \ldots, n\}$ refer to a set of column vectors of weights for encoding, E, and decoding, D, layers, and let T denote vector transposition. The AE changes the n-dimensional column vector $u = [u_1, \ldots, u_n]^T$ into an s-dimensional column vector $h = [h_1, \ldots, h_s]^T$ of hidden features such that $s < n$ by nonlinear uniform transformation of s weighted linear combinations of input where $\sigma(.)$ is a sigmoid function with values from [0, 1], $\sigma(t) = \frac{1}{1+e^{-t}}$.

Our classifier is constructed by stacking AEs, which consist of three hidden layers with a softmax layer for the appearance network. The first hidden layer reduces the input vector to 500 level activators, while the second hidden layer continues the reduction to 300 level activators which are reduced to 100 after the third layer. The softmax layer computes the probability of being malignant or benign through the following equation:

$$p(c;\, W_{o:c}) = \frac{e^{(W_{o:c}^T h^3)}}{e^{\left(\sum_1^c W_{o:c}^T h^3\right)}}, \tag{1.4}$$

where $C = 1, 2$ is the class number, $W_{o:c}$ is the weighting vector for the softmax for class c, and h^3 are the output features from the last hidden layer (the third layer) of the AE. In the second stage, the output probability obtained from the softmax of the appearance and 3D-CNN are fused together and fed to another softmax layer to give the final classification probability.

1.3 Experimental results

To train and test our proposed CADx system, the well-known Lung Image Database Consortium (LIDC) dataset is used. This dataset consists of 1018 thoracic CT scans that have been collected from 1010 different patients from seven different academic centers. After removing the scans with a slice thickness greater than 3 mm and the scans with inconsistent slice spacing, a total of 888 CT scans became available for testing and evaluating our CADx system [18]. The LIDC CT scans are associated with an XML file to provide a good descriptive annotation and radiological diagnosis for the lung lesions, such as segmentation, shape, texture, and malignancy. All this information is provided by four thoracic radiologists in a two-phase image annotation process. In the first phase, each of the four radiologists independently reviewed all the cases and this phase is called the blind read phase, as each opinion is given regardless of the other radiologists. The second phase is the final phase as each radiologist gives their final decision after checking the other three radiologists' decisions, and this phase is called the unblinded phase as all the annotations were made available to all the radiologists before giving their final annotation decision. The radiologists divided the lesions into two groups: nodules and non-nodules. We focused on the nodules $\geqslant$3 mm as they have a malignancy score that varies from 1 for benign to 5 for malignant, and a well-defined contour annotated by the radiologists.

We trained our CAD system on a randomly selected sample of nodules. In order to be sure that the data are almost balanced, we used 413 benign and 314 malignant nodules. For each nodule the combination of the four radiologists' masks is combined to obtain the final nodule mask that we will use in our experiments. A

Table 1.1. Classification results in terms of sensitivity, specificity, accuracy, and AUC for different feature groups.

	Evaluation metrics			
	Sens.	Spec.	Acc.	AUC
Appearance	93.55	87.20	89.91	96.66
CNN	98.92	82.40	89.45	95.73
Comb. features	**91.39**	**94.04**	**92.90**	**96.70**

Table 1.2. Comparison between our proposed system and four other recent nodule classification techniques, in terms of sensitivity, specificity, and accuracy.

		Metric		
		Sensitivity	Specificity	Accuracy
Method	Kumar *et al* [19]	83.35	—	75.01
	Hua *et al* [20]	73.30	78.70	—
	Krewer *et al* [21]	85.71	94.74	90.91
	Jiang *et al* [22]	86.00	88.50	—
	Our system	**91.39**	**94.04**	**92.90**

volume-of-interest (VOI) of size $40 \times 40 \times 40$ mm measured around the center of the nodule's combined mask is extracted for each nodule. The final diagnosis score of each nodule that we decided to work on is evaluated by calculating the average of the diagnosis scores for the four radiologists.

The system is evaluated by randomly dividing the dataset into two parts 70% for training and 30% for testing. The classification accuracy is described in terms of different measurement metrics, namely the specificity, sensitivity, accuracy, and AUC. We reported the accuracy of the appearance model and the 3D-CNN model separately and for the complete fused system to highlight the effect of each model on the overall system (as shown in table 1.1).

1.4 Conclusion

In summary, this chapter proposed a novel CAD system for lung nodule assessment by modeling the nodules' appearance features using a novel higher-order MGRF in addition to local features that are modeled using 3D-CNN to describe the low and high local features. The classification results obtained from a set of 727 nodules collected from 467 patients confirm that the proposed framework holds promise for the early detection of lung cancer. A quantitative comparison with recently developed diagnostic techniques highlights the advantages of the proposed framework over state-of-the-art techniques (table 1.2). These promising results encourage us to model a new shape features using spherical harmonic analysis and include it in the proposed framework to reach the clinically accepted accuracy threshold, which is ⩾95.00%. Moreover, we plan to file an IRB protocol in the future and locally collect data at our site to test our model on subjects that have malignant/benign nodules with biopsy confirmations.

In addition to the lung [23–72], this work could also be applied to various other applications in medical imaging, such as the kidney, heart, prostate, lung, and retina, as well as several non-medical applications [73–77]. One application is renal transplant functional assessment, in particular in developing non-invasive CAD systems for renal transplant function assessment, utilizing different image modalities (e.g. ultrasound, computed tomography (CT), MRI, etc). Accurate assessment of renal transplant function is critically important for graft survival. Although transplantation can improve a patient's wellbeing, there is a potential post-transplantation risk of kidney dysfunction that, if not treated in a timely manner, can lead to the loss of the entire graft and even patient death. In particular, dynamic and diffusion MRI-based systems have been clinically used to assess transplanted kidneys with the advantage of providing information on each kidney separately. For more details about renal transplant functional assessment see [78–102].

The heart is also an important application of this work. The clinical assessment of myocardial perfusion plays a major role in the diagnosis, management, and prognosis of ischemic heart disease patients. Thus, there have been ongoing efforts to develop automated systems for accurate analysis of myocardial perfusion using first-pass images [103–119]. Moreover, the work could be applied to prostate cancer which is the most common cancer in American men and its related mortality rate is the second after lung cancer. Fortunately, the mortality rate can be reduced if prostate cancer is detected in its early stages. Early detection enables physicians to treat prostate cancer before it develops into a clinically significant disease [120–122]. Another application for this work could be the detection of retinal abnormalities. The majority of ophthalmologists depend on visual interpretation for the identification of diseases types. However, inaccurate diagnosis will affect the treatment procedure which may lead to fatal results. Hence, there is a crucial need for computer automated diagnosis systems that yield highly accurate results. Optical coherence tomography (OCT) has become a powerful modality for the non-invasive diagnosis of various retinal abnormalities such as glaucoma, diabetic macular edema, and macular degeneration. The problem with diabetic retinopathy (DR) is that the patient is not aware of the disease until the changes in the retina have progressed to a level that treatment tends to be less effective. Therefore, automated early detection could limit the severity of the disease and assist ophthalmologists in investigating and treating it more efficiently [123–125]. This work can also be applied to other brain abnormalities, such as dyslexia and autism. Dyslexia is one of the most complicated developmental brain disorders that affect children's learning abilities. Dyslexia leads to the failure to develop age-appropriate reading skills despite a normal intelligence level and adequate reading instruction. Neuropathological studies have revealed the abnormal anatomy of some structures, such as the corpus callosum in dyslexic brains. A lot of research has been published in the literature that aims to develop CAD systems for diagnosing such disorders along with other brain disorders [126–145].

For the vascular system [146] this work could also be applied for the extraction of blood vessels, e.g. from phase contrast (PC) magnetic resonance angiography (MRA). Accurate cerebrovascular segmentation using non-invasive MRA is crucial for the early diagnosis and timely treatment of intracranial vascular diseases [131, 132, 147–152].

References

[1] American Cancer Society 2017 *Cancer Facts and figures* https://www.cancer.org/research/cancer-facts-statistics/all-cancer-facts-figures/cancer-facts-figures-2017.html

[2] Brazauskas K A, Ackman J B and Nelson B 2016 Surveillance of actionable pulmonary nodules in children: the potential of thoracic MRI *Insights Chest Dis.* **1** 10

[3] Wu L-M, Xu J-R, Hua J, Gu H-Y, Chen J, Haacke E and Hu J 2013 Can diffusion-weighted imaging be used as a reliable sequence in the detection of malignant pulmonary nodules and masses? *Magn. Reson. Imaging* **31** 235–46

[4] Sun W, Zheng B and Qian W 2016 Computer aided lung cancer diagnosis with deep learning algorithms *Proc. SPIE* **9785** 97850Z

[5] Shen W, Zhou M, Yang F, Yang C and Tian J 2015 Multi-scale convolutional neural networks for lung nodule classification *Int. Conf. on Information Processing in Medical Imaging* (Berlin: Springer), pp 588–99

[6] Likhitkar M V K, Gawande U and Hajari M K O 2014 Automated detection of cancerous lung nodule from the computed tomography images *IOSR J. Comput. Eng.* **16** 05–11

[7] Wei G, Ma H, Qian W, Han F, Jiang H, Qi S and Qiu M 2018 Lung nodule classification using local kernel regression models with out-of-sample extension *Biomed. Signal Process. Control* **40** 1–9

[8] Nishio M and Nagashima C 2017 Computer-aided diagnosis for lung cancer: usefulness of nodule heterogeneity *Acad. Radiol.* **24** 328–36

[9] Wang C, Elazab A, Wu J and Hu Q 2017 Lung nodule classification using deep feature fusion in chest radiography *Computer. Med. Imaging Graph.* **57** 10–8

[10] Dhara A K, Mukhopadhyay S, Dutta A, Garg M and Khandelwal N 2016 A combination of shape and texture features for classification of pulmonary nodules in lung CT images *J. Digit. Imaging* **29** 466–75

[11] Song Q, Zhao L, Luo X and Dou X 2017 Using deep learning for classification of lung nodules on computed tomography images *J. Healthc. Eng.* **2017** 8314740

[12] Shewaye T N and Mekonnen A A 2016 Benign-malignant lung nodule classification with geometric and appearance histogram features, arXiv:1605.08350

[13] Guo N, Yen R-F, El Fakhri G and Li Q 2015 SVM based lung cancer diagnosis using multiple image features in PET/CT *2015 IEEE Nuclear Science Symp. and Medical Imaging Conf. (NSS/MIC)* (Piscataway, NJ: IEEE), pp 1–4

[14] Liu N, Soliman A, Gimel'farb G and El-Baz A 2015 Segmenting kidney DCE-MRI using 1st-order shape and 5th-order appearance priors *Int. Conf. on Medical Image Computing and Computer-Assisted Intervention* (Berlin: Springer), pp 77–84

[15] Blake A, Kohli P and Rother C 2011 *Markov Random Fields for Vision and Image Processing* (Cambridge, MA: MIT Press)

[16] Gimel'Farb G and Farag A 2005 Texture analysis by accurate identification of simple markovian models *Cybern. Syst. Anal.* **41** 27–38

[17] El-Baz A, Gimel'farb G and Suri J S 2015 *Stochastic Modeling for Medical Image Analysis* (Boca Raton, FL: CRC Press)

[18] Armato S G *et al* 2011 The lung image database consortium (LIDC) and image database resource initiative (IDRI): a completed reference database of lung nodules on CT scans *Med. Phys.* **38** 915–31
[19] Kumar D, Wong A and Clausi D A 2015 Lung nodule classification using deep features in CT images *2015 12th Conf. on Computer and Robot Vision (CRV)* (Piscataway, NJ: IEEE), pp 133–8
[20] Hua K-L, Hsu C-H, Hidayati S C, Cheng W-H and Chen Y-J 2015 Computer-aided classification of lung nodules on computed tomography images via deep learning technique *OncoTargets and Therapy* 8 2015–22
[21] Krewer H, Geiger B, Hall L O, Goldgof D B, Gu Y, Tockman M and Gillies R J 2013 Effect of texture features in computer aided diagnosis of pulmonary nodules in low-dose computed tomography *2013 IEEE Int. Conf. on Systems, Man, and Cybernetics (SMC)* (Piscataway, NJ: IEEE), pp 3887–91
[22] Jiang H, Ma H, Qian W, Wei G, Zhao X and Gao M 2017 A novel pixel value space statistics map of the pulmonary nodule for classification in computerized tomography images *2017 39th Annual Int. Conf. of the IEEE Engineering in Medicine and Biology Society (EMBC)* (Piscataway, NJ: IEEE), pp 556–9
[23] Abdollahi B, Civelek A C, Li X-F, Suri J and El-Baz A 2014 PET/CT nodule segmentation and diagnosis: a survey *Multi Detector CT Imaging* ed L Saba and J S Suri (London: Taylor and Francis), ch 30, pp 639–51
[24] Abdollahi B, El-Baz A and Amini A A 2011 A multi-scale non-linear vessel enhancement technique *2011 Annual Int. Conf. of the IEEE Engineering in Medicine and Biology Society, EMBC* (Piscataway, NJ: IEEE), pp 3925–9
[25] Abdollahi B, Soliman A, Civelek A, Li X-F, Gimel'farb G and El-Baz A 2012 A novel Gaussian scale space-based joint MGRF framework for precise lung segmentation *Proc. of IEEE Int. Conf. on Image Processing, (ICIP'12)* (Piscataway, NJ: IEEE), pp 2029–32
[26] Abdollahi B, Soliman A, Civelek A, Li X-F, Gimel'farb G and El-Baz A 2012 A novel 3D joint MGRF framework for precise lung segmentation *Machine Learning in Medical Imaging* (Berlin: Springer), pp 86–93
[27] Ali A M, El-Baz A S and Farag A A 2007 A novel framework for accurate lung segmentation using graph cuts *Proc. of IEEE Int. Symp. on Biomedical Imaging: From Nano to Macro, (ISBI'07)* (Piscataway, NJ: IEEE), pp 908–11
[28] El-Baz A, Beache G M, Gimel'farb G, Suzuki K and Okada K 2013 Lung imaging data analysis *Int. J. Biomed. Imaging* **2013** 1–2
[29] El-Baz A, Beache G M, Gimel'farb G, Suzuki K, Okada K, Elnakib A, Soliman A and Abdollahi B 2013 Computer-aided diagnosis systems for lung cancer: challenges and methodologies *Int. J. Biomed. Imaging* **2013** 1–46
[30] El-Baz A, Elnakib A, Abou El-Ghar M, Gimel'farb G, Falk R and Farag A 2013 Automatic detection of 2D and 3D lung nodules in chest spiral CT scans *Int. J. Biomed. Imaging* **2013** 1–11
[31] El-Baz A, Farag A A, Falk R and La Rocca R 2003 A unified approach for detection, visualization, and identification of lung abnormalities in chest spiral CT scans *International Congress Series* vol 1256 (Amsterdam: Elsevier), pp 998–1004
[32] El-Baz A, Farag A A, Falk R and La Rocca R 2002 Detection, visualization and identification of lung abnormalities in chest spiral CT scan: Phase-I *Proc. of Int. Conf. on Biomedical Engineering (Cairo, Egypt)* **vol 12**

[33] El-Baz A, Farag A, Gimel'farb G, Falk R, El-Ghar M A and Eldiasty T 2006 A framework for automatic segmentation of lung nodules from low dose chest CT scans *Proc. of Int. Conf. on Pattern Recognition, (ICPR'06)* **vol 3** (Piscataway, NJ: IEEE), pp 611–4

[34] El-Baz A, Farag A, Gimel'farb G, Falk R and El-Ghar M A 2011 A novel level set-based computer-aided detection system for automatic detection of lung nodules in low dose chest computed tomography scans *Lung Imaging and Computer Aided Diagnosis* vol 10 (Boca Raton, FL: CRC Press), pp 221–38

[35] El-Baz A, Gimel'farb G, Abou El-Ghar M and Falk R 2012 Appearance-based diagnostic system for early assessment of malignant lung nodules *Proc. of IEEE Int. Conf. on Image Processing, (ICIP'12)* (Piscataway, NJ: IEEE), pp 533–6

[36] El-Baz A, Gimel'farb G and Falk R 2011 A novel 3D framework for automatic lung segmentation from low dose CT images *Lung Imaging and Computer Aided Diagnosis* ed A El-Baz and J S Suri (London: Taylor and Francis), ch 1, pp 1–16

[37] El-Baz A, Gimel'farb G, Falk R and El-Ghar M 2010 Appearance analysis for diagnosing malignant lung nodules *Proc. of IEEE Int. Symp. on Biomedical Imaging: From Nano to Macro (ISBI'10)* (Piscataway, NJ: IEEE), pp 193–6

[38] El-Baz A, Gimel'farb G, Falk R and El-Ghar M A 2011 A novel level set-based CAD system for automatic detection of lung nodules in low dose chest CT scans *Lung Imaging and Computer Aided Diagnosis* vol 1 ed A El-Baz and J S Suri (London: Taylor and Francis), ch 10, pp 221–38

[39] El-Baz A, Gimel'farb G, Falk R and El-Ghar M A 2008 A new approach for automatic analysis of 3D low dose CT images for accurate monitoring the detected lung nodules *Proc. of Int. Conf. on Pattern Recognition, (ICPR'08)* (Piscataway, NJ: IEEE), pp 1–4

[40] El-Baz A, Gimel'farb G, Falk R and El-Ghar M A 2007 A novel approach for automatic follow-up of detected lung nodules *Proc. of IEEE Int. Conf. on Image Processing, (ICIP'07)* **vol 5** (Piscataway, NJ: IEEE), p V–501

[41] El-Baz A, Gimel'farb G, Falk R and El-Ghar M A 2007 A new CAD system for early diagnosis of detected lung nodules *IEEE Int. Conf. on Image Processing, 2007. ICIP 2007* **vol 2** (Piscataway, NJ: IEEE), pp II–461

[42] El-Baz A, Gimel'farb G, Falk R, El-Ghar M A and Refaie H 2008 Promising results for early diagnosis of lung cancer *Proc. of IEEE Int. Symp. on Biomedical Imaging: From Nano to Macro, (ISBI'08)* (Piscataway, NJ: IEEE), pp 1151–4

[43] El-Baz A, Gimel'farb G L, Falk R, Abou El-Ghar M, Holland T and Shaffer T 2008 A new stochastic framework for accurate lung segmentation *Proc. of Medical Image Computing and Computer-Assisted Intervention, (MICCAI'08)* pp 322–30

[44] El-Baz A, Gimel'farb G L, Falk R, Heredis D and Abou El-Ghar M 2008 A novel approach for accurate estimation of the growth rate of the detected lung nodules *Proc. of Int. Workshop on Pulmonary Image Analysis* pp 33–42

[45] El-Baz A, Gimel'farb G L, Falk R, Holland T and Shaffer T 2008 A framework for unsupervised segmentation of lung tissues from low dose computed tomography images *Proc. of British Machine Vision, (BMVC'08)* pp 1–10

[46] El-Baz A, Gimel'farb G, Falk R and El-Ghar M A 2011 3D MGRF-based appearance modeling for robust segmentation of pulmonary nodules in 3D LDCT chest images *Lung Imaging and Computer Aided Diagnosis* ch 3, pp 51–63

[47] El-Baz A, Gimel'farb G, Falk R and El-Ghar M A 2009 Automatic analysis of 3D low dose CT images for early diagnosis of lung cancer *Pattern Recogn.* **42** 1041–51

[48] El-Baz A, Gimel'farb G, Falk R, El-Ghar M A, Rainey S, Heredia D and Shaffer T 2009 Toward early diagnosis of lung cancer *Proc. of Medical Image Computing and Computer-Assisted Intervention, (MICCAI'09)* (Berlin: Springer), pp 682–9

[49] El-Baz A, Gimel'farb G, Falk R, El-Ghar M A and Suri J 2011 Appearance analysis for the early assessment of detected lung nodules *Lung Imaging and Computer Aided Diagnosis* ch 17, pp 395–404

[50] El-Baz A, Khalifa F, Elnakib A, Nitkzen M, Soliman A, McClure P, Gimel'farb G and El-Ghar M A 2012 A novel approach for global lung registration using 3D Markov Gibbs appearance model *Proc. of Int. Conf. Medical Image Computing and Computer-Assisted Intervention, (MICCAI'12) (Nice, France, 1–5 October 2012)* pp 114–21

[51] El-Baz A, Nitzken M, Elnakib A, Khalifa F, Gimel'farb G, Falk R and El-Ghar M A 2011 3D shape analysis for early diagnosis of malignant lung nodules *Proc. of Int. Conf. Medical Image Computing and Computer-Assisted Intervention, (MICCAI'11) (Toronto, Canada, 18–22 September 2011)* pp 175–82

[52] El-Baz A, Nitzken M, Gimel'farb G, Van Bogaert E, Falk R, El-Ghar M A and Suri J 2011 Three-dimensional shape analysis using spherical harmonics for early assessment of detected lung nodules *Lung Imaging and Computer Aided Diagnosis* ch 19, pp 421–38

[53] El-Baz A, Nitzken M, Khalifa F, Elnakib A, Gimel'farb G, Falk R and El-Ghar M A 2011 3D shape analysis for early diagnosis of malignant lung nodules *Proc. of Int. Conf. on Information Processing in Medical Imaging, (IPMI'11) (Monastery Irsee, Germany (Bavaria), 3–8 July 2011)* pp 772–83

[54] El-Baz A, Nitzken M, Vanbogaert E, Gimel'Farb G, Falk R and Abo El-Ghar M 2011 A novel shape-based diagnostic approach for early diagnosis of lung nodules *2011 IEEE Int. Symp. on Biomedical Imaging: From Nano to Macro* (Piscataway, NJ: IEEE), pp 137–40

[55] El-Baz A, Sethu P, Gimel'farb G, Khalifa F, Elnakib A, Falk R and El-Ghar M A 2011 Elastic phantoms generated by microfluidics technology: validation of an imaged-based approach for accurate measurement of the growth rate of lung nodules *Biotechnol. J.* **6** 195–203

[56] El-Baz A, Sethu P, Gimel'farb G, Khalifa F, Elnakib A, Falk R and El-Ghar M A 2010 A new validation approach for the growth rate measurement using elastic phantoms generated by state-of-the-art microfluidics technology *Proc. of IEEE Int. Conf. on Image Processing, (ICIP'10) (Hong Kong, 26–29 September 2010)* pp 4381–3

[57] El-Baz A, Sethu P, Gimel'farb G, Khalifa F, Elnakib A, Falk R and Suri M A E-G 2011 Validation of a new imaged-based approach for the accurate estimating of the growth rate of detected lung nodules using real CT images and elastic phantoms generated by state-of-the-art microfluidics technology *Handbook of Lung Imaging and Computer Aided Diagnosis* vol 1 ed A El-Baz and J S Suri (New York: Taylor and Francis), ch 18, pp 405–20

[58] El-Baz A, Soliman A, McClure P, Gimel'farb G, El-Ghar M A and Falk R 2012 Early assessment of malignant lung nodules based on the spatial analysis of detected lung nodules *Proc. of IEEE Int. Symp. on Biomedical Imaging: From Nano to Macro, (ISBI'12)* (Piscataway, NJ: IEEE), pp 1463–6

[59] El-Baz A, Yuksel S E, Elshazly S and Farag A A 2005 Non-rigid registration techniques for automatic follow-up of lung nodules *Proc. of Computer Assisted Radiology and Surgery, (CARS'05)* **vol 1281** (Amsterdam: Elsevier), pp 1115–20

[60] El-Baz A S and Suri J S 2011 *Lung Imaging and Computer Aided Diagnosis* (Boca Raton, FL: CRC Press)

[61] Soliman A, Khalifa F, Dunlap N, Wang B, El-Ghar M and El-Baz A 2016 An iso-surfaces based local deformation handling framework of lung tissues *2016 IEEE 13th Int. Symp. on Biomedical Imaging (ISBI)* (Piscataway, NJ: IEEE), pp 1253–9

[62] Soliman A, Khalifa F, Shaffie A, Dunlap N, Wang B, Elmaghraby A and El-Baz A 2016 Detection of lung injury using 4D-CT chest images *2016 IEEE 13th Int. Symp. on Biomedical Imaging (ISBI)* (Piscataway, NJ: IEEE), pp 1274–7

[63] Soliman A, Khalifa F, Shaffie A, Dunlap N, Wang B, Elmaghraby A, Gimel'farb G, Ghazal M and El-Baz A 2017 A comprehensive framework for early assessment of lung injury *2017 IEEE Int. Conf. on Image Processing (ICIP)* (Piscataway, NJ: IEEE), pp 3275–9

[64] Shaffie A, Soliman A, Ghazal M, Taher F, Dunlap N, Wang B, Elmaghraby A, Gimel'farb G and El-Baz A 2017 A new framework for incorporating appearance and shape features of lung nodules for precise diagnosis of lung cancer *2017 IEEE Int. Conf. on Image Processing (ICIP)* (Piscataway, NJ: IEEE), pp 1372–6

[65] Soliman A, Khalifa F, Shaffie A, Liu N, Dunlap N, Wang B, Elmaghraby A, Gimel'farb G and El-Baz A 2016 Image-based CAD system for accurate identification of lung injury *2016 IEEE Int. Conf. on Image Processing (ICIP)* (Piscataway, NJ: IEEE), pp 121–5

[66] Soliman A, Shaffie A, Ghazal M, Gimel'farb G, Keynton R and El-Baz A 2018 A novel cnn segmentation framework based on using new shape and appearance features *2018 25th IEEE Int. Conf. on Image Processing (ICIP)* (Piscataway, NJ: IEEE), pp 3488–92

[67] Safta W, Farhangi M M, Veasey B, Amini A and Frigui H 2019 Multiple instance learning for malignant versus benign classification of lung nodules in thoracic screening CT data *2019 IEEE 16th Int. Symp. on Biomedical Imaging (ISBI 2019)* (Piscataway, NJ: IEEE), pp 1220–4

[68] Safta W and Frigui H 2018 Multiple instance learning for benign versus malignant classification of lung nodules in CT scans *2018 IEEE Int. Symp. on Signal Processing and Information Technology (ISSPIT)* (Piscataway, NJ: IEEE), pp 490–4

[69] Shaffie A, Soliman A, Khalifeh H A, Ghazal M, Taher F, Keynton R, Elmaghraby A and El-Baz A 2018 On the integration of CT-derived features for accurate detection of lung cancer *2018 IEEE Int. Symp. on Signal Processing and Information Technology (ISSPIT)* (Piscataway, NJ: IEEE), pp 435–40

[70] Shaffie A, Soliman A, Khalifeh H A, Ghazal M, Taher F, Elmaghraby A, Keynton R and El-Baz A 2019 Radiomic-based framework for early diagnosis of lung cancer *2019 IEEE 16th Int. Symp. on Biomedical Imaging (ISBI 2019)* (Piscataway, NJ: IEEE), pp 1293–7

[71] Shaffie A, Soliman A, Ghazal M, Taher F, Dunlap N, Wang B, Van Berkel V, Gimelfarb G, Elmaghraby A and El-Baz A 2018 A novel autoencoder-based diagnostic system for early assessment of lung cancer *2018 25th IEEE Int. Conf. on Image Processing (ICIP)* (Piscataway, NJ: IEEE), pp 1393–7

[72] Shaffie A *et al* 2018 A generalized deep learning-based diagnostic system for early diagnosis of various types of pulmonary nodules *Technol. Cancer Res. Treat.* **17** 1533033818798800

[73] Ghazal M, Mahmoud A, Shalaby A and El-Baz A 2019 Automated framework for accurate segmentation of leaf images for plant health assessment *Environ. Monit. Assess.* **191** 491

[74] Mahmoud A H 2014 Utilizing radiation for smart robotic applications using visible, thermal, and polarization images *PhD Dissertation* University of Louisville, KY

[75] Mahmoud A, El-Barkouky A, Graham J and Farag A 2014 Pedestrian detection using mixed partial derivative based histogram of oriented gradients *2014 IEEE Int. Conf. on Image Processing (ICIP)* (Piscataway, NJ: IEEE), pp 2334–7

[76] El-Barkouky A, Mahmoud A, Graham J and Farag A 2013 An interactive educational drawing system using a humanoid robot and light polarization *2013 IEEE Int. Conf. on Image Processing* (Piscataway, NJ: IEEE), pp 3407–11
[77] Mahmoud A H, El-Melegy M T and Farag A A 2012 Direct method for shape recovery from polarization and shading *2012 19th IEEE Int. Conf. on Image Processing* (Piscataway, NJ: IEEE), pp 1769–72
[78] Chowdhury A S, Roy R, Bose S, Elnakib F K A and El-Baz A 2012 Non-rigid biomedical image registration using graph cuts with a novel data term *Proc. of IEEE Int. Symp. on Biomedical Imaging: From Nano to Macro, (ISBI'12) (Barcelona, Spain, 2–5 May, 2012)* pp 446–9
[79] El-Baz A, Farag A A, Yuksel S E, El-Ghar M E, Eldiasty T A and Ghoneim M A 2007 Application of deformable models for the detection of acute renal rejection *Deformable Models* (New York: Springer), pp 293–333
[80] El-Baz A, Farag A, Fahmi R, Yuksel S, El-Ghar M A and Eldiasty T 2006 Image analysis of renal DCE MRI for the detection of acute renal rejection *Proc. of IAPR Int. Conf. on Pattern Recognition (ICPR'06) (Hong Kong, 20–24 August, 2006)* pp 822–5
[81] El-Baz A, Farag A, Fahmi R, Yuksel S, Miller W, El-Ghar M A, El-Diasty T and Ghoneim M 2006 A new CAD system for the evaluation of kidney diseases using DCE-MRI *Proc. of Int. Conf. on Medical Image Computing and Computer-Assisted Intervention, (MICCAI'08) (Copenhagen, Denmark, 1–6 October 2006)* pp 446–53
[82] El-Baz A, Gimel'farb G and El-Ghar M A 2008 A novel image analysis approach for accurate identification of acute renal rejection *Proc. of IEEE Int. Conf. on Image Processing, (ICIP'08) (San Diego, California, USA, 12–15 October 2008)* pp 1812–5
[83] El-Baz A, Gimel'farb G and El-Ghar M A 2008 Image analysis approach for identification of renal transplant rejection *Proc. of IAPR Int. Conf. on Pattern Recognition, (ICPR'08) (Tampa, Florida, USA, 8–11 December 2008)* pp 1–4
[84] El-Baz A, Gimel'farb G and El-Ghar M A 2007 New motion correction models for automatic identification of renal transplant rejection *Proc. of Int. Conf. on Medical Image Computing and Computer-Assisted Intervention, (MICCAI'07) (Brisbane, Australia, 29 October–2 November 2007)* pp 235–43
[85] Farag A, El-Baz A, Yuksel S, El-Ghar M A and Eldiasty T 2006 A framework for the detection of acute rejection with dynamic contrast enhanced magnetic resonance imaging *Proc. of IEEE Int. Symp. on Biomedical Imaging: From Nano to Macro, (ISBI'06) (Arlington, Virginia, USA, 6–9 April 2006)* pp 418–21
[86] Khalifa F, Beache G M, El-Ghar M A, El-Diasty T, Gimel'farb G, Kong M and El-Baz A 2013 Dynamic contrast-enhanced MRI-based early detection of acute renal transplant rejection *IEEE Trans. Med. Imaging* **32** 1910–27
[87] Khalifa F, El-Baz A, Gimel'farb G and El-Ghar M A 2010 Non-invasive image-based approach for early detection of acute renal rejection *Proc. of Int. Conf. Medical Image Computing and Computer-Assisted Intervention, (MICCAI'10) (Beijing, China, 20–24 September 2010)* pp 10–8
[88] Khalifa F, El-Baz A, Gimel'farb G, Ouseph R and El-Ghar M A 2010 Shape-appearance guided level-set deformable model for image segmentation *Proc. of IAPR Int. Conf. on Pattern Recognition, (ICPR'10) (Istanbul, Turkey, 23–26 August 2010)* pp 4581–4

[89] Khalifa F, El-Ghar M A, Abdollahi B, Frieboes H, El-Diasty T and El-Baz A 2013 A comprehensive non-invasive framework for automated evaluation of acute renal transplant rejection using DCE-MRI *NMR Biomed.* **26** 1460–70

[90] Khalifa F, El-Ghar M A, Abdollahi B, Frieboes H B, El-Diasty T and El-Baz A 2014 Dynamic contrast-enhanced MRI-based early detection of acute renal transplant rejection *2014 Annual Scientific Meeting and Educational Course Brochure of the Society of Abdominal Radiology, (SAR'14) (Boca Raton, Florida, 23–28 March 2014)* p CID:1855912

[91] Khalifa F, Elnakib A, Beache G M, Gimel'farb G, El-Ghar M A, Sokhadze G, Manning S, McClure P and El-Baz A 2011 3D kidney segmentation from CT images using a level set approach guided by a novel stochastic speed function *Proc. of Int. Conf. Medical Image Computing and Computer-Assisted Intervention, (MICCAI'11) (Toronto, Canada, 18–22 September 2011)* pp 587–94

[92] Khalifa F, Gimel'farb G, El-Ghar M A, Sokhadze G, Manning S, McClure P, Ouseph R and El-Baz A 2011 A new deformable model-based segmentation approach for accurate extraction of the kidney from abdominal CT images *Proc. of IEEE Int. Conf. on Image Processing, (ICIP'11) (Brussels, Belgium, 11–14 September 2011)* pp 3393–6

[93] Mostapha M, Khalifa F, Alansary A, Soliman A, Suri J and El-Baz A 2014 Computer-aided diagnosis systems for acute renal transplant rejection: challenges and methodologies *Abdomen and Thoracic Imaging* ed A El-Baz and L S J Suri (Berlin: Springer), pp 1–35

[94] Shehata M, Khalifa F, Hollis E, Soliman A, Hosseini-Asl E, El-Ghar M A, El-Baz M, Dwyer A C, El-Baz A and Keynton R 2016 A new non-invasive approach for early classification of renal rejection types using diffusion-weighted MRI *2016 IEEE Int. Conf. on Image Processing (ICIP)* (Piscataway, NJ: IEEE), pp 136–40

[95] Khalifa F, Soliman A, Takieldeen A, Shehata M, Mostapha M, Shaffie A, Ouseph R, Elmaghraby A and El-Baz A 2016 Kidney segmentation from CT images using a 3D NMF-guided active contour model *2016 IEEE 13th Int. Symp. on Biomedical Imaging (ISBI)* (Piscataway, NJ: IEEE), pp 432–5

[96] Shehata M, Khalifa F, Soliman A, Takieldeen A, El-Ghar M A, Shaffie A, Dwyer A C, Ouseph R, El-Baz A and Keynton R 2016 3D diffusion MRI-based CAD system for early diagnosis of acute renal rejection *2016 IEEE 13th Int. Symp. on Biomedical Imaging (ISBI)* (Piscataway, NJ: IEEE), pp 1177–80

[97] Shehata M, Khalifa F, Soliman A, Alrefai R, El-Ghar M A, Dwyer A C, Ouseph R and El-Baz A 2015 A level set-based framework for 3D kidney segmentation from diffusion mr images *IEEE Int. Conf. on Image Processing (ICIP), 2015* (Piscataway, NJ: IEEE), pp 4441–5

[98] Khalifa F, Soliman A, Elmaghraby A, Gimel'farb G and El-Baz A 2017 3D kidney segmentation from abdominal images using spatial-appearance models *Comput. Math. Methods Med.* **2017** 1–10

[99] Hollis E, Shehata M, Khalifa F, El-Ghar M A, El-Diasty T and El-Baz A 2016 Towards non-invasive diagnostic techniques for early detection of acute renal transplant rejection: a review *Egyptian J. Radiol. Nucl. Med.* **48** 257–69

[100] Shehata M, Khalifa F, Soliman A, El-Ghar M A, Dwyer A C and El-Baz A 2017 Assessment of renal transplant using image and clinical-based biomarkers *Proc. of 13th Annual Scientific Meeting of American Society for Diagnostics and Interventional Nephrology (ASDIN'17) (New Orleans, LA, 10–12 February 2017)*

[101] Shehata M, Khalifa F, Soliman A, El-Ghar M A, Dwyer A C and El-Baz A 2016 Early assessment of acute renal rejection *Proc. of 12th Annual Scientific Meeting of American Society for Diagnostics and Interventional Nephrology (ASDIN'16) (Phoenix, AZ, USA, 19–21 February 2016)*

[102] Abdeltawab H *et al* 2019 A novel CNN-based CAD system for early assessment of transplanted kidney dysfunction *Sci. Rep.* **9** 5948

[103] Khalifa F, Beache G, El-Baz A and Gimel'farb G 2010 Deformable model guided by stochastic speed with application in cine images segmentation *Proc. of IEEE Int. Conf. on Image Processing, (ICIP'10) (Hong Kong, 26–29 September 2010)* pp 1725–8

[104] Khalifa F, Beache G M, Elnakib A, Sliman H, Gimel'farb G, Welch K C and El-Baz A 2013 A new shape-based framework for the left ventricle wall segmentation from cardiac first-pass perfusion MRI *Proc. of IEEE Int. Symp. on Biomedical Imaging: From Nano to Macro, (ISBI'13) (San Francisco, CA, 7–11 April 2013)* pp 41–4

[105] Khalifa F, Beache G M, Elnakib A, Sliman H, Gimel'farb G, Welch K C and El-Baz A 2012 A new nonrigid registration framework for improved visualization of transmural perfusion gradients on cardiac first–pass perfusion MRI *Proc. of IEEE Int. Symp. on Biomedical Imaging: From Nano to Macro, (ISBI'12) (Barcelona, Spain, 2–5 May 2012)* pp 828–31

[106] Khalifa F, Beache G M, Firjani A, Welch K C, Gimel'farb G and El-Baz A 2012 A new nonrigid registration approach for motion correction of cardiac first-pass perfusion MRI *Proc. of IEEE Int. Conf. on Image Processing, (ICIP'12) (Lake Buena Vista, Florida, 30 September–3 October 2012)* pp 1665–8

[107] Khalifa F, Beache G M, Gimel'farb G and El-Baz A 2012 A novel CAD system for analyzing cardiac first-pass MR images *Proc. of IAPR Int. Conf. on Pattern Recognition (ICPR'12) (Tsukuba Science City, Japan, 11–15 November 2012)* pp 77–80

[108] Khalifa F, Beache G M, Gimel'farb G and El-Baz A 2011 A novel approach for accurate estimation of left ventricle global indexes from short-axis cine MRI *Proc. of IEEE Int. Conf. on Image Processing, (ICIP'11) (Brussels, Belgium, 11–14 September 2011)* pp 2645–9

[109] Khalifa F, Beache G M, Gimel'farb G, Giridharan G A and El-Baz A 2011 A new image-based framework for analyzing cine images *Handbook of Multi Modality State-of-the-Art Medical Image Segmentation and Registration Methodologies* vol 2 ed A El-Baz, U R Acharya, M Mirmedhdi and J S Suri (New York: Springer), ch 3, pp 69–98

[110] Khalifa F, Beache G M, Gimel'farb G, Giridharan G A and El-Baz A 2012 Accurate automatic analysis of cardiac cine images *IEEE Trans. Biomed. Eng.* **59** 445–55

[111] Khalifa F, Beache G M, Nitzken M, Gimel'farb G, Giridharan G A and El-Baz A 2011 Automatic analysis of left ventricle wall thickness using short-axis cine CMR images *Proc. of IEEE Int. Symp. on Biomedical Imaging: From Nano to Macro, (ISBI'11) (Chicago, IL, 30 March–2 April 2011)* pp 1306–9

[112] Nitzken M, Beache G, Elnakib A, Khalifa F, Gimel'farb G and El-Baz A 2012 Accurate modeling of tagged CMR 3D image appearance characteristics to improve cardiac cycle strain estimation *2012 19th IEEE Int. Conf. on Image Processing (ICIP)* (Orlando, FL: IEEE), pp 521–4

[113] Nitzken M, Beache G, Elnakib A, Khalifa F, Gimel'farb G and El-Baz A 2012 Improving full-cardiac cycle strain estimation from tagged CMR by accurate modeling of 3D image appearance characteristics *2012 9th IEEE Int. Symp. on Biomedical Imaging (ISBI)* (Barcelona: IEEE), pp 462–5

[114] Nitzken M J, El-Baz A S and Beache G M 2012 Markov–Gibbs random field model for improved full-cardiac cycle strain estimation from tagged CMR *J. Cardiovasc. Magn. Reson.* **14** 1–2

[115] Sliman H, Elnakib A, Beache G, Elmaghraby A and El-Baz A 2014 Assessment of myocardial function from cine cardiac MRI using a novel 4D tracking approach *J. Comput. Sci. J. Comput. Sci.* **7** 169–73

[116] Sliman H, Elnakib A, Beache G M, Soliman A, Khalifa F, Gimel'farb G, Elmaghraby A and El-Baz A 2014 A novel 4D PDE-based approach for accurate assessment of myocardium function using cine cardiac magnetic resonance images *Proc. of IEEE Int. Conf. on Image Processing (ICIP'14) (Paris, France, 27–30 October 2014)* pp 3537–41

[117] Sliman H, Khalifa F, Elnakib A, Beache G M, Elmaghraby A and El-Baz A 2013 A new segmentation-based tracking framework for extracting the left ventricle cavity from cine cardiac MRI *Proc. of IEEE Int. Conf. on Image Processing, (ICIP'13) (Melbourne, Australia, 15–18 September 2013)* pp 685–9

[118] Sliman H, Khalifa F, Elnakib A, Soliman A, Beache G M, Elmaghraby A, Gimel'farb G and El-Baz A 2013 Myocardial borders segmentation from cine MR images using bi-directional coupled parametric deformable models *Med. Phys.* **40** 1–13

[119] Sliman H, Khalifa F, Elnakib A, Soliman A, Beache G M, Gimel'farb G, Emam A, Elmaghraby A and El-Baz A 2013 Accurate segmentation framework for the left ventricle wall from cardiac cine MRI *Proc. of Int. Symp. on Computational Models for Life Science, (CMLS'13) (Sydney, Australia, 27–29 November 2013)* **vol 1559** pp 287–96

[120] Reda I, Ghazal M, Shalaby A, Elmogy M, AbouEl-Fetouh A, Ayinde B O, AbouEl-Ghar M, Elmaghraby A, Keynton R and El-Baz A 2018 A novel ADCS-based CNN classification system for precise diagnosis of prostate cancer *2018 24th Int. Conf. on Pattern Recognition (ICPR)* (Piscataway, NJ: IEEE), pp 3923–8

[121] Reda I, Khalil A, Elmogy M, Abou El-Fetouh A, Shalaby A, Abou El-Ghar M, Elmaghraby A, Ghazal M and El-Baz A 2018 Deep learning role in early diagnosis of prostate cancer *Technol. Cancer Res. Treat.* **17** 1533034618775530

[122] Reda I, Ayinde B O, Elmogy M, Shalaby A, El-Melegy M, El-Ghar M A, El-fetouh A A, Ghazal M and El-Baz A 2018 A new CNN-based system for early diagnosis of prostate cancer *2018 IEEE 15th Int. Symp. on Biomedical Imaging (ISBI 2018)* (Piscataway, NJ: IEEE), pp 207–10

[123] Eladawi N, Elmogy M, Ghazal M, Helmy O, Aboelfetouh A, Riad A, Schaal S and El-Baz A 2018 Classification of retinal diseases based on OCT images *Front. Biosci.* **23** 247–64

[124] ElTanboly A, Ismail M, Shalaby A, Switala A, El-Baz A, Schaal S, Gimel'farb G and El-Azab M 2017 A computer-aided diagnostic system for detecting diabetic retinopathy in optical coherence tomography images *Med. Phys.* **44** 914–23

[125] Sandhu H S, El-Baz A and Seddon J M 2018 Progress in automated deep learning for macular degeneration *JAMA Ophthalmol.* **136** 1366–67

[126] Dombroski B, Nitzken M, Elnakib A, Khalifa F, El-Baz A and Casanova M F 2014 Cortical surface complexity in a population-based normative sample *Transl. Neurosci.* **5** 17–24

[127] El-Baz A, Casanova M, Gimel'farb G, Mott M and Switala A 2008 An MRI-based diagnostic framework for early diagnosis of dyslexia *Int. J. Comput. Assist. Radiol. Surg.* **3** 181–9

[128] El-Baz A, Casanova M, Gimel'farb G, Mott M, Switala A, Vanbogaert E and McCracken R 2008 A new CAD system for early diagnosis of dyslexic brains *Proc. Int. Conf. on Image Processing (ICIP'2008)* (Piscataway, NJ: IEEE), pp 1820–3

[129] El-Baz A, Casanova M F, Gimel'farb G, Mott M and Switwala A E 2007 A new image analysis approach for automatic classification of autistic brains *Proc. IEEE Int. Symp. on Biomedical Imaging: From Nano to Macro (ISBI'2007)* (Piscataway, NJ: IEEE), pp 352–5

[130] El-Baz A, Elnakib A, Khalifa F, El-Ghar M A, McClure P, Soliman A and Gimel'farb G 2012 Precise segmentation of 3-D magnetic resonance angiography *IEEE Trans. Biomed. Eng.* **59** 2019–29

[131] El-Baz A, Farag A, Gimel'farb G, El-Ghar M A and Eldiasty T 2006 Probabilistic modeling of blood vessels for segmenting MRA images *18th Int. Conf. on Pattern Recognition (ICPR'06)* **vol 3** (Piscataway, NJ: IEEE), pp 917–20

[132] El-Baz A, Farag A A, Gimel'farb G, El-Ghar M A and Eldiasty T 2006 A new adaptive probabilistic model of blood vessels for segmenting MRA images *Medical Image Computing and Computer-Assisted Intervention–MICCAI 2006* vol 4191 (Berlin: Springer), pp 799–806

[133] El-Baz A, Farag A A, Gimel'farb G and Hushek S G 2005 Automatic cerebrovascular segmentation by accurate probabilistic modeling of TOF-MRA images *Medical Image Computing and Computer-Assisted Intervention–MICCAI 2005* (Berlin: Springer), pp 34–42

[134] El-Baz A, Farag A, Elnakib A, Casanova M F, Gimel'farb G, Switala A E, Jordan D and Rainey S 2011 Accurate automated detection of autism related corpus callosum abnormalities *J. Med. Syst.* **35** 929–39

[135] El-Baz A, Farag A and Gimelfarb G 2005 Cerebrovascular segmentation by accurate probabilistic modeling of TOF-MRA images *Image Analysis* vol 3540 (Berlin: Springer), pp 1128–37

[136] El-Baz A, Gimel'farb G, Falk R, El-Ghar M A, Kumar V and Heredia D 2009 A novel 3D joint Markov–Gibbs model for extracting blood vessels from PC–MRA images *Medical Image Computing and Computer-Assisted Intervention–MICCAI 2009* vol 5762 (Berlin: Springer), pp 943–50

[137] Elnakib A, El-Baz A, Casanova M F, Gimel'farb G and Switala A E 2010 Image-based detection of corpus callosum variability for more accurate discrimination between dyslexic and normal brains *IEEE Int. Symp. on Biomedical Imaging: From Nano to Macro (ISBI'2010)* (Piscataway, NJ: IEEE), pp 109–12

[138] Elnakib A, Casanova M F, Gimel'farb G, Switala A E and El-Baz A 2011 Autism diagnostics by centerline-based shape analysis of the corpus callosum *Proc. IEEE Int. Symp. on Biomedical Imaging: From Nano to Macro (ISBI'2011)* (Piscataway, NJ: IEEE), pp 1843–6

[139] Elnakib A, Nitzken M, Casanova M, Park H, Gimel'farb G and El-Baz A 2012 Quantification of age-related brain cortex change using 3D shape analysis *2012 21st Int. Conf. on Pattern Recognition (ICPR)* (Piscataway, NJ: IEEE), pp 41–4

[140] Nitzken M, Casanova M, Gimel'farb G, Elnakib A, Khalifa F, Switala A and El-Baz A 2011 3D shape analysis of the brain cortex with application to dyslexia *2011 18th IEEE Int. Conf. on Image Processing (ICIP)* (Brussels: IEEE), pp 2657–60

[141] El-Gamal F E-Z A, Elmogy M M, Ghazal M, Atwan A, Barnes G N, Casanova M F, Keynton R and El-Baz A S 2017 A novel CAD system for local and global early diagnosis of Alzheimer's disease based on PIB-PET scans *2017 IEEE Int. Conf. on Image Processing (ICIP)* (Piscataway, NJ: IEEE), pp 3270–4

[142] Ismail M M, Keynton R S, Mostapha M M, ElTanboly A H, Casanova M F, Gimel'farb G L and El-Baz A 2016 Studying autism spectrum disorder with structural and diffusion magnetic resonance imaging: a survey *Front. Human Neurosci.* **10** 211

[143] Alansary A *et al* 2016 Infant brain extraction in T_1-weighted MR images using BET and refinement using LCDG and MGRT models *IEEE J. Biomed. Health Inform.* **20** 925–35

[144] Asl E H, Ghazal M, Mahmoud A, Aslantas A, Shalaby A, Casanova M, Barnes G, Gimel'farb G, Keynton R and El-Baz A 2018 Alzheimer's disease diagnostics by a 3D deeply supervised adaptable convolutional network *Front. Biosci.* **23** 584–96

[145] Dekhil O *et al* 2019 A personalized autism diagnosis CAD system using a fusion of structural MRI and resting-state functional MRI data *Front. Psychiatry* **10** 392

[146] Mahmoud A, El-Barkouky A, Farag H, Graham J and Farag A 2013 A non-invasive method for measuring blood flow rate in superficial veins from a single thermal image *Proc. of the IEEE Conf. on Computer Vision and Pattern Recognition Workshops* (Piscataway, NJ: IEEE), pp 354–9

[147] Shalaby A, Mahmoud A, Ghazal M, Suri J S and El-Baz A 2018 2 segmentation of blood vessels using magnetic resonance angiography images *Cardiovascular Imaging and Image Analysis* (Boca Raton, FL: CRC Press), pp 23–42

[148] Chowdhury A S, Rudra A K, Sen M, Elnakib A and El-Baz A 2010 Cerebral white matter segmentation from MRI using probabilistic graph cuts and geometric shape priors *ICIP* (Piscataway, NJ: IEEE), pp 3649–52

[149] Gebru Y, Giridharan G, Ghazal M, Mahmoud A, Shalaby A and El-Baz A 2018 Detection of cerebrovascular changes using magnetic resonance angiography *Cardiovascular Imaging and Image Analysis* (Boca Raton, FL: CRC Press), pp 1–22

[150] Mahmoud A, Shalaby A, Taher F, El-Baz M, Suri J S and El-Baz A 2018 Vascular tree segmentation from different image modalities *Cardiovascular Imaging and Image Analysis* (Boca Raton, FL: CRC Press), pp 43–70

[151] Taher F, Mahmoud A, Shalaby A and El-Baz A 2018 A review on the cerebrovascular segmentation methods *2018 IEEE Int. Symp. on Signal Processing and Information Technology (ISSPIT)* (Piscataway, NJ: IEEE), pp 359–64

[152] Kandil H, Soliman A, Fraiwan L, Shalaby A, Mahmoud A, ElTanboly A, Elmaghraby A, Giridharan G and El-Baz A 2018 A novel MRA framework based on integrated global and local analysis for accurate segmentation of the cerebral vascular system *2018 IEEE 15th Int. Symp. on Biomedical Imaging (ISBI 2018)* (Piscataway, NJ: IEEE), pp 1365–8

Chapter 2

Capsule networks for lung cancer screening

Aryan Mobiny, Supratik Moulik, Naveen Garg, Carol C Wu and Hien V Nguyen

Lung cancer has been the leading cause of cancer-related deaths in past years. A major challenge in lung cancer screening is the detection of lung nodules from computed tomography (CT) scans. State-of-the-art approaches in automated lung nodule classification use deep convolutional neural networks (CNNs). However, these networks require a large number of training samples to generalize well. This chapter investigates the use of capsule networks (CapsNets) as an alternative to CNNs. We show that CapsNets significantly outperform CNNs when the number of training samples is small. To increase the computational efficiency, we introduce a consistent dynamic routing mechanism that results in 3× speed-up of CapsNet. Finally, we show that the original image reconstruction method of CapsNets performs poorly on volumetric lung nodule data. We recommend an efficient alternative, called the convolutional decoder, that yields lower reconstruction error and higher classification accuracy.

2.1 Introduction

Lung cancer has been consistently ranked as the leading cause of cancer-related death all around the world in past years, accounting for more than one-quarter (26%) of all cancer-related deaths [1]. The stage at which diagnosis is made largely determines the overall prognosis of the patient. The five-year relative survival rate is over 50% in early-stage disease, while survival rates drop to less than 5% for late-stage disease [1]. Lung cancer screening of high-risk individuals, which is designed to detect the disease at an early stage, has been shown in the National Lung Screening Trial (NLST) to reduce lung cancer mortality by 20% [2]. The main challenge in lung cancer screening is detecting lung nodules [2, 3]. Radiologist fatigue, increasing workload, and stringent turnaround-time requirements are just a few of the factors which negatively affect the detection rate of lung nodules. Many studies have documented the occurrence of diagnostic errors in clinical practice, caused by many different contributing factors which can generally be divided into person-specific

doi:10.1088/978-0-7503-2540-0ch2

(such as satisfaction of search, etc), nodule-specific (small size, low density), and environment-specific issues (e.g. inadequate equipment, staff shortages, excess workload, etc) [4, 5].

Computer-aided diagnosis (CAD) systems aim to improve the radiologist's performance in terms of diagnostic accuracy and speed [6]. The role of CAD systems in lung nodule detection and screening has been demonstrated over the years [7, 8], as well as their role in distinguishing benign from malignant nodules [6, 9]. However, the automated identification of nodules from non-nodules is quite challenging mainly due to the large variation in size, shape, margins, and density of the nodules [10]. The nodules can also occur in different locations (such as peri-fissural, subpleural, endobronchial, perivascular), contributing to the diversified contextual environment around the nodule tissue [11].

The performance of a conventional CAD system depends heavily on the intermediate image processing stages (such as extracting hand-crafted morphological and statistical features) which are both time-consuming and subjective [12]. In recent years, deep learning technology has attracted considerable interest in the computer vision and machine learning community [13–15]. Deep neural networks (DNNs) have the advantage of automatically capturing the image's higher level features directly from the raw input data. This leads to powerful features tuned to specific tasks of medical image analysis [16–19]. In particular, convolutional neural networks (CNNs) [14, 20, 21] are the state-of-the-art methods in lung nodule classification. In the context of pulmonary nodule classification in computed tomography (CT) images, the study in [22] introduced models of a deep belief network and a convolutional neural network that outperform the conventional hand-crafted features. Setio *et al* [23] proposed a multiview convolutional network for lung nodule detection. Most recently, the study in [24] shows that deep networks, trained on a hospital-scale dataset of 42 290 computed tomography scans, achieve more than 94% area under curve on in lung nodule detection tasks. Therefore, the current trend shows that many researchers are working on designing deep networks which are more suitable for their tasks. This leads to more complex models with a huge number of parameters and hyper-parameters to be tuned, which makes the overall network harder to optimize. This motivates the development of new techniques to address the fundamental limitations of the current CNN structures.

One fundamental drawback of CNNs is the way they route information between layers. Routing is the mechanism of relaying information from one layer to the next layer in the network. CNNs currently perform routing via pooling layers, most commonly being max-pooling and average pooling. However, pooling is a naive way of routing as it discards information about the precise location and pose of the entity within the region, which can be valuable for classification purposes. This gives a limited translation invariance in which a feature can move slightly within the pooling window and still does not change the network's output [25].

Moreover, while CNNs are translation invariant (and partially rotational invariant when using data augmentation), they are unable to identify the position of one object *relative* to another [26, 27]. They can only identify if the object exists in a certain region or not. Therefore, this makes it difficult to correctly identify objects with spatial relationships between features [25]. For example, a set of randomly assembled face parts might look like a face to a CNN as it sees all the key features.

Recently, Sabour *et al* [28] introduced a new architecture called capsule network (CapsNet for short) to address CNNs' shortcomings. The idea is to encode the relative relationships (e.g. locations, scales, orientations) between local parts and the whole object. Encoding these relationships equips the model with a built-in understanding of the three-dimensional space. This makes CapsNets more *invariant to viewpoint* which enables them to recognize objects from different viewpoints not seen in the training data [29]. Sabour *et al* [28] successfully used this algorithm for training the network on hand-written images of digits (MNIST) and achieved state-of-the-art performance. In [30], Hinton introduces matrix capsules with expected-maximization (EM) routing to encode the relationship between entities. Bahadori [31] proposes a novel variation of capsule networks, called spectral capsule networks, that is more stable than the capsule network with EM routing, and converges faster as well. Multi-scale CapsNet [32] is another variation of capsule networks which employs a two-stage processing for extracting and encoding the hierarchy of features. It also uses a modified dropout to improve the robustness of the network and achieves competitive performance on the FashionMNIST and CIFAR-10 datasets.

CapsNets has also been adopted into various tasks and fields. CapsuleGAN [33] is proposed as a generative model which uses a CapsNet discriminator to replace the standard CNN. Siamese CapsNet [34] is introduced as a variant utilized in a pairwise learning task. Capsule networks have been recently used in medical image analysis tasks and achieved remarkable results. Afshar *et al* [35] utilized a modified version of CapsNet for the brain tumor classification task in MRI images. Lalonde *et al* [36] proposed a convolutional–deconvolutional capsule network, which expands capsule networks to segment pathological lungs from low dose CT scans. These studies show the potential of CapsNet to scale to large and volumetric images.

2.2 Capsule network

2.2.1 Capsule computation

A capsule is defined as a group of neurons whose outputs form an *activation vector*. They predict the presence and the pose parameters of a particular object at a given pixel location. The direction of an activation vector captures the object's pose information, such as location and orientation, while the length (a.k.a norm or magnitude) of the activation vector represents the probability that an object of interest exists. For instance, if we rotate an image, the activation vectors also change accordingly, but their lengths stay the same. This property is usually referred to as *equivariance*. Figure 2.1 illustrates the way CapsNets route information from one layer to another layer, using face detection as an example. The length of the activation vector from a lower-level capsule ($\mathbf{u}_1, \mathbf{u}_2, \ldots, \mathbf{u}_I$) encodes the existence probability of its corresponding entity (e.g. eyes, nose, and mouth). The direction of the vector encodes various properties of the entity, such as its size, orientation, position, etc.

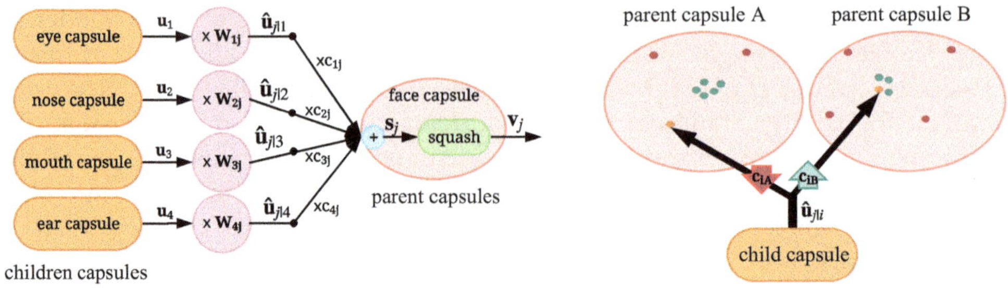

Figure 2.1. Connections between the child and parent capsules in a face detection example. Left: Each child capsule encodes the detailed information about the lower-level entities (such as nose, mouth, etc) in its output $\mathbf{u}_i$. Then every child predicts the output of the parent capsule. In our example, the mouth capsule tries to answer: 'what is the face going to look like given the pose of the mouth'. It makes this prediction by computing the dot-product of a transformation matrix ($\mathbf{W}_{3j}$) with its own activation vector, $\mathbf{u}_3$. Right: Routing by agreement—dynamic routing will ensure that a child capsule will send information to the parent capsules that *agree* with its prediction. In other words, if several child capsules point at the same pose of the face, then there must be a face there. © [2019] IEEE. Reprinted, with permission, from [25].

The relationship between the ith capsule in a lower layer and jth capsule in the next higher layer is encoded using a linear transformation matrix $\mathbf{W}_{ij}$. The information is propagated as: $\hat{\mathbf{u}}_{j|i} = \mathbf{W}_{ij}\mathbf{u}_i$. The vector $\hat{\mathbf{u}}_{ij}$ represents the belief of the ith capsule in a lower layer about the jth capsule in the higher layer. In our example, $\hat{\mathbf{u}}_{j|1}$ represents the predicted pose of the face according to the detected pose of the nose. During the training, the network will gradually learn a transformation matrix for each capsule pair to encode the corresponding part–whole relationship.

2.2.2 Dynamic routing

Having computed the prediction vectors, the lower-level capsules then route their information to parent capsules that agree the most with their predictions. The mechanism that ensures that the outputs of the child capsules are sent to the proper parent capsules is called *dynamic routing*. Let c_{ij} denote the routing coefficient from the ith capsule in the lower layer to the jth capsule in the higher layer, where $\sum_j c_{ij} = 1$ and $c_{ij} \geqslant 0, \quad \forall j$. When $c_{ij} = 1$, all information from the ith capsule will be sent to the jth capsule, whereas when $c_{ij} = 0$ there is no information flowing between the two capsules. The dynamic routing method iteratively tunes the c_{ij} coefficients and routes the child capsules' outputs to the appropriate capsule in the next layer so that they obtain a cleaner input, thus determining the pose of the objects more accurately.

The right panel of figure 2.1 shows a lower-level capsule (e.g. nose capsule) making a decision to send its output to the parent capsules. This decision is made by adjusting the routing coefficients, c_{ij}, that will be multiplied by the prediction vectors before sending it to high-level capsules. CapsNets compute the parent capsules' activation vector ($\mathbf{v}_j$) and routing coefficients as follows:

$$\mathbf{v}_j = \frac{||\mathbf{s}_j||^2}{1 + ||\mathbf{s}_j||^2} \frac{\mathbf{s}_j}{||\mathbf{s}_j||}, \quad \mathbf{s}_j = \sum_i c_{ij} \hat{\mathbf{u}}_{j|i}, \tag{2.1}$$

$$c_{ij} = \frac{\exp(b_{ij})}{\sum_k \exp(b_{ik})}, \quad b_{ij} \leftarrow b_{ij} + \hat{\mathbf{u}}_{j|i} \cdot \mathbf{v}_j. \tag{2.2}$$

The output of each parent capsule $\mathbf{v}_j$ is computed as the weighted sum of all predictions from child capsules (i.e. $\mathbf{s}_j$), then passed through a *squash* non-linearity. Squashing makes sure that the output vector has a length of no more than 1 (so that its length can be interpreted as the probability of a given feature being detected by the capsule) without changing its direction. Each parent capsule receives predictions ($\hat{\mathbf{u}}_{j|i}$) from all child capsules. These vectors are represented by points in figure 2.1. The dynamic routing mechanism will increase the routing coefficient to parent capsule j by a factor of $\hat{\mathbf{u}}_{j|i} \cdot \mathbf{v}_j$ whose value increases for the similar vectors. Thus a child capsule will send more information to the parent capsule whose output $\mathbf{v}_j$ is more similar to its prediction $\hat{\mathbf{u}}_{j|i}$.

2.2.3 Capsule network architecture

The original capsule network contains two main parts, the encoder and decoder, depicted in the first two figures of [28]. The encoder contains three layers: two convolution layers and one fully connected layer. The first layer is a standard convolution layer with 256 filters of size 9 × 9 and stride 1, followed by ReLU activation. The next layer is a convolutional capsule layer called the PrimaryCaps layer. Capsules are arranged in 32 channels (commonly referred to as 32 capsule types) where each primary capsule applies eight convolutional filters of size 9 × 9 and stride 2 to the input volume. Therefore, each primary capsule sees the outputs of all 256 (the whole input depth) × 81 (that fall inside the 9 × 9 filter) units of the first convolutional layer. In this setting, all PrimaryCaps in each of the 32 channels share their weights with each other and each capsule outputs an eight-dimensional vector of activations. The last layer is called the DigitCaps layer which has one 16D capsule per class. Routing takes place between these capsules and all PrimaryCaps, encoding the input into a 16-dimensional activation vector of instantiation parameters. The lengths of these prediction vectors are used to determine the predicted class.

The decoder tries to reconstruct the input from the final capsules, which will force the network to preserve as much information from the input as possible across the whole network. This effectively works as a regularizer that reduces the risk of over-fitting and helps generalize to new samples. In the decoder, the 16D outputs of the final capsules are all masked out (set to zero) except for the ones corresponding to the target (while training) or predicted (while testing) class. They proposed using a three-layer feed-forward neural network with 512, 1024, and 784 units to reconstruct the input image.

2.3 Fast capsule network

2.3.1 Consistent dynamic routing

Dynamic routing has been shown to improve the classification accuracy of CapsNet [28]. However, this operation is computationally expensive and does not scale well to high dimensional data, such as 3D CT scans with a large number of pixels. We propose a consistent dynamic routing mechanism to address this problem. Specifically, we force all capsules in the PrimaryCaps layer corresponding to the same pixels to have the same routing coefficients:

$$c_{ij} = c_{kj}, \quad \forall\, i, k \in \mathcal{S} = \{i, k \mid \text{loc}(i) = \text{loc}(k)\}, \tag{2.3}$$

where loc() is the function converting a capsule index to its pixel location. This strategy will dramatically reduce the number of routing coefficients. For example, the original CapsNet has 32 capsules for each pixel location in the PrimaryCaps layer. The proposed method will, therefore, reduce the number of routing coefficients by a factor of 32. The iterative routing procedure is a bottleneck of CapsNets. Through reducing the number of routing operations, we expect to dramatically increase the network's efficiency. There are many possible ways to enforce the constraint in equation (2.3). In this chapter, we use a simple strategy that allows only one capsule at each pixel location. To compensate for the reduction of the number of capsules, we increase the dimension of each capsule to 256D instead of 8D as in the original CapsNet. Our results show that the proposed architecture achieves similar classification accuracy, and is 3× faster than CapsNet.

2.3.2 Convolutional decoder

CapsNet uses an additional reconstruction loss as a regularization to prevent overfitting during learning the network's parameters [28]. This encourages the digit capsules to encode as much information from the input as possible. The reconstruction is done by feeding 16D output of the final capsules to a three-layer feed-forward neural network. Unfortunately, our experiments show that lung nodule data cannot be reconstructed well from the final capsules. This could be due to the high visual variability within the data. To this end, we propose a different reconstruction mechanism to serve as the training regularization. Instead of using the masked outputs of the NoduleCaps, we used the PrimaryCaps prediction vectors ($\hat{\mathbf{u}}_{j|i}$) only for the target (or predicted) class. For the example in figure 2.2, it is a $8 \times 8 \times 16$ tensor. We also concatenated the one-hot-encoded target (predicted) vector replicated over the space to form a final tensor of $8 \times 8 \times 18$ as the decoder's input. This tensor is then fed to two consecutive fractionally strided convolution layers (also known as deconvolution [37] or transposed convolution layers) with 16 and 1 filters of size 4×4 and stride 2. This structure has many fewer parameters (about 5K) and significantly outperforms the feed-forward network in the reconstruction task. Figure 2.3 shows examples of reconstructed images using CapsNet and the proposed method.

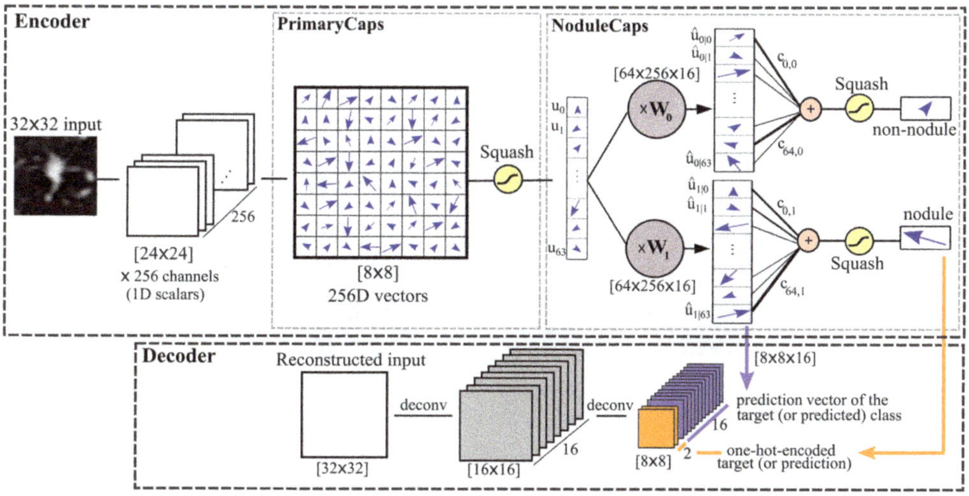

Figure 2.2. Visual representation of fast capsule network for lung nodule classification. Reprinted by permission from Springer Nature: [29] © (2018).

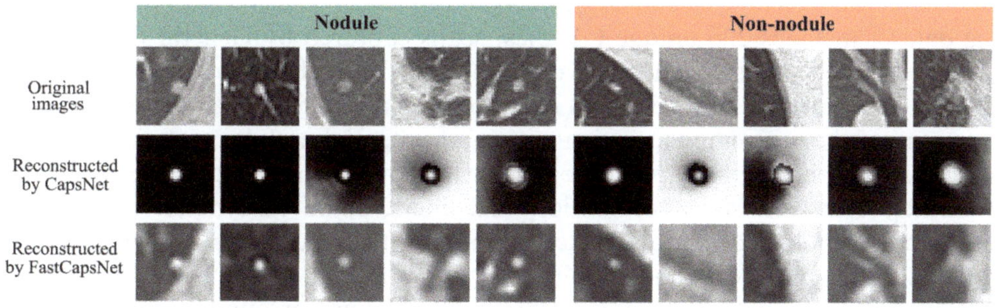

Figure 2.3. Sample images of nodules (left) and non-nodules (right) and their reconstructions using the original CapsNet (middle row) and the FastCapsNet (bottom row). Reprinted by permission from Springer Nature: [29] © (2018).

2.3.3 Loss function

Similar to [28], we used margin loss to force the activation vector of the top-level capsule k ($k \in \{0, 1\}$) to have a large length if and only if the target class (nodule or non-nodule) is present in the image. The total margin loss is the sum of the losses for each NoduleCap and is computed as

$$L_{\text{margin}} = \sum_k [T_k \max(0, m^+ - ||\mathbf{v}_k||)^2 + \lambda(1 - T_k) \max(0, ||\mathbf{v}_k|| - m^-)^2], \tag{2.4}$$

where $T_k = 1$ iff class k is present, and $m^+ = 0.9$, $m^- = 0.1$, and $\lambda = 0.5$ as set in [28]. The sum of squared differences between the input and reconstructed images is used as the reconstruction loss and the total loss is computed as

$$L_{\text{Total}} = L_{\text{margin}} + \alpha L_{\text{reconstruction}}, \tag{2.5}$$

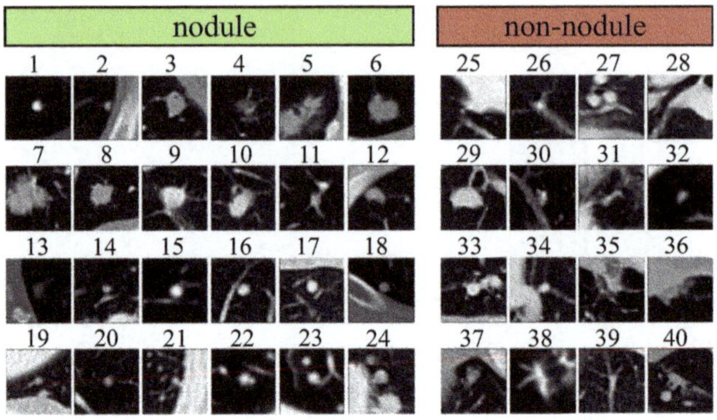

Figure 2.4. Sample images of nodules (left) and non-nodules (right) selected from our dataset. Each image is a slice along a 2D axial plane in the middle of the volume.

where α is set to 0.0005 to scale down the reconstruction loss so that it does not dominate the margin loss during training.

2.4 Dataset

The dataset includes 226 unique CT chest scans captured by General Electric and Siemens scanners at a single hospital on a single day. The data were preprocessed by automated segmentation software in order to identify structures to the organ level. From within the segmented lung tissue, a set of potential nodule points is generated based on the size and shape of regions within the lung which exceed the air Hounsfield unit (HU) threshold. Additional filters, based on symmetry and other common morphological characteristics, are applied to decrease the false positive rate while maintaining very high sensitivity.

Bounding boxes with at least eight voxels of padding surrounding the candidate nodules are cropped and resized to $32 \times 32 \times 32$ pixels. Each generated candidate is reviewed and annotated by at least one board-certified radiologist. From all the generated images (about 7400 images), around 56% were labeled as nodules and the rest non-nodules. The radius of the detected nodules ranges from 3 to 15 mm with an average of 5 ($\pm$1.86) mm. The differences in scan protocol for the various chest studies yields a slice thickness ranging from 0.625–2.5 mm. In each case, an attempt was made to get as close to isotropic as possible while adhering to slice thickness multiples of 0.625 mm. For example, most studies have an in-plane resolution of approximately 0.7×0.7 mm; in this case, linear interpolation was used to convert the data to 0.625 mm slice thickness (voxel dimension of $0.7 \times 0.7 \times 0.625$ mm^3). Figure 2.4 shows examples of extracted candidates and the corresponding labels provided by radiologists. These images illustrate the highly challenging task of distinguishing nodules from non-nodule lesions. The first reason is that the pulmonary nodules come with large variations in shape, size, type, etc (see 1–24 in figure 2.4).

In figure 2.4, examples of solitary (1), subpleural (2), cavitary (3), and ground-glass (4) nodules are depicted. (5) is a more complicated sample containing a mixed solid and ground-glass nodule with irregular margins. While nodules are commonly known as spherical lesions, they also often have a non-spherical shape (12–13) and irregular margins. These irregularities can be caused by vessels and/or spiculations (6–11). Other objects and tissues might also appear in the nodule samples, such as single or multiple blood vessels (14–17), the chest wall (18–19), lung recess (19), etc. Moreover, one nodule image can also contain several nodules of different shapes and sizes (21–24).

The second reason which hinders the identification process is non-nodule candidates mimicking the morphological appearance of real pulmonary nodules. Calcification (30), short vessels (31–34), scarring (35), infection (36–37), vessels with motion artifacts mimicking a ground-glass nodule (38), and septical thickening (39). Some images might also contain a nodule, but centered on another tissue (such as a vessel in (40)) and so is labeled as non-nodule. For all these reasons, the detection and classification of lung nodules is a challenging task, even for experienced radiologists.

2.5 Experiments

2.5.1 2D capsule network

Figure 2.2 provides an illustration of the proposed architecture, which consists of three different layers. To prepare the required 2D images, we used the middle slices of the 3D volumes along the x-axis (as the x-axis contains more information according to the radiologist's feedback). The first layer is a 3D convolution layer with 256 filters of size 9 and stride 1. Given our 32×32 pixel inputs, this layer outputs a $24 \times 24 \times 256$ tensor, which is the basic features extracted from the input image. The next layer is the PrimaryCaps layer which applies 256 convolutional filters on the input to obtain an $8 \times 8 \times 256$ tensor. We consider this tensor to be $8 \times 8 = 64$ capsules, each with 256D. This results in only one capsule at each pixel, therefore effectively enforcing consistent dynamic routing. These vectors will then be passed through a squashing non-linearity to obtain the final output of the lower-level capsules (i.e. $\mathbf{u}_i$). The proposed architecture is a departure from the original CapsNet, which divides the tensor into $8 \times 8 \times 32 = 2048$ capsules, each of 8D, resulting in 32 capsules for each pixel location. While the total number of parameters of the two networks is the same, our network drastically reduces the number of PrimaryCaps from 2048 to 64, thereby decreasing the number of voting coefficients by 32 times.

In the final layer, called NoduleCaps, 256D output from the PrimaryCaps layer are multiplied with its own 256×16 transformation matrix which maps the output to the 16D space (results in $\hat{\mathbf{u}}_{j|i}$). Finally, the routing parameter tunes the coupling coefficients and decides the amount of contribution they make to the NoduleCaps. During training, the coefficients are initialized uniformly, meaning that the output from the PrimaryCaps layer is sent equally to all the capsules in the NoduleCaps layer. Then the routing between the two layers is learned iteratively.

2.5.2 3D capsule network

The 3D version of the proposed architecture is structurally similar to the explained 2D version. In the first two layers, 2D convolutions are replaced by 3D convolution operators capturing the cross-correlation of the voxels. The number and size of the filters and the strides are the same as before. This results in an $8 \times 8 \times 8$ volume of primary capsules, each sees the output of all $256 \times 9 \times 9 \times 9$ units of the previous convolution layer. Therefore, our proposed faster architecture gives 512 PrimaryCaps, compared to 23 328 of the original network. This will limit the number of required routing coefficients, help the dynamic routing perform faster and perform significantly better. NodulesCaps are the same as in the 2D network, fully connected to PrimaryCaps with the dynamic routing happening in the middle. Similar to the proposed 2D FastCapsNet, the decoder takes the prediction vectors of all PrimaryCaps (only the ones routed to the correct class) and concatenates it with the one-hot-encoded label of the target to form a tensor of shape $8 \times 8 \times 8 \times 18$. It then reconstructs the input from this tensor by applying two consecutive 3D fractionally strided convolution layers with 16 and 1 filters, respectively. Obviously, a feed-forward architecture would not scale well for reconstructing the 3D images (it requires $32 \times 32 \times 32$ output units which drastically increases the number of parameters).

2.6 Results and discussion

The 2D version of the proposed faster CapsNet was trained and compared to two well-known deep network architectures, AlexNet [14] and ResNet-50 [20], as well as the original Capsule network. Trying both 2D and 3D architectures helps in testing the network's performance in both settings, as well as enabling us to quantify the contribution of the third dimension. All analyses are performed using a desktop machine equipped with 128 GB of memory, four NVidia GTX 1080 with 8 GB of video memory each, and an Intel Xeon CPU 2.40 GHz with 16 cores.

The test prediction results are presented in table 2.1. The capsule networks achieve relatively lower error rates compared to AlexNet and ResNet. FastCapsNet has fewer parameters than other models, thus is more than three times faster than the

Table 2.1. Comparison of the performance, number of trainable parameters (M is for millions), and required training time per epoch of the deep networks.

	Precision	Recall	Error rate	#Params	sec/epoch
Automated software	73.65	82.13	25.34	—	—
2D AlexNet	88.09	85.52	13.09	7.6M	6.9
2D ResNet-50	89.14	85.52	12.51	23.5M	16.3
2D CapsNet	89.44	85.98	12.16	7.4M	18.8
2D FastCapsNet	**89.71**	**87.41**	**11.45**	5.8M	6.2
3D AlexNet	91.05	87.92	10.42	7.8M	175.1
3D ResNet-50	90.51	**90.42**	9.58	48.2M	341.5
3D FastCapsNet	**91.84**	89.11	**9.52**	52.2M	320.0

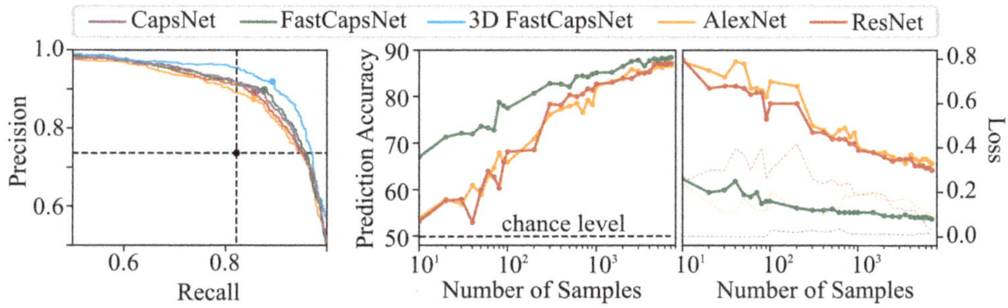

Figure 2.5. Left: Test precision–recall curves. Center: Test prediction accuracy of models trained on a different number of training samples. Right: Train (dashed) and test (solid) loss of models trained on a different number of training samples. Reprinted by permission from Springer Nature: [29] © (2018).

regular CapsNet in both training and test runs. For 3D images, the 3D implementation of the original CapsNet failed to converge. The prediction accuracy remains close to chance level with the validation loss increasing gradually. However, our proposed 3D FastCapsNet converges relatively fast (reaching less than 20% test loss after only three training epochs).

The precision–recall curves of the models are presented in the left panel of figure 2.5, confirming the superior performance of the proposed FastCapsNets compared to the other models. The 3D FastCapsNet performs significantly better than the rest, beating the 2D version by almost 2% accuracy, indicating the contribution of the third dimension. We also trained the 2D models using different numbers of training samples. The prediction accuracy and loss values of different models are presented in the middle and right panel of figure 2.5, respectively. The capsule network performs comparatively more robustly. For a very small number of samples, AlexNet and ResNet-50 go almost to chance level while the capsule network remains at about 70%.

2.7 Conclusions

The observations made in this chapter show that CapsNet is a promising alternative to CNN. Experimental results demonstrate that CapsNets compare favorably to CNNs when the training size is large, but significantly outperform CNNs on small datasets. This is particularly helpful when the system must learn from small amounts of data, which is often the case in medical settings where data collection is either expensive (due to the requirement for highly trained experts), or time-consuming (due to the multiple repetitions of an experiment). We showed that, by modifying the routing mechanism, we can speed up CapsNets by three times while maintaining the same accuracy.

References

[1] Siegel R L, Miller K D and Jemal A 2017 Cancer statistics, 2017 *CA Cancer J. Clin.* **67** 7–30

[2] The National Lung Screening Trial Research Team 2011 Reduced lung-cancer mortality with low-dose computed tomographic screening *N. Engl. J. Med.* **2011** 395–409

[3] Horeweg N, Scholten E T, de Jong P A, van der Aalst C M, Weenink C, Lammers J-W J, Nackaerts K, Vliegenthart R, ten Haaf K and Yousaf-Khan U A 2014 Detection of lung cancer through low-dose CT screening (NELSON): a prespecified analysis of screening test performance and interval cancers *Lancet Oncol.* **15** 1342–50

[4] Brady A, Laoide R Ó, McCarthy P and McDermott R 2012 Discrepancy and error in radiology: concepts, causes and consequences *Ulster Med. J.* **81** 3

[5] Brady A P 2016 Error and discrepancy in radiology: inevitable or avoidable? *Insights Imaging* **8** 171–82

[6] Shewaye T N and Mekonnen A A 2016 Benign-malignant lung nodule classification with geometric and appearance histogram features, arXiv:1605.08350

[7] Awai K, Murao K, Ozawa A, Komi M, Hayakawa H, Hori S and Nishimura Y 2004 Pulmonary nodules at chest CT: effect of computer-aided diagnosis on radiologists detection performance *Radiology* **230** 347–52

[8] Sahiner B *et al* 2009 Effect of CAD on radiologists' detection of lung nodules on thoracic CT scans: analysis of an observer performance study by nodule size *Acad. Radiol.* **16** 1518–30

[9] Lee S L A, Kouzani A Z and Hu E J 2010 Random forest based lung nodule classification aided by clustering *Computer. Med. Imaging Graph.* **34** 535–42

[10] Dou Q, Chen H, Yu L, Qin J and Heng P-A 2017 Multilevel contextual 3-D CNNs for false positive reduction in pulmonary nodule detection *IEEE Trans. Biomed. Eng.* **64** 1558–67

[11] Firmino M, Morais A H, Mendoça R M, Dantas M R, Hekis H R and Valentim R 2014 Computer-aided detection system for lung cancer in computed tomography scans: review and future prospects *Biomed. Eng. Online* **13** 41

[12] Shen W, Zhou M, Yang F, Yu D, Dong D, Yang C, Zang Y and Tian J 2017 Multi-crop convolutional neural networks for lung nodule malignancy suspiciousness classification *Pattern Recogn.* **61** 663–73

[13] LeCun Y, Bengio Y and Hinton G 2015 Deep learning *Nature* **521** 436–44

[14] Krizhevsky A, Sutskever I and Hinton G E 2012 ImageNet classification with deep convolutional neural networks *NIPS'12 Proc. of the 25th Int. Conf. on Neural Information Processing Systems - Volume 1* pp 1097–105

[15] Donahue J, Anne Hendricks L, Guadarrama S, Rohrbach M, Venugopalan S, Saenko K and Darrell T 2015 Long-term recurrent convolutional networks for visual recognition and description *Proc. of the IEEE Conf. on Computer Vision and Pattern Recognition* pp 2625–34

[16] Xu Y, Mo T, Feng Q, Zhong P, Lai M, Eric I and Chang C 2014 Deep learning of feature representation with multiple instance learning for medical image analysis *2014 IEEE Int. Conf. on Acoustics, Speech and Signal Processing (ICASSP)* (Piscataway, NJ: IEEE), pp 1626–30

[17] Ghesu F C, Krubasik E, Georgescu B, Singh V, Zheng Y, Hornegger J and Comaniciu D 2016 Marginal space deep learning: efficient architecture for volumetric image parsing *IEEE Trans. Med. Imaging* **35** 1217–28

[18] Greenspan H, van Ginneken B and Summers R M 2016 Guest editorial deep learning in medical imaging: overview and future promise of an exciting new technique *IEEE Trans. Med. Imaging* **35** 1153–9

[19] Bar Y, Diamant I, Wolf L, Lieberman S, Konen E and Greenspan H 2015 Chest pathology detection using deep learning with non-medical training *2015 IEEE 12th Int. Symp. on Biomedical Imaging (ISBI)* (Piscataway, NJ: IEEE), pp 294–7

[20] He K, Zhang X, Ren S and Sun J 2016 Deep residual learning for image recognition *Proc. of the IEEE Conf. on Computer Vision and Pattern Recognition* pp 770–8

[21] Mobiny A, Moulik S and Van Nguyen H 2017 Lung cancer screening using adaptive memory-augmented recurrent networks, arXiv:1710.05719

[22] Hua K-L, Hsu C-H, Hidayati S C, Cheng W-H and Chen Y-J 2015 Computer-aided classification of lung nodules on computed tomography images via deep learning technique *OncoTargets Ther.* **8** 2015–22

[23] Setio A A A, Ciompi F, Litjens G, Gerke P, Jacobs C, van Riel S J, Wille M M W, Naqibullah M, Sánchez C I and van Ginneken B 2016 Pulmonary nodule detection in CT images: false positive reduction using multi-view convolutional networks *IEEE Trans. Med. Imaging* **35** 1160–9

[24] Ardila D *et al* 2019 End-to-end lung cancer screening with three-dimensional deep learning on low-dose chest computed tomography *Nat. Med.* **25** 954–61

[25] Mobiny A, Lu H, Nguyen H V, Roysam B and Varadarajan N 2019 Automated classification of apoptosis in phase contrast microscopy using capsule network *IEEE Trans. Med. Imaging* https://ieeexplore.ieee.org/document/8720196

[26] Cohen T and Welling M 2016 Group equivariant convolutional networks *Int. Conf. on Machine Learning* pp 2990–9

[27] Worrall D E, Garbin S J, Turmukhambetov D and Brostow G J 2017 Harmonic networks: deep translation and rotation equivariance *Proc. IEEE Conf. on Computer Vision and Pattern Recognition (CVPR)* **vol 2** (Piscataway, NJ: IEEE)

[28] Sabour S, Frosst N and Hinton G E 2017 Dynamic routing between capsules *Advances in Neural Information Processing Systems* pp 3856–66

[29] Mobiny A and Van Nguyen H 2018 Fast CapsNet for lung cancer screening, Medical Image Computing and Computer Assisted Intervention – MICCAI 2018 (Lecture Notes in Computer Science vol 11071) (Cham: Springer)

[30] Sabour S, Frosst N and Hinton G 2018 Matrix capsules with EM routing *6th Int. Conf. on Learning Representations, ICLR*

[31] Bahadori M T 2018 Spectral capsule networks *Proc. ICLR*

[32] Xiang C, Zhang L, Zou W, Tang Y and Xu C 2018 MS-CapsNet: a novel multi-scale capsule network *IEEE Signal Process. Lett.* **25** 1850–4

[33] Jaiswal A, AbdAlmageed W and Natarajan P 2018 CapsuleGAN: generative adversarial capsule network, arXiv:1802.06167

[34] Neill J O 2018 Siamese capsule networks, arXiv:1805.07242

[35] Afshar P, Plataniotis K N and Mohammadi A 2019 Capsule networks for brain tumor classification based on MRI images and coarse tumor boundaries *ICASSP 2019-2019 IEEE Int. Conf. on Acoustics, Speech and Signal Processing (ICASSP)* (Piscataway, NJ: IEEE), pp 1368–72

[36] LaLonde R and Bagci U 2018 Capsules for object segmentation, arXiv:1804.04241

[37] Zeiler M D, Krishnan D, Taylor G W and Fergus R 2010 Deconvolutional networks *2010 IEEE Conf. on Computer Vision and Pattern Recognition (CVPR)* (Piscataway, NJ: IEEE), pp 2528–35

Chapter 3

Quantitative malignancy recognition of lung cancer using non-invasive image modalities

Chung-Ming Lo

3.1 Introduction

Currently, lung cancer is the most common cancer worldwide. Although various medications and therapies have been developed, the death rate is still high [1, 2]. Like in other cancers, a possible reason for this phenomenon is the high prevalence of late-stage cancers. That is, the cancers are not detected earlier. One way to reduce the late detection is lung cancer screening using low-dose computed tomography to find early-stage peripheral lung cancers [3]. However, computed tomography cannot detect endobronchial lesions. Therefore, bronchoscopic examination plays a necessary role as an imaging modality in diagnosing endobronchial/tracheal lesions [4, 5].

About 85% of lung cancers are non-small-cell lung cancer (NSCLC) [4, 5]. Among these, 80% are adenocarcinomas (ACs) and squamous cell carcinomas (SCCs). The differentiation by type in the clinic leads to the following different treatment strategies. Patients with advanced lung ACs tend to have mutations of the epidermal growth factor receptor (EGFR) which respond well to EGFR-tyrosine kinase inhibitors (EGFR-TKIs) but SCCs do not [6–8]. Cytotoxic chemotherapy or radiotherapy have been the standard treatments to deal with SCCs in the past and recently immune checkpoint blockade therapy has gradually become the new standard to treat advanced SCC with a high expression of programmed death ligand 1 (PD-L1). Consequently, patients with different types of lung cancer should undergo different treatment. The determination of the correct histological type is the key starting point.

An immunohistochemical (IHC) panel is commonly used to determine the histological type, however, this takes a couple of days. For endobronchial lesions, bronchoscopic biopsy can be used as a convenient way to acquire tumor tissue and diagnose the pathological type. The limitation is that only a small amount of tissue is extracted. Due to the heterogeneity of malignant tissues, uncertainty is associated

doi:10.1088/978-0-7503-2540-0ch3

with this invasive procedure. During cancer detection, bronchoscopic imaging techniques are convenient to detect abnormalities. An accompany diagnosis of histological type using bronchoscopy would be helpful in determining staging and subsequent treatment. Both traditional white-light bronchoscopy (WLB) and autofluorescent imaging (AFI) may have the potential ability to detect and diagnose endobronchial premalignant lesions in the bronchial mucosa [6–8]. The extent of the mass and the resection margins can be also estimated simultaneously [9]. In the literature, the comparison of AFI and WLB showed higher detection rates and sensitivities but variable specificity [10]. Inter-observer variability should be reduced to make these approaches more practical [9].

Machine-learning based automatic classification has been widely used for medical images. After image preprocessing, such as contrast enhancement or color analysis, meaningful diagnostic features from bronchoscopy can be extracted and combined to generate a classification model. Each case is given a probability indicating the likelihood of it being a certain type. Analyzing the whole tumor area with so-called computer-aided diagnosis (CAD) would be more objective and efficient.

A previous CAD system was developed to classify normal mucosa and lung tumors using WLB [11] and achieved an accuracy of 80%. In this study, we further extend the application to differentiate cancer types using WLB and AFI. In the experiment, via bronchoscopy, textures in multiple color channels of RGB are separately quantified to classify ACs and SCCs. The hue–saturation–value (HSV) color space translates the color component, making it more intuitive to provide a better color interpretation, such as the results mentioned in medical applications. The proposed method may facilitate the physicians' decision making in a clinical environment.

3.2 Materials and methods

3.2.1 Patient information

This study analyzing bronchoscopy images was approved by the institutional review board of Shuang Ho Hospital (New Taipei City, Taiwan). Due to its retrospective nature, informed consent from patients was waived. From September 2015 to April 2017, 70 patients at Shuang Ho Hospital were examined under BF-F260 (Olympus Optical, Tokyo, Japan). Among the 70 cases, 36 had normal mucosa findings while 34 had neoplastic findings using WLB and AFI. The pathological diagnosis of the 34 abnormal neoplastic cases was determined by bronchoscopic biopsies and a pathologist. In the image observations, only 23 endobronchial tumors were clearly recognized with WLB and AFI without confounding by bleeding. Other cases were difficult to interpret using human observation. Additionally, two SCCs, two unknown carcinomas, and one tracheal tumor were excluded due to small size. Finally, the enrolled tumor database included 12 ACs (patients aged 42–83 years) and 11 SCCs (for WLB, only 10; patients aged 50–90 years). The AC and SCC samples are shown in figures 3.1 and 3.2. The tumor areas that appeared in the WLB or AFI were determined and delineated by a physician as regions of interest (ROIs).

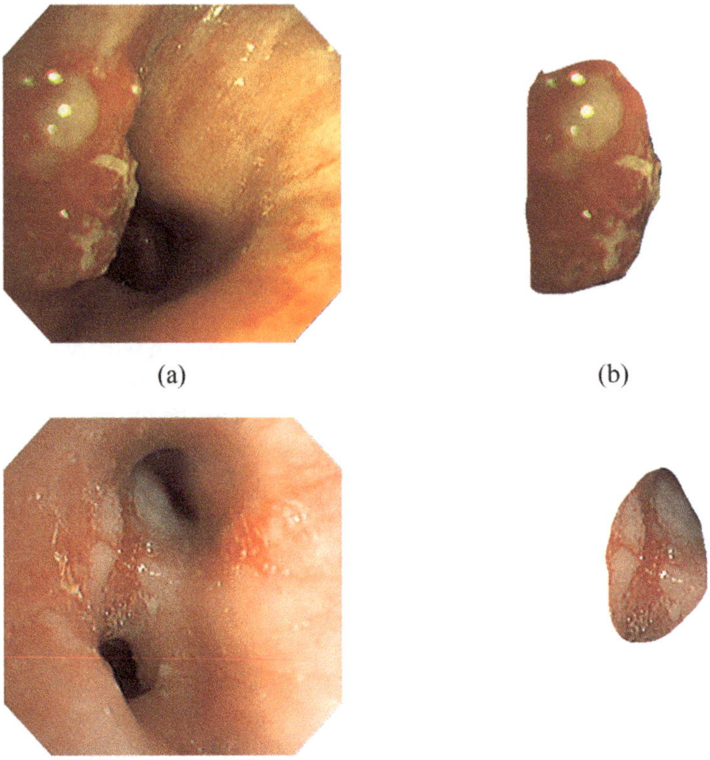

(a) (b)

(c) (d)

Figure 3.1. Samples of (a) adenocarcinomas in white-light bronchoscopy, (b) the corresponding tumor area and (c) squamous cell carcinomas in white-light bronchoscopy, (d) the corresponding tumor area.

3.2.2 Multichannel features

Medical images include various image appearances according to the tissue properties and how they are interpreted [12–14]. Tissues such as skin, fat, and bone can be differentiated by the rate of absorption of radiation in x-ray imaging or computed tomography. Different tissues have different reflecting echoes, which is the basic theory of ultrasound. These imaging modalities generate a gray-scale representation of organs inside the human body because they are determined by signal intensity. Compared to gray-scale images, the bronchoscopy images used in detecting lung cancer in this study have visible light as the illuminance source. These color images are composed of multi-channels, i.e. the standard red (R), green (G), and blue (B).

Day-to-day imaging examinations in hospitals mostly generate gray-scale images, which belong to the remit of the radiology department. Thus, previous CAD systems have quantified the image features of ultrasound, magnetic resonance imaging, and so on [15, 16]. Gray-scale images have only one channel, i.e. the brightness. In most situations, the diagnostic information extracted from the gray-sale is already sufficient for medical decision making, such as the differentiation of benign and malignant [15–19]. In this study, the proposed CAD systems use image features extracted from multiple channels to classify different lung cancer types. The

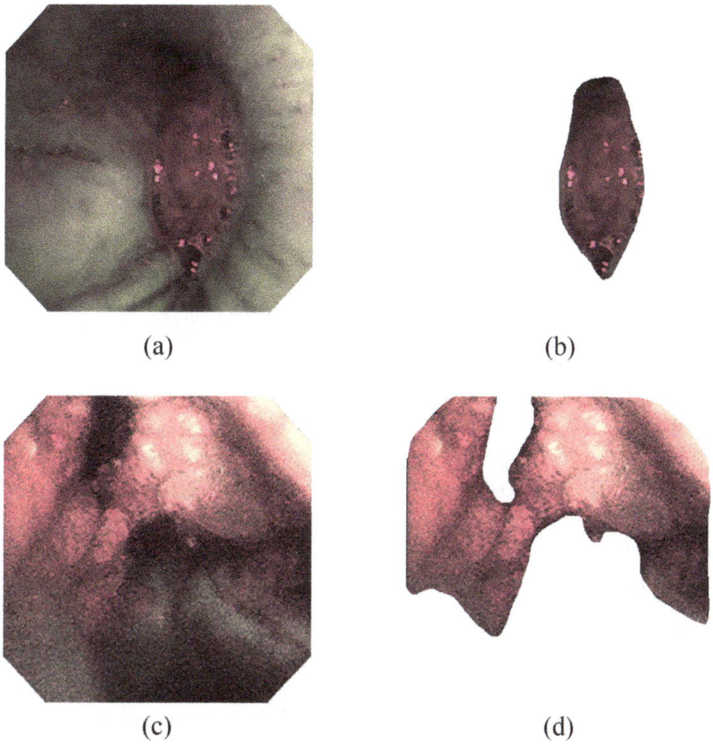

Figure 3.2. Samples of (a) adenocarcinomas in autofluorescent imaging, (b) the corresponding tumor area and (c) squamous cell carcinomas in autofluorescent imaging, (d) the corresponding tumor area.

bronchoscopy images generated from WLB and AFI are in color. Therefore, calculating quantitative image features from multiple channels rather than the conventional gray-scale is the main purpose of the experiment. In addition, the original standard RGB is not suitable for describing color. In order to extract meaningful color features for tissue characterization, the color space transformation is performed first to convert RGB to hue (H), saturation (S), and value (V). After that, textural features are individually extracted from the H, S, and V channels for the pattern recognition of lung cancers.

3.2.2.1 HSV transformation

As mentioned previously, unlike other medical images, bronchoscopy generates color images when using either WLB or AFI. Also, in clinical examinations, physicians have to detect abnormalities according to the color characteristics of tissues. Since color information plays such an important role, the use of color space substantially affects the classification result. The RGB color space is the original color space used by image capture modules and the JPEG format. However, it is not intuitive to describe color using the RGB composition. A better color space used to describe color is HSV [20]. HSV was proposed to imitate human perception. When the physician detects abnormal tissues from background tissues, they must depend greatly on hue, saturation, and brightness. Hue means the main color such as red or

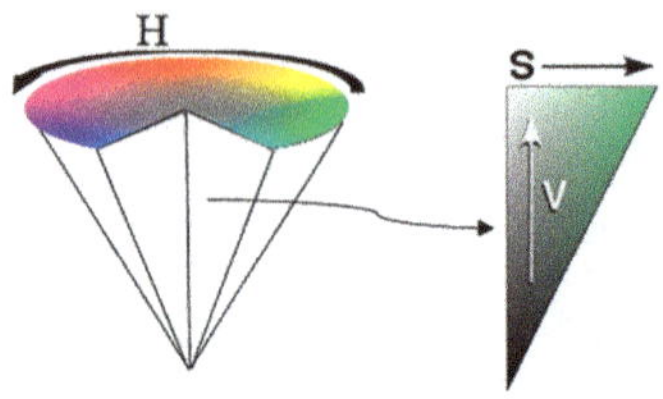

Figure 3.3. The HSV color space presents hue (H), saturation (S), and value (V).

yellow. Saturation indicates how rich the hue is, and brightness can tell us the level of luminance. Figure 3.3 shows the shape of the HSV color space.

3.2.2.2 Textural features

Pattern recognition in medical images always depends on the correlations between pixels, that is texture analyses [15, 16]. Texture is a second-order statistic, which means feature generation involving two or more pixels together rather than a lone pixel. Previous studies in the literature have used textural features to classify tissues in ultrasound or other imaging modalities [15, 16]. Here, the texture features were extracted from three channels (H, S, V) and combined to present the differences between malignant types.

The target tissues were just the tumor area, which was delineated by the physicians who carried out the bronchoscopy. Next, the gray-level co-occurrence matrix (GLCM) [21] was used to describe the joint frequencies of pair-wise pixel combinations. Because color images have three channels, the GLCM was individually applied to three channels. The whole delineated area was scanned to generate co-occurrence matrices $P = [p(i,j|d,\theta)]$ showing the frequencies of two adjacent pixels at a distance d and a direction θ. As per the equation listed below, the two gray-scale pixel values were i and j. Four offset directions, $\theta = 0°, 45°, 90°$, and $135°$, were used to find the correlations between the two adjacent pixels, as shown in figure 3.4. To achieve rotation invariance, these four directions were combined in the matrix. The statistics of the matrix listed below are the 14 GLCM textural features:

$$\text{Autocorrelation} = \sum_i \sum_j (p_x - \mu_x)(p_y - \mu_y)/\sigma_x\sigma_y; \tag{3.1}$$

$$\text{Contrast} = \sum_n n^2 \left\{ \sum_i \sum_j p(i,j) \right\},\ |i - j| = n; \tag{3.2}$$

$$\text{Correlation} = \frac{\sum_i \sum_j (i - \mu_x)(j - \mu_y)p(i,j)}{\sigma_x\sigma_y}; \tag{3.3}$$

$$\text{Cluster prominence} = \sum_i \sum_j (i + j - \mu_x - \mu_y)^4 p(i,j); \tag{3.4}$$

$$\text{Cluster shading} = \sum_i \sum_j (i + j - \mu_x - \mu_y)^3 p(i,j); \tag{3.5}$$

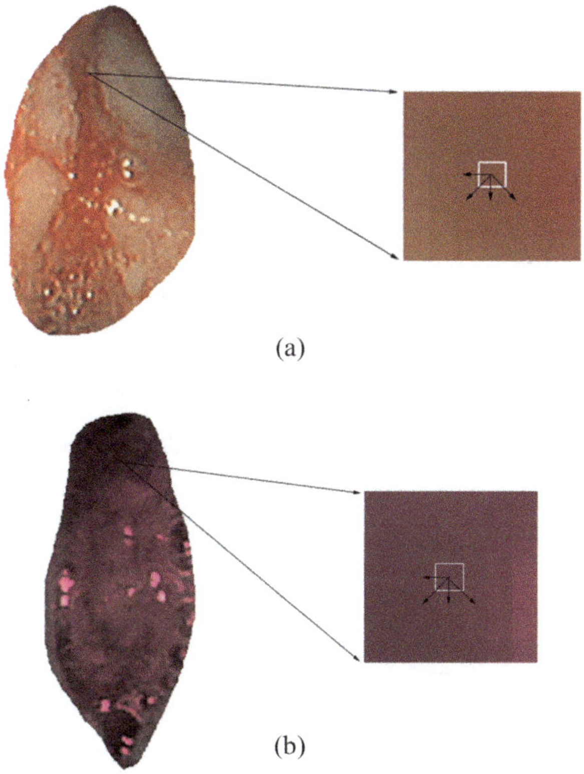

Figure 3.4. Texture features are correlations between adjacent pixels in (a) white-light bronchoscopy and (b) autofluorescent imaging.

$$\text{Dissimilarity} = \sum_i \sum_j p(i, j)|i - j|; \tag{3.6}$$

$$\text{Energy} = \sum_i \sum_j p(i, j)^2; \tag{3.7}$$

$$\text{Entropy} = -\sum_i \sum_j p(i, j)\log(p(i, j)); \tag{3.8}$$

$$\text{Homogeneity} = -\sum_i \sum_j \frac{1}{1 + i - j} p(i, j); \tag{3.9}$$

$$\text{Difference variance} = \sum_i i^2 p_{x-y}(i); \tag{3.10}$$

$$\begin{aligned} \text{Difference entropy} &= -\sum_i p_{x+y}(i)\log(p_{x+y}(i)); \\ &\times \frac{HXY - HXY1}{\max\{HX, HY\}} \\ HXY &= \text{Entropy} = -\sum_i \sum_j p(i, j)\log(p(i, j)), \end{aligned} \tag{3.11}$$

$$\text{Information measure of correlation} = HXY1 = -\sum_i\sum_j p(i,j)\log(p_x(i)p_y(j)) \quad (3.12)$$
$$HX = \text{entropy of } p_x,$$
$$HY = \text{entropy of } p_y;$$

$$\text{Inverse difference normalized} = \sum_i\sum_j \frac{1}{1+|i-j|}p(i,j); \text{ and} \quad (3.13)$$

$$\text{Inverse difference moment} = \sum_i\sum_j \frac{1}{1+(i-j)^2}p(i,j); \quad (3.14)$$

where μ_x, μ_y, σ_x, and σ_y are the means and standard deviations of the distributions of $p(i,j|d,\theta)$:

$$\mu_x = \sum_i i\sum_j p(i,j), \quad \mu_y = \sum_j j\sum_i p(i,j) \quad (3.15)$$

and

$$\sigma_x^2 = \sum_i (i-u_x)^2\sum_j p(i,j), \quad \sigma_y^2 = \sum_j (j-u_y)^2\sum_i p(i,j). \quad (3.16)$$

3.2.2.3 Statistical analysis

Quantitative texture features were extracted from three channels. To determine whether they had diagnostic ability, these features were evaluated to determine if they were statistically significant in the differentiation of cancer type. The Kolmogorov–Smirnov test [22] was first used to evaluate if the texture features were normally distributed. Features having normal or non-normal distributions were then tested using the corresponding Student's t-test [22] and Mann–Whitney U-test [22]. The features with a p-value of <0.05 show a statistically significant difference. Texture features were also combined in the binary logistic regression model [23]. Using backward elimination, the most relevant feature combination can be selected during the elimination process.

Due to the limited size of the collected database, the leave-one-out cross-validation method [24, 25] was used to validate the generalization ability of the prediction model. With k cases, in each iteration $k-1$ are used for training and the remaining case was used to test the trained model. Using a biopsy-proven result as the ground truth of the cancer type, each case was given a malignancy probability. With different thresholds, five performance indices, including the accuracy, sensitivity, specificity, positive predictive value (PPV), and negative predictive value (NPV), were obtained. The probability formula combined selected features to indicate the likelihood of being a certain type of cancer:

$$P = \frac{1}{1+e^{-(c_1\times x_1+c_2\times x_2+\cdots+c_n\times x_n+c_0)}}. \quad (3.17)$$

Performance index comparisons were evaluated using the chi-squared test in SPSS software (version 16 for Windows; SPSS, Chicago, IL, USA). The trade-offs between sensitivity and specificity under different thresholds were illustrated using the receiver operating characteristic (ROC) curve. A_z, the area under an ROC curve, was also evaluated using a bivariate chi-squared test in the ROCKIT software (C Metz, University of Chicago, Chicago, IL, USA).

3.2.3 Result

3.2.3.1 White-light bronchoscopy

From HSV color space, every channel has 14 GLCM textural features. In the test results, as shown in table 3.1, the significant features ($p < 0.05$) are correlation, cluster prominence, cluster shading, and difference variance in the S channel, and cluster prominence and cluster shading in the V channel. The logistic regression classifier selected correlation (S), difference variance (S), and cluster shading (V) to generate the prediction model and achieve an accuracy of 86% (19/22), a sensitivity of 90% (9/10), a specificity of 83% (10/12), a PPV of 82% (9/11), and an NPV of 91% (10/11). The AUC was 0.82. Only one SCC was misclassified.

3.2.3.2 Autofluorescent imaging

Two kinds of bronchoscopy images were used in the experiment to automatically classify malignant types. Same as WLB texture features, 42 AFI texture features were tested first. The information measure of the correlation in S and correlation in V had significant p-values <0.05 as shown in table 3.2. By combining these two features in the logistic regression classifier, the model achieved an accuracy of 83% (19/23), a sensitivity of 73% (8/11), a specificity of 92% (11/12), and $A_z = 0.82$. A further experiment was carried out using RGB features, and the information measure of the correlation in R and G were significant. Combining the features achieved an accuracy of 57% (13/23), a sensitivity of 73% (8/11), a specificity of 42% (5/12), and $A_z = 0.67$. Obviously, HSV performed better than RGB, in particular for specificity (p-value = 0.009 4) and only one AC was misclassified.

Table 3.1. Significant textural features in the hue–saturation–value (HSV) color space tested by the Student's *t*-test.

	AC	SCC	
Texture feature	Mean ± SD	Mean ± SD	p
Correlation (S)	0.987 ± 0.004	0.979 ± 0.004	<0.001[a]
Cluster prominence (S)	1589.937 ± 818.998	738.032 ± 433.412	<0.01[a]
Cluster shading (S)	130.865 ± 66.141	64.554 ± 36.635	<0.01[a]
Difference variance (S)	20.257 ± 9.692	12.559 ± 6.827	<0.05[a]
Cluster prominence (V)	298.707 ± 206.022	143.151 ± 80.896	<0.05[a]
Cluster shade (V)	−32.370 ± 20.906	−16.407 ± 8.691	<0.05[a]

[a] A p-value <0.05 indicates a statistically significant difference.

AC, adenocarcinoma; SCC, squamous cell carcinoma; S, saturation; V, value; SD, standard deviation.

Table 3.2. Significant HSV textural features and corresponding p-values evaluated using Student's t-test.

	AC	SCC	
Feature	Mean ± SD	Mean ± SD	p-value
Information measure of correlation (S)	−0.854 ± 0.015	−0.821 ± 0.039	<0.05[a]
Correlation (V)	0.984 ± 0.003	0.976 ± 0.013	<0.05[a]

[a] A p-value <0.05 indicates a statistically significant difference.
AC, adenocarcinoma; SCC, squamous cell carcinoma; S, saturation; V, value; SD, standard deviation.

3.2.4 Discussion

Currently, bronchoscopy is widely used in detecting and taking biopsies of endobronchial lesions of lung cancer. If physicians could obtain an initial classification of carcinomas using only bronchoscopy images, their practical use in clinical contexts would be much greater. Therefore, this study proposed using quantitative image features to generate a prediction model for a rapid and accurate assessment of malignancies. Based on the color textures in the HSV color space, the proposed CAD system can generate more objective diagnoses with less inter-observer variability than was reported in the previous literature as the diagnosis limitation. Using WLB, the CAD system achieved an accuracy of 86% (19/22), a sensitivity of 90% (9/10), a specificity of 83% (10/12), a PPV of 82% (9/11), and an NPV of 91% (10/11). AFI had better sensitivity and specificity to clinically detect early endobronchial lesions. In our result, using GLCM textural features from HSV images achieved an accuracy of 83% (19/23), a sensitivity of 73% (8/11), and a specificity of 92% (11/12), which was better than the results achieved using RGB features.

The HSV model separates the brightness component (V) of a color from its chrominance components (H and S). Previously, Sural *et al* used HSV to develop a workflow in image segmentation and color histogram generation. The HSV features achieved substantial improvement in content based image retrieval [26]. For medical images, HSV has also shown its comparably better ability in the definition of existing trauma colors than RGB [27]. HSV transformation is not a time-consuming or computation intensive process. Using the HSV color texture, an initial assessment of tissue malignancy using bronchoscopy images can be an alternative approach to the histological examination of biopsy specimens. Clinical physicians could obtain rapid results before a final pathological diagnosis is available. This alternative procedure could facilitate physician availability for more severe and urgent lung cancer patients.

Although this study did not collect many cases, the experiments using WLB and AFI to classify malignant lung tumors is the first study exploring the ability of the image processing and logistic regression classifier. We showed that both WLB and AFI can achieve accuracies higher than 80%. A previous CAD system achieved a similar accuracy (83% versus 80%) in classifying normal mucosa and tumors using WLB [18]. It also demonstrates the strong potential for the use of image features to classify different types of tumors. In future studies, automatic lesion detection should be added to improve the practical use of the proposed CAD system. While carrying out bronchoscopy, physicians could detect more possible abnormalities and perform a rapid assessment of malignancy and subsequent treatment. Also, combining WLB and AFI may achieve higher accuracy, although the clinical use is not so practical.

3.3 Conclusion

This study proposed using WLB and AFI image features to classify different malignant types. HSV transformation and texture features were used to strengthen the classification ability. Both WLB and AFI achieved a diagnostic accuracy higher than 80%, which can provide an assessment suggestion to physicians in clinical use.

References

[1] Ferlay J *et al* 2015 Cancer incidence and mortality worldwide: sources, methods and major patterns in GLOBOCAN 2012 *Int. J. Cancer* **136** E359–86

[2] Fitzmaurice C *et al* 2017 Global, regional, and national cancer incidence, mortality, years of life lost, years lived with disability, and disability-adjusted life-years for 32 cancer groups, 1990 to 2015: a systematic analysis for the global burden of disease study *JAMA Oncol.* **3** 524–48

[3] National Lung Screening Trial Research Team 2011 Reduced lung-cancer mortality with low-dose computed tomographic screening *N. Engl. J. Med.* **365** 395–409

[4] Zaric B *et al* 2011 Autofluorescence imaging videobronchoscopy in the detection of lung cancer: from research tool to everyday procedure *Expert Rev. Med. Dev.* **8** 167–72

[5] Zaric B *et al* 2013 Diagnostic value of autofluorescence bronchoscopy in lung cancer *Thorac. Cancer* **4** 1–8

[6] Lam S, MacAulay C, leRiche J C and Palcic B 2000 Detection and localization of early lung cancer by fluorescence bronchoscopy *Cancer* **89** 2468–73

[7] Hirsch F R *et al* 2001 Fluorescence versus white-light bronchoscopy for detection of preneoplastic lesions: a randomized study *J. Natl. Cancer Inst.* **93** 1385–91

[8] Sharma D, Newman T G and Aronow W S 2015 Lung cancer screening: history, current perspectives, and future directions *Arch. Med. Sci.* **11** 1033–43

[9] Kennedy T C, Lam S and Hirsch F R 2001 Review of recent advances in fluorescence bronchoscopy in early localization of central airway lung cancer *Oncologist* **6** 257–62

[10] Sun J *et al* 2011 The value of autofluorescence bronchoscopy combined with white light bronchoscopy compared with white light alone in the diagnosis of intraepithelial neoplasia and invasive lung cancer: a meta-analysis *J. Thorac. Oncol.* **6** 1336–44

[11] Benz M, Rojas-Solano J R, Kage A, Wittenberg T, Munzenmayer C and Becker H D 2010 Computer-assisted diagnosis for white light bronchoscopy: first results *CHEST* **138** 433A

[12] Chang R-F, Lee C-C and Lo C-M 2019 Quantitative diagnosis of rotator cuff tears based on sonographic pattern recognition *PLoS One* **14** e0212741

[13] Lo C-M, Hung P-H and Hsieh K L-C 2019 Computer-aided detection of hyperacute stroke based on relative radiomic patterns in computed tomography *Appl. Sci.* **9** 1668

[14] Moon W K *et al* 2018 Quantitative breast density analysis using tomosynthesis and comparison with MRI and digital mammography *Comput. Methods Programs Biomed.* **154** 99–107

[15] Hsieh K L-C, Chen C-Y and Lo C-M 2017 Radiomic model for predicting mutations in the isocitrate dehydrogenase gene in glioblastomas *Oncotarget* **8** 45888
[16] Hsieh K L-C, Chen C-Y and Lo C-M 2017 Quantitative glioma grading using transformed gray-scale invariant textures of MRI *Comput. Biol. Med.* **83** 102–8
[17] Moon W K, Chen I-L, Chang J M, Shin S U, Lo C-M and Chang R-F 2017 The adaptive computer-aided diagnosis system based on tumor sizes for the classification of breast tumors detected at screening ultrasound *Ultrasonics* **76** 70–7
[18] Hsieh K L-C, Lo C-M and Hsiao C-J 2017 Computer-aided grading of gliomas based on local and global MRI features *Comput. Methods Programs Biomed.* **139** 31–8
[19] Hsieh K L-C, Tsai R-J, Teng Y-C and Lo C-M 2017 Effect of a computer-aided diagnosis system on radiologists' performance in grading gliomas with MRI *PLoS One* **12** e0171342
[20] Oliveira R B, Mercedes Filho E, Ma Z, Papa J P, Pereira A S and Tavares J M R 2016 Computational methods for the image segmentation of pigmented skin lesions: a review *Comput. Methods Programs Biomed.* **131** 127–41
[21] Haralick R M, Shanmuga K and Dinstein I 1973 Textural features for image classification *IEEE Trans. Syst. Man Cybern.* **Smc3** 610–21
[22] Field A P 2009 *Discovering Statistics Using SPSS* 3rd edn (Los Angeles, CA: SAGE)
[23] Hosmer D W 2000 *Applied Logistic Regression* 2nd edn (New York: Wiley)
[24] Alpaydin E 2004 *Introduction to Machine Learning* (Cambridge, MA: MIT Press)
[25] Refaeilzadeh P, Tang L and Liu H 2009 Cross-validation *Encyclopedia of Database Systems* (Berlin: Springer), pp 532–8
[26] Sural S, Qian G and Pramanik S 2002 Segmentation and histogram generation using the HSV color space for image retrieval *Proc. of Int. Conf. on Image Processing, 2002* **vol 2** (Piscataway, NJ: IEEE), p I–II
[27] Georgieva L, Dimitrova T and Angelov N 2005 RGB and HSV colour models in colour identification of digital trauma images *Proc. of the Int. Conf. CompSysTech*

Chapter 4

Epidemiology of lung cancer

Meng-Hua Tao

4.1 Descriptive epidemiology of lung cancer

Lung cancer has been the most common cancer in the world for several decades. In 2018, lung cancer accounted for approximately 2.1 million new cases worldwide (1 368 524 men and 725 353 women), representing approximately 12.0% of all new cancer cases [1, 2]. There are still more lung cancer cases in very high human development index (HDI) and high HDI regions than in medium and low HDI regions of the world [2]. Worldwide, lung cancer is the leading cause of cancer death in men and the second leading cause of cancer death in women, with about 1.8 million individuals dying from the disease in 2018, that is, 18.4% of all cancer deaths [2].

Worldwide, lung cancer incidence is generally higher in men than in women, and the magnitude of the difference varies between two- to nine-fold. Among men, lung cancer was the most common cancer in the world in 2018, with the highest incidence rates in Micronesia/Polynesia, Eastern and Western Europe, and Eastern Asia [2]. In addition, worldwide, lung cancer is the third most frequent cancer in women; the highest lung cancer incidence rates, over 24.0 per 100 000 per year, are observed in North America, Northern and Western Europe, and Australia/New Zealand [1, 2]. Notably, lung cancer incidence rates in Chinese women are higher than the rates among women in several European countries despite their lower smoking prevalence [1, 2]. In many developed countries, the age-standardized incidence (standardized to the World Standard Population) of lung cancer has decreased steeply in men compared to a rising trend in incidence among women over the past three decades [2]. Given the variations of trend by gender, lung cancer incidence rates are converging in men and women in the United States (US) and several European countries. In the US, the lung cancer incidence rate is higher among young women (less than 50 years old) than among young men, particularly among non-Hispanic whites and Hispanics [3], and this cannot be fully explained by gender differences in smoking behavior.

doi:10.1088/978-0-7503-2540-0ch4

The geographical and temporal variations in the incidence of lung cancer are to a large extent determined by past exposure to tobacco smoking and the relative maturity of the tobacco epidemic in a given country [4–7]. An increase in tobacco consumption is paralleled several decades later by an increase in the incidence of lung cancer; similarly, a decrease in consumption is followed by a decrease in incidence. In populations that are not exposed to tobacco smoke or industrial lung carcinogens, the age-adjusted incidence rate of lung cancer is generally low (less than 5 per 100 000 per year) [2, 8].

Many developing countries have still not experienced the worst consequences of the tobacco epidemic, as cigarette smoking became widespread only during the last 30 years. China is inhabited by one-fifth of the world's population, and thus determines to a great extent the cancer burden at a global level. It was estimated that the lung cancer incidence in China would increase by 27% in men and 38% in women from the year 2000 to 2005, due mostly to changes in cancer risk (cigarette smoking), as well as to some degree alterations of population size and age structure [9]. According to GLOBOCAN 2018, around 774 323 lung cancer cases were diagnosed in China in 2018, and 824 965 lung cancer cases are predicted in 2020 [10], a higher prediction of new cases than previous estimates [11]. If current incidence rates and trends prevail, it is estimated that the number of new lung cancer cases in China will increase to 1 097 788 by 2030 [10]. The full effects of increased tobacco consumption are expected to occur in the next few decades. It has been estimated that worldwide smoking caused 11.5% (6.4 million) of global deaths from all causes in 2015 [12], while by around 2030, worldwide deaths from tobacco will most likely increase to approximately 10 million of 60 million deaths from all causes, with the majority of the increase taking palace in Asia, Africa, and South America [13].

The main histological types of lung cancer are squamous cell carcinoma, small cell carcinoma, adenocarcinoma, and large cell carcinoma. Over the last 20 years, the distribution of the histological types of lung cancer has been changing. The proportion of squamous cell carcinoma, the previously predominant type, has declined for both sexes in many countries since the 1970s, whereas during the same period of time the incidence rates of adenocarcinoma have been increasing, particularly in women [14–16]. The possible explanations for the increase of lung adenocarcinoma include changes in the composition and patterns of tobacco consumption (deeper inhalation of low-nicotine and tar tobacco smoke), air pollution, and improvements of diagnostic techniques [15, 17].

Largely due to improvements in the diagnosis and treatment of lung cancer, the one year relative survival of lung cancer patients has been improved in some countries. In the US, the one year lung cancer survival rate increased from 37% in 1975–9 to 45% in 2008–11 [18]. However, lung cancer continues to have one of the lowest five year survival rates among all malignancies around the world. The five year survival of lung cancer ranged from 10% to 20% for most geographical areas, both in the developed and developing worlds [19, 20]. Because the early disease is typically asymptomatic, only 16% of lung cancers are diagnosed at the local stage, for which the five year survival rate is 56% [19]. Data from these reports suggested the importance of early diagnosis and adequate treatment procedures for lung cancer survival and prognosis.

4.2 Risk factors of lung cancer

4.2.1 Tobacco

Tobacco smoking is the main cause of lung cancer in most human populations. The carcinogenic effect of tobacco smoke on the lung was demonstrated in the 1950s and has been recognized by public health and regulatory authorities since the mid-1960s [21]. Compared to never-smokers, continuous smokers have 10–20 fold higher risk of development of lung cancer. The overall relative risk reflects the contribution of the different aspects of tobacco smoking, including average consumption, duration of smoking, time since quitting, age at start, type of tobacco product, and inhalation pattern. Numerous epidemiological studies have consistently shown the relative contributions of duration and amount of cigarette smoking in excess lung cancer risk, and there is an exposure–response relationship between cigarette smoking and lung cancer risk [21, 22]. Similar patterns of causal relationship have been shown for smoking of cigars, cigarillos, pipes, bidi, hookah, water pipe, khii yoo, and other types of tobacco products with lung cancer risk, indicating the carcinogenic effect of these products [21, 23, 24].

An important aspect of tobacco-related lung carcinogenesis is the effect of cessation of smoking. Cessation of smoking at 60 years of age can reduce the lifetime risk of lung cancer by 40%, cessation at 50, 40, and 30 years of age decreases the risk by 60%, 80%, and 90%, respectively [21]. However, a small excess risk of lung cancer likely persists even in long-term quitters throughout their lifetime [21, 25].

4.2.2 Second-hand smoke

Second-hand smoke (SHS), also known as environmental tobacco smoke (ETS), is composed of both mainstream smoke (exhaled) and side-stream smoke emitted by the burning cigarette. Various carcinogens have been identified in SHS, including benzene, benzo[a]pyrene, 1,3-butadiene, and many others [21]. The collective epidemiologic evidence and biological plausibility suggest a causal association between SHS and lung cancer risk in never-smokers, after taking into account the possible confounding effects of active smoking, diet, or other factors, and of possible reporting bias [21, 26, 27]. It has been estimated that never-smokers exposed to SHS have about 20%–30% excess risk of lung cancer [21, 27]. The effect of SHS appears to be present from both household exposure, mainly from the spouse, and workplace exposure [21, 26, 27], while little evidence showed an association between childhood SHS exposure and lung cancer in adulthood [28].

4.2.3 Diet, obesity, and physical activity

There is limited evidence for the protective effects of vegetable and fruit consumption against lung cancer [29, 30]. Isoflavones, a class of phytoestrogens, are found in soybeans, legumes, grains, and vegetables. Epidemiologic evidence has suggested that a high intake of foods containing isoflavones may decrease the risk of lung cancer in never-smokers [30, 31]. Despite many studies on the consumption of other foods, such as cereals, pulses, meat, fish, eggs, milk, and dairy products, there is limited and inconsistent evidence to allow a judgment regarding the evidence of a carcinogenic or protective effect [30]. In addition, no conclusive evidence has shown a protective effect of antioxidant vitamins such as vitamin C against lung cancer [30].

Many observational studies have shown a decreased risk of lung cancer with increased dietary intake of carotenoids, in particular β-carotene, and a clear dose–response relationship is apparent from cohort studies [30, 32]. A similar relationship has also been reported between serum or plasma carotenoid concentrations and lung cancer [30, 32]. In contrast to the observational studies, several large-scale randomized clinical trials designed to investigate the effects of β-carotene supplements failed to prove the protective association. In a large randomized prevention study with smokers, the results suggested an increased lung cancer risk in the current smokers who were treated with β-carotene supplements [33], while another trial with workers exposed to asbestos and heavy smokers did not find any difference of risk between the treated and the control groups [34]. In addition, there is an interaction between β-carotene, smoking, and genotype [35]. More convincing evidence showed that high-dose β-carotene supplements cause lung cancer in current and former smokers [30].

Epidemiologic studies from areas with high exposure to arsenic consistently reported a significant increased risk of lung cancer with high cumulative exposure to arsenic in drinking water [30, 36, 37]. There is insufficient evidence of an excess risk of lung cancer from alcohol drinking [30, 38–40]. Because drinking and smoking are strongly associated, residual confounding from tobacco smoking might have biased the association. Additionally, recent systematic reviews did not observe clear associations between alcohol consumption and lung cancer risk in never-smokers [41, 42].

Anthropometric factors including height, waist circumference, and body mass index (BMI) have been studied with regard to risk of lung cancer in epidemiological studies [30, 43–46]. Several meta-analyses have reported a reverse association between BMI and lung cancer risk [47, 48]. However, this association has a high potential to be caused by inadequate adjustment for tobacco smoking, as smoking is strongly related to lower BMI, and by other residual confounding variable [30]. A recent meta-analysis focusing on never-smokers found a 23% reduction of lung cancer risk for excess body weight (BMI $\geqslant$25), and the inverse association persisted in never-smoking women but not in men [49]. Meanwhile, results from certain studies suggested that physical activity may lower lung cancer risk in both men and women [30, 50–52], but the potential residual confounding by tobacco smoking could not be eliminated for this inverse finding. Although the relationship between physical activity, BMI, and smoking makes the evidence difficult to explain, there is limited evidence of decreased lung cancer risk associated with either high BMI or physical activity.

4.2.4 Occupational exposures

The important role of occupational exposures in the carcinogenesis of lung neoplasm has been well established in reports dating back to the 1950s. The risk of lung cancer is increased among workers employed in several industries and occupations. Evidence for the carcinogenicity of many occupational agents has been reviewed by the International Agency for Research on Cancer (IARC) Monographs Program since 1972, and multiple lung carcinogens have been classified. Of these, asbestos, arsenic, and combustion fumes are several of the most important occupational causes [53, 54]. It has been established that occupational agents are responsible for an estimated 5%–10% of lung cancers in industrialized countries.

Arsenic and inorganic arsenic compounds, including arsenic trioxide, arsenite, and arsenate, have been known as a lung carcinogen since the late 1960s [54, 55]. Inhalation of arsenic-containing particulates is the primary route of occupational exposure. Historically, the occupational exposure to arsenic mainly occurred among workers employed in hot smelting of non-ferrous metal; other industries or industrial activities exposed to arsenic are coal-fired power plants, battery assembly, preparation of or work with pressure-treated wood, glass-manufacture, electronics industry, fur handlers, manufacturers of sheep-dip compounds and pesticides, and vineyard workers [54, 55].

The first evidence of elevated risk of lung cancer following inhalation of asbestos fibers dates back to the 1950s. Since then, numerous epidemiological studies have demonstrated the positive association of lung cancer with occupational exposure to asbestos. All different forms of asbestos, including chrysotile, rocidolite, amosite, tremolite, actinolite, and anthophyllite, are carcinogenic to the human lung [54], although there are still controversies on whether chrysotile asbestos has lower potency than other forms of asbestos, and whether the potency of long and thin asbestos fibers may be higher than short and thick ones. Strict regulations governing exposure or bans on asbestos exposure have been applied in many countries since the 1970s; however, worldwide a substantial number of workers are still exposed, mainly in the construction industry. In many low- and medium-resource countries with high production and/or consumption of asbestos [56], occupational asbestos exposure remains widespread, and is responsible for a large number of occupationally related lung cancers [53, 54].

4.2.5 Ionizing radiation

There is conclusive evidence that exposure to ionizing radiation increases the risk of lung cancer [57]. Although atomic bomb survivors and patients treated with radiotherapy for ankylosing spondylitis or breast cancer have been reported to have a moderately increased risk of lung cancer, studies of nuclear industry workers exposed to relatively low levels provided little evidence of an increased risk of lung cancer [57, 58]. Underground miners exposed to radioactive radon and its decay products, which emit α-particles, have been consistently found to have increased risk for lung cancer [59, 60]. In addition, several studies showed an increased risk of lung cancer in miners who smoke compared to never-smoking miners, with both a possibly additive and a potentially synergistic and multiplicative interaction [61, 62]. Since radon exposure continues to be an occupational concern in underground work and mining around the world, more longitudinal and quantitative evaluations of occupationally exposed workers are needed to improve our understanding of the carcinogenic effects of radon.

For the general population, indoor exposure to radon and its decay products has been considered as the largest component of environmental radiation in many areas of the world. Pooled and meta-analyses of case-control studies conducted in Europe and North America have consistently reported a positive association between residential radon exposure and lung cancer [63–67], and the exposure–response relationship is linear without evidence of a threshold [65]. The available evidence also suggests that residential radon exposure is responsible for 10%–15% of the lung cancer burden, making it the second leading cause of lung cancer, particularly in never-smokers without exposure to occupational carcinogens [66].

4.2.6 Environmental air pollution

Indoor air pollution has been thought to be responsible for the increased risk of lung cancer experienced by never-smoking women who are living in several regions of China and other Asian countries. The evidence is strongest for coal burning in poorly ventilated houses, burning of wood and other solid fuels, as well as fumes from high-temperature cooking using unrefined vegetable oils such as rapeseed oil [68, 69]. The positive association of lung cancer risk with indoor air pollution from solid fuels has also been found in populations with less extreme exposure, such as populations in Central and Eastern Europe and Mexico [69, 70].

In October 2013, IARC officially classified outdoor air pollution and particulate matter (PM) from outdoor air pollution as carcinogens to humans (Group 1), and concluded that outdoor air pollution and PM cause lung cancer [71]. Based on 18 studies, a recent meta-analysis reported that a 10 $\mu g\ m^{-3}$ increase in the $PM_{2.5}$ and PM_{10} concentrations were significantly associated with increased meta-relative risk (RR) of lung cancer (RR = 1.09, 95% CI, and 1.04–1.14, and RR = 1.08, 95% CI, and 1.00–1.17, respectively) [72]. More meta-analyses were further conducted to quantify the magnitude of the risk of lung cancer associated with outdoor air pollution. The positive association of $PM_{2.5}$ with lung cancer may also vary by smoking status, with a stronger association among never-smokers [73] or former smokers [72]. In some countries, outdoor air pollution may be particularly important for vulnerable populations as more evidence has demonstrated the disparity by socioeconomic status or race/ethnicity in burden of air pollution exposure [74].

4.2.7 Infection

The role of infection in lung carcinogenesis has been examined but much remains unknown. Patients with pulmonary tuberculosis have been found to have excess risk of lung cancer, although it is still not clear whether the excess risk is due to the chronic inflammatory status of the lung parenchyma or to the specific action of the *Mycobacterium* [75, 76]. *Chlamydia pneumonia* is a common cause of acute respiratory infection. Using serology to define previous *Chlamydia* infection, several epidemiologic studies have reported a higher risk of lung cancer associated with positive serology compared to those with negative serology [77]. A meta-analysis of 12 studies showed a positive association between *C. pneumonia* infection and risk of lung cancer in both retrospective and prospective studies [78]. The detail mechanism of the reported association remains unknown, and *C. pneumonia* infection may also act synergistically with tobacco smoking to increase lung cancer risk. Further studies are needed to better understand the role of *C. pneumonia* infection in the etiology of lung cancer.

Previous studies with inconsistent results have evaluated whether chronic infection by certain viruses, such as human papillomavirus (HPV), human immunodeficiency virus (HIV), or JC virus, can increase the risk of lung cancer [79]. A recent meta-analysis showed a strong association of HPV infection with lung cancer risk, and a marginal association between HPV 16/18 genotypes and lung adenocarcinoma (OR = 3.69, 95% CI, 0.99–13.71) [80]. However, previous studies were mainly conducted in Chinese populations, and it is still unclear whether similar associations are present in other populations.

4.2.8 Genetic factors

There is a genetic component to the development of lung cancer; this positive association may be related to host susceptibility, with or without exposure to tobacco smoke and other potential risk factors, or an individual's responsiveness to biological therapies. A positive familial history of lung cancer has been found to be a risk factor in some studies. Gauderman *et al* [81] suggested that inheritance of a major gene, in conjunction with tobacco smoking, might account for more than 50% of cases diagnosed below age 60. Using family linkage approaches, a pooled analysis of high-risk pedigrees identified a major susceptibility locus to chromosome 6q23–25 [82].

In addition to the possible effect of relatively rare genes with high penetrance, there have also been many studies on candidate low-penetrance susceptibility genes that are involved in the metabolism of tobacco or other carcinogens, DNA repair, and cell cycle control. There is accumulated evidence suggesting an increased risk of lung cancer associated with the rare variant of several genes (e.g. *GSTM1* and *GSTT1*) [83]. However, for most genes, results have been mixed and do not allow conclusions on the presence or absence of an effect [83]. This may be due to methodological limitations in the available studies and low statistical power. With the availability of high-density genotyping and large sample size, genome-wide association studies (GWAS) in different populations have identified 45 susceptibility loci associated with the risk of lung cancer [84]. Genetic polymorphisms are likely to act by modifying the effect of the risk factors of lung cancer, such as tobacco smoking, occupational exposures, and air pollution. Numerous studies including genome-wide studies have been conducted to investigate the possible gene–environmental interactions in the field of lung cancer. The first genome-wide gene–smoking interaction study identified significant interactions between two single nucleotide polymorphisms (SNPs) (rs1316298 and rs4589502) and smoking on lung cancer risk in a Chinese population [85]. More studies with large sample size and well-characterized information on environmental exposures are needed to understand the mechanisms of the etiology of lung cancer.

There is strong evidence for stepwise accumulation in lung carcinogenesis of genetic and molecular alterations, including allelic losses, chromosomal instability, mutations in both proto-oncogenes and tumor-suppressor genes, epigenetic events, and expression alterations [86].

4.3 Lung cancer in never-smokers

Although tobacco smoking is the predominant risk factor of lung cancer, there are a distinct proportion of patients who develop the disease without a history of tobacco smoking. Approximately 15%–25% of lung cancer cases worldwide occur in never-smokers [87–89], and recent data further suggests the incidence of lung cancer in never-smokers to be increasing in a number of countries, even after controlling for gender and race/ethnicity [90–92]. Women are more likely than men to have non-smoking-associated lung cancer regardless of geographic variations [89]. The highest incidence has been observed in East and South Asia, where 60%–80% of women with lung cancer are never-smokers [93, 94]; whereas approximately 20% of lung cancer in women and 6% in men are never-smokers in the US [88, 93]. The histology is predominantly adenocarcinoma, often with a high frequency of driver mutations such as the epidermal growth factor (*EGFR*) and human EGF receptor 2 (*HER2*), and the echinoderm microtubule-associated protein-like 4 and anaplastic lymphoma kinase (*EML4–ALK*) rearrangement which respond well to targeted therapies [94–96].

If considered as a separate entity, lung cancer in never-smokers ranks as the seventh leading cause of cancer-related death worldwide, and is a top-ten cause of death in the US [89]. In the US, 17 000–26 000 lung cancer deaths are estimated to occur in never-smokers every year [97]. It was estimated that never-smoking men had higher death rates from lung cancer than women in the US [87, 98], with age-standardized mortality rates ranging from 32.3 to 13.8 per 100 000 in men and 16.5 to 10.5 per 100 000 in women. The mortality rates from lung cancer among never-smoking African Americans were higher than in Caucasians for both men and women [87].

4.4 Screening

The prognosis for lung cancer patients is dismal. Although important progress has been made both in the medical and surgical treatment of lung cancer, most patients still succumb to the disease. The main explanation is that patients are diagnosed at a late stage of the natural history of the disease, most patients have unresectable, metastatic disease; and even among patients considered resectable, 60% eventually relapse [99]. There have been substantial efforts in developing and implementing screening strategies such as chest x-ray and/or sputum cytology to detect early-stage lung cancers; however, a meta-analysis of seven trials found no difference in lung cancer mortality when comparing screening with chest x-rays and sputum cytology to chest x-rays alone [100]. Recent results from a large clinical trial also showed that annual screening using chest x-rays did not reduce lung cancer mortality compared to usual care [101].

The emergence of newer methods, such as low-dose computed tomography (LDCT) scans and molecular markers in sputum, provide the possibility of detecting lung cancer at earlier, more operable stages in high-risk populations. CT technology has the potential to detect pulmonary nodules smaller than 5 mm, and the introduction of LDCT has enabled examination of the entire lung in one breath-hold and increased the number of detected nodules [102]. The National Lung Screening Trial (NLST), a randomized trial to determine the effectiveness of lung cancer screening in high-risk individuals, recently showed that compared to the chest x-ray group, lung cancer screening with LDCT significantly reduced lung cancer mortality by up to 20% among current or former heavy smokers (⩾30 pack-year history; <15 years since cessation for ex-smokers) [103]. Subsequently, the US Preventive Services Task Forces (USPSTF), National Comprehensive Cancer Network, and a number of professional organizations recommended screening for lung cancer with LDCT in high-risk persons. The USPSTF guidelines recommend lung cancer screening in adults aged 55–80 years who have a 30 pack-year smoking history and currently smoke or have quit within the past 15 years [104]. Moreover, from 2015, Medicare [105], the Affordable Care Act [106], and most private insurance companies began to provide coverage for the annual screening for lung cancer with LDCT.

4.5 Conclusion

As the most important cancer epidemic of the twentieth century, lung cancer will likely continue to be a major public health problem in the current century. Considerable efforts are being made in the public and private domains to develop more effective therapeutic approaches; however, most lung cancer patients still succumb to poor prognosis. There have been substantial efforts in developing and implementing screening strategies to detect the disease at an early stage. In the US, it was estimated that 6.8 million Americans were eligible for LDCT screening, while only 3.9% of eligible individuals reported receiving screening for lung cancer with LDCT in 2015 [107]. Studies are needed to identify various barriers to adoption of the lung cancer screening guidelines, which will promote successfully implementing this important public health prevention strategy outside a trial setting. Moreover, the incidence of never-smoking lung cancer has been increasing rapidly, while little is known about the relevance of LDCT screening for never-smokers and its effectiveness [108, 109]. The most recent data suggested that LDCT screening can help to detect a significant number of lung cancers at a very early stage in never-smokers [108], and another retrospective cohort study of never-smoking Korean women found that only female never-smokers with an initial LDCT image showing 'suspicious malignancy' need annual LDCT screening [109]. Future research is needed to comprehensively evaluate the value of using LDCT screening in never-smokers. In addition, the potential risks associated with screening, such as accumulation of radiation exposures from multiple screening procedures and additional invasive procedures followed for false-positive patients, need to be evaluated. More studies are needed to determine the optimal duration and frequency of LDCT screening in both asymptomatic high-risk populations and never-smoking populations, as well as to improve the sensitivity and specificity of LDCT screening.

Until now, primary prevention remains the main weapon against this neoplasm, and the control of tobacco smoking is by far the most important strategy of lung cancer prevention. In some populations, the decreased incidence of the disease can be attributable to reduced consumption of tobacco. Much, however, remains to be done, in particular among women and the young, as well as in developing countries, such as China and India. Reduction in exposure to occupational and environmental carcinogens (in particular indoor pollution and radon), and an increase in the consumption of fruits and vegetables are additional preventive opportunities.

Due to the increased number of cases, lung cancer in never-smokers has been an increasingly prominent public health issue. Current known risk factors, including second-hand smoking, occupational exposure to carcinogens, air pollution, and residential exposure to radon cannot explain more than a minor proportion of these cases. Dietary, infection, and molecular factors are currently receiving more attention, and more well-established studies are needed to improve our understanding of the etiology of lung cancer in never-smokers.

References

[1] American Cancer Society 2018 *Global Cancer Facts and Figures* 4th edn (Altanta, GA: American Cancer Society)

[2] Bray F, Ferlay J, Soerjomataram I, Siegel R L, Torre L A and Jemal A 2018 Global cancer statistics 2018: GLOBOCAN estimates of incidence and mortality worldwide for 36 cancers in 185 countries *CA Cancer J. Clin.* **68** 394–424

[3] Jemal A *et al* 2018 Higher lung cancer incidence in young women than young men in the United States *N. Engl. J. Med.* **378** 1999–2009

[4] Jemal A, Center M M, DeSantis C and Ward E M 2010 Global patterns of cancer incidence and mortality rates and trends *Cancer Epidemiol. Biomarker Prev.* **19** 1893–907

[5] Ferlay J *et al* 2018 Cancer incidence and mortality patterns in Europe: estimates for 40 countries and 25 major cancers in 2018 *Eur. J. Cancer* **103** 356–87

[6] Chen W *et al* 2017 Cancer incidence and mortality in China, 2013 *Cancer Lett.* **401** 63–71

[7] Chen W *et al* 2016 Cancer statistics in China, 2015 *CA Cancer J. Clin.* **66** 115–32

[8] Parkin D M 2004 International variation *Oncogene* **23** 6329–40

[9] Yang L, Parkin D M, Ferlay J, Li L and Chen Y 2005 Estimates of cancer incidence in China for 2000 and projections for 2005 *Cancer Epidemiol. Biomarker Prev.* **14** 243–50

[10] Global Cancer Observatory 2018 International Agency for Research on Cancer http://gco.iarc.fr (Accessed: 20 June 2019)

[11] Chen W Q, Zheng R S and Zeng H M 2011 Bayesian age-period-cohort prediction of lung cancer incidence in China *Thorac. Cancer* **2** 149–55

[12] GBD 2015 Tobacco Collaborators 2017 Smoking prevalence and attributable disease burden in 195 countries and territories, 1990–2015: a systematic analysis from the Global Burden of Disease Study 2015 *Lancet* **389** 1885–906

[13] Peto R, Lopez A D, Boreham J, Thun M and Heath C Jr 1994 *Mortality from Smoking in Developed Countries 1950–2000* (Oxford: Oxford University Press)

[14] Meza R, Meernik C, Jeon J and Cote M L 2015 Lung cancer incidence trends by gender, race and histology in the United States, 1973–2010 *PLoS One* **10** e0121323

[15] Lortet-Tieulent J, Soerjomataram I, Ferlay J, Rutherford M, Weiderpass E and Bray F 2014 International trends in lung cancer incidence by histological subtype: adenocarcinoma stabilizing in men but still increasing in women *Lung Cancer* **84** 13–22

[16] Kinoshita F L, Ito Y and Nakayama T 2016 Trends in lung cancer incidence rates by histological type in 1975–2008: a population-based study in Osaka, Japan *J. Epidemiol.* **26** 579–86

[17] CDC 2004 *Surgeon General's 2004 Report: The Health Consequences of Smoking* (Rockville, MD: US Department of Health and Human Services)

[18] Miller K D *et al* 2016 Cancer treatment and survivorship statistics, 2016 *CA Cancer J. Clin.* **66** 271–89

[19] American Cancer Society 2019 *Cancer Facts and Figures* (Atlanta, GA: American Cancer Society)

[20] Allemani C *et al* 2018 Global surveillance of trends in cancer survival 2000–14 (CONCORD-3): analysis of individual records for 37 513 025 patients diagnosed with one of 18 cancers from 322 population-based registries in 71 countries *Lancet* **391** 1023–75

[21] IARC 2004 Tobacco smoke and involuntary smoking *IARC Monographs on the Evaluation of Carcinogenic Risks of Chemicals to Humans* vol 83 (Lyon: IARC Press)

[22] IARC 1986 Tobacco smoking *IARC Mongraphs on the Evaluation of the Carcinogenic Risk of Chemicals to Human* vol 86 (Lyon: IARC Press)

[23] Akl E A, Gaddam S, Gunukula S K, Honeine R, Jaoude P A and Irani J 2010 The effects of waterpipe tobacco smoking on health outcomes: a systematic review *Int. J. Epidemiol.* **39** 834–57

[24] Pednekar M S, Gupta P C, Yeole B B and Hébert J R 2011 Association of tobacco habits, including bidi smoking, with overall and site-specific cancer incidence: results from the Mumbai cohort study *Cancer Causes Control* **22** 859–68

[25] Nakamura K, Huxley R, Ansary-Moghaddam A and Woodward M 2009 The hazards and benefits associated with smoking and smoking cessation in Asia: a meta-analysis of prospective studies *Tob. Control* **18** 345–52

[26] Samet J M *et al* 2009 Lung cancer in never smokers: clinical epidemiology and environmental risk factors *Clin. Cancer Res.* **15** 5626–45

[27] Kim C H *et al* 2014 Exposure to secondhand tobacco smoke and lung cancer by histological type: a pooled analysis of the International Lung Cancer Consortium (ILCCO) *Int. J. Cancer* **135** 1918–30

[28] Boffetta P, Tredaniel J and Grecco A 2002 Risk of childhood cancer and adult lung cancer after childhood exposure to passive smoke: a meta-analysis *Environ. Health Perspect.* **108** 73–82

[29] International Agency for Research on Cancer 2003 Fruit and vegetables *IARC Handbooks of Cancer Prevention* vol 8 (Lyon: IARC Press)

[30] World Cancer Research Fund/American Institute for Cancer Research 2004 Food, Nutrition, Physical Activity, and Cancer: a Global Perspective. Continuous Update Project Expert Report 2018

[31] Lam T K *et al* 2009 Cruciferous vegetable consumption and lung cancer risk: a systematic review *Cancer Epidemiol. Biomarker Prev.* **18** 184–95
[32] Gallicchio L *et al* 2008 Carotenoids and the risk of developing lung cancer: a systematic review *Am. J. Clin. Nutr.* **88** 372–83
[33] Albanes D *et al* 1996 Alpha-tocopherol and beta-carotene supplements and lung cancer incidence in the alpha-tocopherol, beta-carotene cancer prevention study: effects of base-line characteristics and study compliance *J. Natl. Cancer Inst.* **88** 1560–70
[34] Omenn G S *et al* 1996 Risk factors for lung cancer and for intervention effects in CARET, the Beta-Carotene and Retinol Efficacy Trial *J. Natl. Cancer Inst.* **88** 1550–9
[35] Woodson K *et al* 1999 Effect of vitamin intervention on the relationship between GSTM1, smoking, and lung cancer risk among male smokers *Cancer Epidemiol. Biomarkers Prev.* **8** 965–70
[36] Smith A H, Marshall G, Roh T, Ferreccio C, Liaw J and Steinmaus C 2018 Lung, bladder, and kidney cancer mortality 40 years after arsenic exposure reduction *J. Natl. Cancer Inst.* **110** 241–9
[37] Bardach A E *et al* 2015 Epidemiology of chronic disease related to arsenic in Argentina: a systematic review *Sci. Total Environ.* **538** 802–16
[38] Wakai K *et al* 2007 Alcohol drinking and lung cancer risk: an evaluation based on a systematic review of epidemiologic evidence among the Japanese population *Jpn. J. Clin. Oncol.* **37** 168–74
[39] Li Y, Yang H and Cao J 2011 Association between alcohol consumption and cancers in the Chinese population—a systematic review and meta-analysis *PLoS One* **6** e18776
[40] Bagnardi V *et al* 2015 Alcohol consumption and site-specific cancer risk: a comprehensive dose-response meta-analysis *Br. J. Cancer* **112** 580–93
[41] García-Lavandeira J A, Ruano-Ravina A and Barros-Dios J M 2016 Alcohol consumption and lung cancer risk in never smokers *Gac. Sanit.* **30** 311–7
[42] Bagnardi V *et al* 2011 Alcohol consumption and lung cancer risk in never smokers: a meta-analysis *Ann. Oncol.* **22** 2631–9
[43] Renehan A G, Soerjomataram I and Leitzmann M F 2010 Interpreting the epidemiological evidence linking obesity and cancer: a framework for population-attributable risk estimations in Europe *Eur. J. Cancer* **46** 2581–92
[44] Koh W P, Yuan J M, Wang R, Lee H P and Yu M C 2010 Body mass index and smoking-related lung cancer risk in the Singapore Chinese Health Study *Br. J. Cancer* **102** 610–4
[45] Yang L *et al* 2009 Body mass index and mortality from lung cancer in smokers and nonsmokers: a nationally representative prospective study of 220,000 men in China *Int. J. Cancer* **125** 2136–43
[46] Kabat G C, Kim M, Hunt J R, Chlebowski R T and Rohan T E 2008 Body mass index and waist circumference in relation to lung cancer risk in the Women's Health Initiative *Am. J. Epidemiol.* **168** 158–69
[47] Yang Y *et al* 2013 Obesity and incidence of lung cancer: a meta-analysis *Int. J. Cancer* **132** 1162–9
[48] Li X *et al* 2015 Association of body mass index with chromosome damage levels and lung cancer risk among males *Sci. Rep.* **5** 9458
[49] Zhu H and Zhang S 2018 Body mass index and lung cancer risk in never smokers: a meta-analysis *BMC Cancer* **18** 635

[50] Leitzmann M F *et al* 2009 Prospective study of physical activity and lung cancer by histologic type in current, former, and never smokers *Am. J. Epidemiol.* **169** 542–53
[51] Emaus A and Thune I 2011 Physical activity and lung cancer prevention *Recent Results Cancer Res.* **186** 101–33
[52] Schmid D, Ricci C, Behrens G and Leitzmann M F 2016 Does smoking influence the physical activity and lung cancer relation? A systematic review and meta-analysis *Eur. J. Epidemiol.* **31** 1173–90
[53] Kamp D W 2009 Asbestos-induced lung disease:an update *Transl. Res.* **153** 143–52
[54] IARC 2011 Arsenic, metals, fibres, and dusts *IARC Monographs on the Evaluation of Carcinogenic Risks to Humans* vol 100C (Lyon: IARC Press)
[55] IARC 1987 Overall evaluation of carcinogenicity: an updating of IARC monographs volumes 1 to 42 *IARC Monographs on the Evaluation of the Carcinogenic Risk of Chemicals to Humans Suppl 7* (Lyon: IARC Press)
[56] Leong S L, Zainudin R, Kazan-Allen L and Robinson B W 2015 Asbestos in Asia *Respirology* **20** 548–55
[57] IARC 2000 Ionizing radiation. Part 1: x- and gamma (γ)-radiation, and neutrons *IARC Monographs on the Evaluation of Carcinogenic Risks to Humans* vol 75 (Lyon: IARC Press)
[58] Wakeford R 2009 Radiation in the workplace—a review of studies of the risks of occupational exposure to ionising radiation *J. Radiol. Prot.* **29** A61–79
[59] IARC 2001 Ionizing radiation. Part 2: Some internally deposited radionuclides *IARC Monographs on the Evaluation of Carcinogenic Risks to Humans* vol 78 (Lyon: IARC Press)
[60] Field R W 2010 Environmental factors in cancer: radon *Rev. Environ. Health* **25** 23–31
[61] Leuraud K *et al* 2011 Radon, smoking and lung cancer risk: results of a joint analysis of three European case-control studies among uranium miners *Radiat. Res.* **176** 375–87
[62] Schnelzer M, Hammer G P, Kreuzer M, Tschense A and Grosche B 2010 Accounting for smoking in the radon-related lung cancer risk among German uranium miners: results of a nested case-control study *Health Phys.* **98** 20–8
[63] Field R W *et al* 2006 An overview of the North American residential radon and lung cancer case-control studies *J. Toxicol. Environ. Health* **69** 599–631
[64] Gray A, Read S, McGale P and Darby S 2009 Lung cancer deaths from indoor radon and the cost effectiveness and potential of policies to reduce them *BMIJ* **338** a3110
[65] Darby S *et al* 2005 Radon in homes and risk of lung cancer: collaborative analysis of individual data from 13 European case-control studies *BMIJ* **330** 223
[66] Torres-Durán M, Barros-Dios J M, Fernández-Villar A and Ruano-Ravina A 2014 Residential radon and lung cancer in never smokers. A systematic review *Cancer Lett.* **345** 21–6
[67] Rodríguez-Martínez Á, Torres-Durán M, Barros-Dios J M and Ruano-Ravina A 2018 Residential radon and small cell lung cancer. A systematic review *Cancer Lett.* **426** 57–62
[68] IARC 2010 Household use of solid fuels and high-temperature frying *IARC Monographs on the Evaluation of Carcinogenic Risks to Humans* vol 95 (Lyon: IARC Press)
[69] Hosgood H D 3rd *et al* 2011 Household coal use and lung cancer: systematic review and meta-analysis of case-control studies, with an emphasis on geographic variation *Int. J. Epidemiol.* **40** 719–28
[70] Lissowska J *et al* 2005 Lung cancer and indoor pollution from heating and cooking with solid fuels: the IARC international multicentre case-control study in Eastern/Central Europe and the United Kingdom *Am. J. Epidemiol.* **162** 326–33

[71] *The International Agency for Research on Cancer* 2013 *IARC: Outdoor Air Pollution a Leading Environmental Cause of Cancer Deaths* https://iarc.fr/wp-content/uploads/2018/07/pr221_E.pdf (Accessed: 11 Feburary 2019)

[72] Hamra G B *et al* 2014 Outdoor particulate matter exposure and lung cancer: a systematic review and meta-analysis *Environ. Health Perspect.* **122** 906–11

[73] Yang W S, Zhao H, Wang X, Deng Q, Fan W Y and Wang L 2016 An evidence-based assessment for the association between long-term exposure to outdoor air pollution and the risk of lung cancer *Eur. J. Cancer Prev.* **25** 163–72

[74] Boehmer T K, Foster S L, Henry J R, Woghiren-Akinnifesi E L and Yip F Y 2013 Residential proximity to major highways—United States, 2010 *MMWR Suppl.* **62** 46–50

[75] Liang H Y *et al* 2009 Facts and fiction of the relationship between preexisting tuberculosis and lung cancer risk: a systematic review *Int. J. Cancer* **125** 2936–44

[76] Wu C Y *et al* 2011 Pulmonary tuberculosis increases the risk of lung cancer: a population-based cohort study *Cancer* **117** 618–24

[77] Littman A J, Jackson L A and Vaughan T L 2005 Chlamydia pneumoniae and lung cancer: epidemiologic evidence *Cancer Epidemiol. Biomarkers Prev.* **14** 773–8

[78] Zhan P *et al* 2011 Chlamydia pneumoniae infection and lung cancer risk: a meta-analysis *Eur. J. Cancer* **47** 742–7

[79] Rezazadeh A, Laber D A, Ghim S J, Jenson A B and Kloecker G 2009 The role of human papilloma virus in lung cancer: a review of the evidence *Am. J. Med. Sci.* **338** 64–7

[80] Zhai K, Ding J and Shi H Z 2015 HPV and lung cancer risk: a meta-analysis *J. Clin. Virol.* **63** 84–90

[81] Gauderman W J, Morrison J L, Carpenter C L and Thomas D C 1997 Analysis of gene-smoking interaction in lung cancer *Genet. Epidemiol.* **14** 199–214

[82] Bailey-Wilson J E *et al* 2004 A major lung cancer susceptibility locus maps to chromosome 6q23-25 *Am. J. Hum. Genet.* **75** 460–74

[83] Spitz M R, Wu X, Wilkinson A and Wei Q 2006 Cancer of the lung *Cancer Epidemiology and Prevention* 3rd edn ed D Schottenfeld and J F Raumeni (Oxford: Oxford University Press)

[84] Bossé Y and Amos C I 2018 A decade of GWAS results in lung cancer *Cancer Epidemiol. Biomarker Prev.* **27** 363–79

[85] Zhang R *et al* 2014 A genome-wide gene–environment interaction analysis for tobacco smoke and lung cancer susceptibility *Carcinogenesis* **35** 1528–35

[86] Gazdar A, Franklin W A, Brambilla E, Hainaut P, Yokota J and Harris C C 2004 Genetic and molecular alterations *Pathology and Genetics Tumors of the Lung, Pleura, Thymus and Heart* ed W D Travis, E Brambilla, H K Muller-Hermelink and C C Harris (Lyon: IARC Press)

[87] Thun M J *et al* 2008 Lung cancer occurrence in never-smokers: an analysis of 13 cohorts and 22 cancer registry studies *PLoS Med.* **5** e185

[88] Siegel R L, Miller K D and Jemal A 2019 Cancer statistics *CA Cancer J. Clin.* **69** 7–34

[89] Couraud S, Zalcman G, Mileron B, Morin F and Souquet P J 2012 Lung cancer in never smokers—a review *Eur. J. Cancer* **48** 1299–311

[90] Jenks S 2016 Is lung cancer incidence increasing in never-smokers? *J. Natl. Cancer Inst.* **108** 3–4

[91] Cufari M E *et al* 2017 Increasing frequency of non-smoking lung cancer: presentation of patients with early disease to a tertiary institution in the UK *Eur. J. Cancer* **84** 55–9

[92] Park J Y and Jang S H 2016 Epidemiology of lung cancer in Korea: recent trends *Tuberc. Respir. Dis.* **79** 58–69

[93] Sun S, Schiller J H and Gazdar A F 2007 Lung cancer in never smokers—a different disease *Nat. Rev. Cancer* **7** 778–90

[94] Torok S *et al* 2011 Lung cancer in never smokers *Future Oncol.* **7** 1195–211

[95] Okazaki I, Ishikawa S, Ando W and Sohara Y 2016 Lung adenocarcinoma in never smokers: problems of primary prevention from aspects of susceptible genes and carcinogens *Anticancer Res.* **36** 6207–24

[96] Chapman A M, Sun K Y, Ruestow P, Cowan D M and Madl A K 2016 Lung cancer mutation profile of EGFR, ALK, and KRAS: meta-analysis and comparison of never and ever smokers *Lung Cancer* **102** 122–34

[97] Rivera G A and Wakelee H 2016 Lung cancer in never smokers *Adv. Exp. Med. Biol.* **893** 43–57

[98] Thun M J, Henley S J, Burns D, Jemal A, Shanks T G and Calle E E 2006 Lung cancer death rates in lifelong nonsmokers *J. Natl. Cancer Inst.* **98** 691–9

[99] Mountain C F 1997 Revisions in the international system for staging lung cancer *Chest* **111** 1710–7

[100] Manser R L, Irving L B, Stone C, Byrnes G, Abramson M and Campbell D 2004 Screening for lung cancer *Cochrane Database Syst. Rev.* **1** CD001991

[101] Oken M M *et al* 2011 Screening by chest radiograph and lung cancer mortality: the Prostate, Lung, Colorectal, and Ovarian (PLCO) randomized trial *JAMA* **306** 1865–73

[102] Diederich S, Wormanns D and Heindel W 2001 Low-dose CT: new tool for screening lung cancer? *Eur. Radiol.* **11** 1916–24

[103] Aberle D R *et al* 2011 Reduced lung-cancer mortality with low-dose computed tomographic screening *N. Engl. J. Med.* **365** 395–409

[104] Moyer V AU.S. Preventive Services Task Force 2014 Screening for lung cancer: US Preventive Services Task Force recommendation statement *Ann. Intern. Med.* **160** 330–8

[105] CMS 2015 *Decision Memo for Screening for Lung Cancer with Low Dose Computed Tomography (LDCT) (CAG-00439N)* https://cms.gov/medicare-coverage-database/details/nca-decision-memo.aspx?NCAId=274 (Accessed: 7 May 2019)

[106] US Department of Health and Human Services 2010 *Patient Protection and Affordable Care Act, 2010* https://healthcare.gov/where-can-i-read-the-affordable-care-act/ (Accessed: 7 May 2019)

[107] Lewis J A *et al* 2015 Low-dose CT lung cancer screening practices and attitudes among primary care providers at an academic medical center *Cancer Epidemiol. Biomarkers Prev.* **24** 664–70

[108] Kang H R *et al* 2019 Role of low-dose computerized tomography in lung cancer screening among never-smokers *J. Thorac. Oncol.* **14** 436–44

[109] Kim H Y *et al* 2018 Lung cancer screening with low-dose CT in female never smokers: retrospective cohort study with long-term national data follow-up *Cancer Res. Treat.* **50** 748–56

Chapter 5

Use of biomarkers in lung cancer diagnosis, prognosis, and treatment

Saima Shakil Malik, Nosheen Masood and Iqra

5.1 Introduction

Lung cancer is the principal cause of cancer-related mortality and morbidity all over the world. Non-small-cell lung cancer (NSCLC) was found to be the most common lung cancer subtype (85%), with a 16% over 5 year overall survival rate, without any significant improvement for several decades [1]. The poor lung cancer prognosis may be attributed to disease diagnosis at an advanced stage, a lack of complete treatment/therapy, and shorter survival times at advanced stages [2, 3]. Until now, NSCLCs were treated based on tumor staging. Surgery alone was considered as the standard of care for NSCLC cases with stage I–IIIA, subsequently resulting in survival rates ranging from 23% to 33% and then 89% in stages IIIA, IIB, and IA, respectively [4]. It was evident that after surgical resection of localized NSCLC, adjuvant chemotherapy could increase the survival rate at five years by approximately 5% and is now recommended for all resected cases except for stage IA patients [5]. A combination of platinum based chemotherapy and thoracic-radiotherapy is usually used in the treatment of stage IIIB NSCLCs [6]. Until recently stage IV NSCLC cases were entirely treated with chemotherapy without any histology or biomarker related selection [7]. The therapeutic potential of lung cancer diagnosis and treatment has been of great interest in the past few years, specifically from the perspectives of targeted/personalized therapies and immunotherapies. The notion of targeted/personalized medicine has grown immensely with predictive biomarker integration, giving the potential to recognize cases that can derive the maximum advantage and least toxicity from various treatments, such as chemotherapy/immunotherapy, or personalized medicine based on individual tumor profiling. Now, targeted therapy/personalized medicine has become part of routine practise in lung cancer treatment, specifically at the advanced stages. In this chapter we will discuss the potential of genomic,

doi:10.1088/978-0-7503-2540-0ch5

proteomic, metabolic, and immunotherapeutic markers along with targeted therapy/personalized medicine in lung cancer diagnosis, prognosis, and treatment.

5.2 Histological subtypes and respective personalized medicine

In the past, the foremost step in the direction of personalized medicine for NSCLC treatment was taken by considering histological types. In the early 2000s, the standard of care among advanced NSCLC cases was a combination of chemotherapy with a platinum compound, for example cisplatin/carboplatin and a third-generation drug such as vinorelbine/gemcitabine, or some taxane compound such as docetaxel/paclitaxel [8, 9]. Phase III clinical trials had shown the comparable efficacy of these pairs with little variance in their toxicity profiles [10–14]. Later, a combination of three phase III randomized-non-inferiority clinical trials compared cisplatin/pemetrexed to cisplatin/gemcitabine in chemotherapy-naïve stage IIIB/IV NSCLC cases with a performance status of 0–1 [15]. The overall survival for cisplatin/pemetrexed was found to be non-inferior to cisplatin/gemcitabine with a hazard ratio of 0.94. However, according to histological types overall survival was reported to be significantly longer with cisplatin/pemetrexed compared to cisplatin/gemcitabine among a sub-group of adenocarcinoma cases (12.6 months versus 10.9 months) and large cell carcinoma cases (10.4 months versus 6.7 months). However, a significantly shorter overall survival was observed for another sub-group of squamous cell carcinoma cases with cisplatin/pemetrexed (9.4 months) in comparison to cisplatin/gemcitabine (10.8 months) [16]. Therefore, the pemetrexed and cisplatin combination was approved as first-line treatment for advanced NSCLC and restricted to non-squamous histologies. Similarly, pemetrexed monotherapy was restricted to maintenance therapy [17] and second-line treatment [18].

The differences among the survival rates of previously untreated NSCLC cases were compared in a clinical trial using carboplatin/paclitaxel chemotherapy with or without bevacizumab. Survival rates were significantly higher for a combination of carboplatin/paclitaxel with bevacizumab 15 mg kg^{-1} [19]. Similar combinations were tried in another phase III clinical trial with a range of bevacizumab concentrations (7.5 mg kg^{-1} and 15 mg kg^{-1}) until progression and were found to have significantly higher ($P = 0.001$) progression free survival [20].

Two different phase III trials measured the efficacy of necitumumab according to histological type among NSCLC cases. In one of the trials no difference in overall and progression free survival was observed among previously untreated, stage IV non-squamous NSCLC cases who received either the pemetrexed/cisplatin doublet alone, or in combination with necitumumab [21].

A second trial was conducted with squamous cell carcinoma cases where significantly improved overall survival was observed with cisplatin/gemcitabine (11.5 months versus 9.9 months). Therefore, necitumumab approval has been restricted to squamous NSCLC treatment [22]. Recently, cisplatin/gemcitabine in combination with necitumumab was found to be well tolerated by squamous NSCLC cases. Moreover, this combination was reported to have clinically expressive treatment benefits and better progression free survival in first-line treatment [23].

5.3 Available screening assays to detect molecular alterations and genetic rearrangements

Lung cancer can be screened via many different molecular assays available commercially in the market that are specific, sensitive, efficient, cost effective, use less sample, and identify all targets of clinical importance. The major types of non-germline mutations in lung cancer are translocations, inversions, change in copy or exon number, deletions, insertions, duplications, point mutations, and single nucleotide variations. The most common mutations found in EGFR are: in exon 19 with deletions of 15-bp, 18-bp, 9-bp, 12-bp, 24-bp, and 27-bp, L858R mutation, and insertions of 15-bp and 18-bp; in exon 20 with insertion of S768 and T790M mutation; in exon 18 with mutations of E709 and G719; and in exon 21 with mutations of L861Q, T854, and L858R. The various modes of screening technologies depend on which mutational analysis is to be performed. If EGFR has to be detected it can be screened via pyrosequencing, high resolution melt analysis (HRMA), next generation sequencing (NGS), or Sanger sequencing, or targeted via SNaPShot, Therascreen *EGFR* Kit, Cobas EGFR Mutation Test, or Agena MassARRAY Oncocarta panel (these are all commercially available). The screening method can identify all the mutations in the EGFR gene that are already reported or are novel, whereas the targeted method can only detect hotspot or known mutations [24]. Some of these assays are discussed in detail in this chapter (see figure 5.1).

5.3.1 Screening assays for EFGR

5.3.1.1 Sanger sequencing

Sanger sequencing is also known as sequencing by chain termination. Extension of primers is stopped using ddNTP. The ingredients of the PCR reaction include adenine, cytosine, guanine, and thymine nucleotides, ddNTP, DNA polymerase, and primers for sequencing. The resulting PCR product contains fragments of DNA

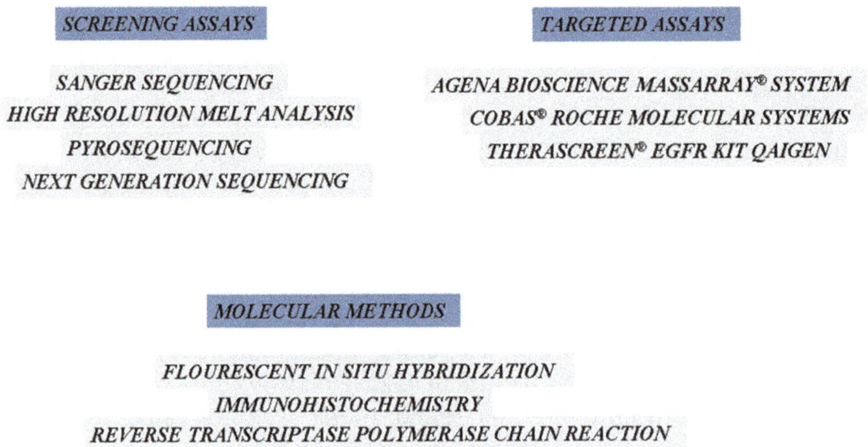

Figure 5.1. Different assays that can be used to detect genetic mutations/variation in lung cancer patients.

with different sizes which are later separated by electrophoresis. This technique can detect a variety of mutations but is unable to detect copy number variations, has reduced sensitivity, and is non-scalable [25].

5.3.1.2 High resolution melt analysis

HRMA is a sensitive, rapid, and cheap method of mutational screening that is usually followed by sequencing. Real-time PCR is used and melt analysis is performed. The whole procedure is usually provided by the manufacturer. The basic science lies in melting DNA, changing double stranded DNA into single stranded. The mutated DNA will melt at a temperature different to nonmutated single stranded DNA. The difference in temperature will determine the mutation followed by sequencing [25].

5.3.1.3 Pyrosequencing

In this method particular base additions are detected by inorganic pyrophosphate that are identified by chemiluminescence. It is also called sequencing by synthesis and is sensitive and quick. Pyrophosphate is released during the extension of the primer and each time it is added at the 3′ end light is emitted and a pyrogram is formed. This is more sensitive compared to Sanger sequencing and is able to detect below 5% mutation in the tumor compared to Sanger, which requires at least 10%–20% in the sample. It can easily detect SNVs but not copy number and structural changes.

5.3.1.4 Next generation sequencing

NGS has the ability to screen for a large number of mutations in multiple patients at one time. It is used for expressed sequences, exome analysis, and whole genome screening. Variations in NGS methodology can be found but the basic principle is the same. A library is constructed by random fragmentation using PCR-sequencing and annealing the fragments with a linker that helps in PCR amplification [26]. Different chemistries of sequencing are used by different platforms, for example Illumina uses termination by reversible dye [27], Ion PGM uses a technique somewhat similar to pyrosequencing, and single molecule real-time sequencing (SMRT) is used by Pacific Biosciences [28]. NGS focuses on clinically relevant genes in cancer in a more applicable, efficient, and affordable manner [29]. NGS requires small amounts of material (biopsy or cytological) and can detect multiple targets of interest. However, the only drawback associated with NGS is in the use of PCR, as this technique has its own flaws, such as false mutations [30].

5.3.2 Targeted assays

Therascreen®, Cobas®, SNaPShot, and MassARRAY are all mutation detection kits that are available on the market from different brands and are used for EGFR mutational screening. Other than EGFR, KRAS and BRAF mutations can be identified by targeted assays. Specialized kits are available for KRAS mutations in the 12th, 13th, and 61st codon, including 19 mutations. Similarly, the V600 variation of the BRAF gene can also be assayed through commercially available kits. The beauty of these assays lies in the multiplex option for the detection of multiple mutations of hotspot regions in one assay. The only drawback associated with these techniques is that they are unable to detect novel mutations, although they are highly sensitive and require a lot less initial material compared to other techniques [31].

5.3.2.1 Agena Bioscience Massarray® system

This technique is available to identify 215 somatic mutations in different tumor suppressor and oncogenes, such as TP53, PTPRD, PTEN, PTCH1, PIK3CA, NTRK3, NTRK2, NTRK1, NRF2, NOTCH1, MET, STK11, MAP2K1, JAK2, EGFR4, ERBB2, EPHA5, EPHA3, DDE2, AKT1, ALK, BRAF, NRAS, KRAS, and EGFR. The main principle of this technique is the amplification of DNA using PCR with an allele specific primer. The PCR product is evaluated using the 'matrix-assisted laser desorption/ionization time-of-flight' MALDI-TOF principle [31].

5.3.2.2 Cobas® EGFR mutation test

This is a real-time PCR technique using allele specific primers and detects exon 21 substitution mutation L858R and exon 19 deletion in the EGFR gene. They are used for patients treated with erlotinib in lung cancer trials to compare with platinum based chemotherapy [32]. In addition, this technique can identify EGFR exon 18–21 mutations including 41 sites.

5.3.2.3 Therascreen® EGFR kit

This is also a real-time PCR based assay that can screen deletions of exons 18 and 19, L861Q and L858R mutations in exon 21, insertions at three sites, T790M and S7681 in exon 20, in exon 19 a total of 19 deletions, and in exon 18 G719X mutations. Scorpions and the ARMS principle are used in this technique. Fluorescence is released because of the separation between the quencher and fluorophore due to binding of the ARMS amplicon with the Scorpion primer.

5.4 Molecular methods used to detect mutations

The above-mentioned techniques are sensitive and highly efficient, but they have their own drawbacks, as they are unable to identify the copy number and structural mutations. Different molecular assays are used to detect such mutations and some of them are explained below.

5.4.1 Fluorescence *in situ* hybridization (FISH)

In clinical practice FISH is used to identify exon or copy number changes, inversions, or rearrangements. This technique is very efficient in detecting RET, ROS1, and ALK mutations without any information regarding the translocation partner. The sequence on the target DNA is bound to a specific sequence on the DNA using two probes. Fluorescent dye is attached to the probes which allows detection. ALK mutation detection is difficult as both inversion as well as translocation is present on one arm of the chromosome, therefore the 'ALK break apart FISH' technique is used for this purpose. A lot of expertize is required to interpret its results and FISH is an expensive technique compared to other molecular methods [33].

5.4.2 Immunohistochemistry (IHC)

IHC is mostly used for ALK screening. Normally ALK is not present in the lung, but due to some mutation such as rearrangement, the ALK protein is formed constitutively and this leads to its overexpression [33, 34]. The 'Gold FISH' test has been used to compare to IHC, utilizing different antibody clones (SP8, ALKO1, ALK1, D5F3, 5A4) [35, 36]. The technique of IHC leads to staining of protein and labeling as negative (0), weak (1), moderate (2), or strong (3). Results are positive if a 1–3 score has been found and negative in the case of 0 [37]. Rearrangements in RET and ROS1 can also be screened using IHC [38] and results are similar to FISH or RTPCR. In relation to EGFR, three IHC tests are available, for total ECFR, phosphorylated EFGR, and mutant specific EFGR. The first two are not used alone any longer due to some complications, while the third type screens for exon 19 deletion of 15-bp and L858R mutation in exon 21.

5.4.3 Reverse transcriptase polymerase reaction (RTPCR)

ALT, RET, and ROS1 translocations can be screened using RTPCR in addition to IHC and FISH. Information regarding the translocation partner is required in this technique and is efficient and precise when combined with sequencing to detect the exact variant [36].

There are hundreds of molecular techniques available for the detection of lung cancer and subsequent treatment. The choice of methodology depends on the clinical requirements, whether it is for detection or for personalized medicine. The basic precision lies in the choice of screening, as cancer is a heterogeneous disease and the best way is to multiplex and identify many mutations in different genes at once.

5.5 Genomic markers

Conventionally the only treatment strategy was to identify the patient through symptoms that are visible and then administer whatever treatment seemed best and wait for a positive or negative response. This methodology leads to highly elevated levels of death rate and most of the patients do not even survive the treatment and die within one year of diagnosis [39]. This provided the concept that although phenotypically patients are the same, genetically they are different and have differences in the metabolizing activity of different compounds [40]. With the advent of new techniques and mutational screening, these conventional methods have been replaced by targeted therapies and provide a new concept of personalized medicine.

5.5.1 EFGR-TKI

One of the strategies to treat cancer is using tyrosine kinase inhibitors (TKI). The protein family of EFGR, such as HER1–4, when overexpressed, activates the KRAS and phosphoinositide 3-kinase/protein kinase B (PI3K/AKT) resulting in cell division and growth, causing lung cancer and many other cancers as well. EGFR has an ATP receptor site that can be blocked by TKI leading to blockage of the EGFR homodimer to receive ATP, which is required for phosphorylation into phosphotyrosine and prevent overexpression of EFGR. Proliferation and cell survival mechanisms regulated by STAT/JAK, ERK/RAS, and AKT/PI3K are activated due to phosphorylation and structural changes in EFGR [41]. In the case of lung cancer, elevated gene copy number and higher expression of EFGR has been reported in clinical reports with inconsistent results [42] and drugs that inhibit the activity of EFGR have opened new horizons for mutation identification [43]. It has been found that exons 18, 19, 20, and 21, which are associated with tyrosine kinase activity, are the most commonly mutated sites. Among these exons, deletion mutation at E 746-A 750 occurred in approximately 45%, while substitution mutation at L858R has a 40%–45% occurrence rate. Nearly 10% of mutations are rare in the case of all the EFGR mutations reported, such as 1% are insertions in exon 19, 4% are insertions in exon 20, 1%–2% are L861 and L861Q point mutations in exon 21, and 3% are G719X mutations in exon 18 [44–47]. Depending on the type of mutation the treatment strategy may differ as some mutations may be associated with ALK or KRAS rearrangements and they may have a relation to histology of bronchioloalveola or adenocarcinoma [48]. EFGR mutational rates in North America are about 15%–20% compared to Western Europe with about 10%–15%, and are highest in Asians with about 45%–50%, and most of these individuals are women and non-smokers [49–52]. Afatinib, erlotinib, and gefitinib are the three most commonly used first generation drugs and the second generation drugs are neratinib and afatinib. The most recent third-generation drug is osimertinib. All of these are administered according to the EFGR mutational spectrum by a strategy known as personalized targeted therapy because EFGR-TKI sensitivity depends on the type of mutation. Response rates of 70%–100% have been observed in patients with deletion of exon 19 compared to L858R mutation and deletion in exon 19 with a response rate of 20%–67% [44, 53, 54]. Insertions in exon 20 show resistance to TKI therapy, whereas common mutations such as G719X or L861Q showed good efficiency of EFGR-TKI therapy as well as the drug afatinib compared to rare mutations of EFGR [42, 45, 54]. Among patients with T790M mutation rociletinib and osimertinib, the two inhibitors of EFGR, have shown promising results and are known as third-generation EFGE inhibitors.

5.5.2 Analplastic lymphoma kinase

Among lung cancer patients, screening of ALK revealed that it forms a fusion protein with KIF5B or EML4 (echinoderm microtubule associated protein like 4) due to chromosomal rearrangements, whereas normally they are involved in neuron formation and microtubule development [38, 55, 56]. Lung cancer tumors that have

KRAS and EFGR wild type genotype, in patients who are light smokers and young, have been found to have 3%–5% ALK rearrangement so helping oncologists to identify high risk populations. For such patients crizotinib, which targets MET, ROS1, and ALK by inhibiting them, has shown a nearly 60% response rate in phase I to III trials. Crizotinib has also been found to inhibit TKI [57]. However, a large number of patients developed resistance to crizotinib in one year of therapy [35, 58–62]. Inhibitors of ALK are reported to have a 5-year overall survival rate, whereas lorlatinib encompassing ALK-ROS1 mutations in lung cancer may treat some ALK mutations that are resistant and is in phase II clinical trials. Depending on the mutation (ALKF1174X or ALKI1171X) ceritinib or alectinib is administered to the patients as both respond differently to these mutations.

5.5.3 KRAS

Feedback regulation of KRAS is affected due to loss in activity of GTPase if there are rare mutations in codon 61 or 13 or frequent mutations in codon 12 [63]. Due to this feedback regulation the PI3K and ERK/MEK/BRAF pathways are activated leading to enhanced proliferation of cells [64]. It has been shown that mutations in KRAS were associated with short overall survival and do not affect progression free survival [65, 66]. Contradictory reports were found regarding the association of G12V and codon 13 mutations and lung cancer throughout the literature, some observing significant association while others found no association [13, 67–71]. Therefore, whether KRAS can be used for prognosis is still under debate. In the case of colorectal cancer KRAS mutations are well defined and strongly associated with drug response, but not in the case of lung cancer as monoclonal anti-EFGR antibodies do not respond in adenocarcinoma [72]. Once mutations in KRAS occur, BRAF activates ERK and MEK protein by phosphorylation resulting in apoptosis, angiogenesis, proliferation, and differentiation [73]. Approximately 1.6% of smokers and 1.8% of non-smokers had these mutations in lung cancer patients. V600E is the most common mutation followed by D594G mutation [74]. The prognostic value of BRAF is still unclear due to contradictory reports throughout the literature [75–78].

5.5.4 Antibody mediated treatment

All the methods explained above are based on genetic screening followed by personalized medicine and all the drugs cause their effect by quenching the energy molecule ATP, leading to inhibition of the gene. In the case of lung cancer, antibody treatment has a different mode of action. The T cell mediated response is initiated, that destroys cancerous cells by activating the immune system of the body. Two important proteins of this cascade are activated, i.e. PD-1 'programmed cell death protein 1' and PDL1 'programmed death ligand 1'. In cancer cells PDL1 is overexpressed leading to an insufficient immune system of body. In the case of antibody treatment, the PD-1 receptor is blocked leading to an enhanced defense system of the body. This strategy seems to work but it does not last long, as there are multiple pathways involved in the body's defense system, and others are activated and start to work, such as '2, 3-dioxygenase and indoleamine-pyrrole increase for starvation of tryptophan for T cells, galectin-9 with hepatitis A virus cellular receptor 2, CD155 with T cell immunoreceptor with Ig and ITIM domains, CD80/CD86 binding with cytotoxic T-lymphocyte-associated protein 4' [79–81]. The current chemotherapeutic drugs in use follow a similar technique. Pembrolizumab (the most recent drug approved in 2017) and nivolumab target the PD-1 receptor while atezolizumab targets the PDL1 ligand [82–84]. Pembrolizumab is the most promising drug, as reported by the literature, that effects the PDL1 ligand [9]. Many studies have compared the effect of pembrolizumab with docetaxel and found a 111% increased median survival time in the two groups. Similar results were found when compared to other chemotherapeutic drugs [9, 85]. The drawbacks associated with the use of pembrolizumab may be the resistance, and as it encounters the body's defense mechanism other mechanisms associated with the immune system may have adverse effects on the body [86].

5.6 Proteomic markers

Proteomics is an important method for identifying biomarkers and therapeutic agents for carcinoma treatment. Mass spectroscopy and two-dimensional gel-electrophoresis are the two most widely used techniques for protein identification. However, currently, multiple protein analysis in one reaction is the most demanding field, which can identify many crucial protein mutations in lung cancer patients and lead to better responses to therapy, as the protein is the actual modulator behind activities rather than the transcript [87]. Lung cancer is the most common cause of cancer-related death, due to late diagnosis. There are a number of proteins that may be used as prognostic factors, such as tumor liberated protein that is a nearly 100 K Dalton protein used as a blood biomarker [88] and is effective for stage I patients. Tumor liberated protein is present in interstitial lung fibrosis and has the ability to elicit a specific immune response, therefore it may be utilized as an anticancer vaccine. Currently, research is ongoing to produce this protein for initiating antibody response and to make it an effective vaccine for anticancer treatment. The micro-environment of lung cancer has proinflammatory cytokines and inflammatory cells due to inflammation at the site. Due to this condition acute phase reactant proteins are formed and are used in the identification of different types of cancer. The group of these APRPs includes apolipoprotein A1, serum-amyloid A (SAA), and haptoglobin (Hp) β-chain [89, 90]. The major role of Hp is cell migration, angiogenesis, and removal of free plasma hemoglobins. Although it may be used as a good prognostic factor, sometimes the results are mixed with other respiratory diseases [89]. SAA is involved in the formation of an enzyme that degrades the extracellular matrix, the formation of an immune response at the site of inflammation, and cholesterol transfer towards the liver. It is also involved in metastasis of lung cancer through MMP9 expression by macrophages and serves as prognostic factor [91]. Similarly, ApoA1 is decreased in response to increased SAA1 and SAA2, therefore it may be considered as a potential marker [40].

Other protein biomarkers that may be used as prognostic factors are as follows. PGK1 is a good predictor of patient survival independent of stage because it is dependent on oxygen tension and higher levels depict aggressive hypoxic cancers. ANXA-3 is a calcium and phospholipid binding protein that promotes angiogenesis and leads to metastasis [92]. Increased levels of S100A11 showed increased TNM stages and lymph-node positivity [93, 94]. A few genes involved in the reorganization of the cytoskeletal framework may also be used as a prognostic factor of lung cancer. Cytokeratins and nonmuscle-myosin IIA are found to be associated with lung cancer prognosis. The former protein has many isoforms, such as CK7, CK8, CK18, and CK19, which are found to be elevated in carcinoma [95–97]. PHP-14 is known to inhibit the invasion and migration of cancerous cells in knocked down cell lines. Similarly calmodulin, thymosin $\beta 4$, thymosin $\beta 10$, and cofilin 1 are all cytoskeletal proteins that have now been proved to be good prognostic markers in lung cancer [98].

For lung cancer treatment, chemotherapy alone is not sufficient for patients and a variety of treatments need to be given leading to poor survival outcomes, but with the identification of protein markers personalized medicine may be given to patients to rule out irrelevant drugs and their side effects.

5.7 Metabolic markers

5.7.1 Metabolomics

The study of metabolite identification along with their qualitative and quantitative analysis that constitutes the metabolome of a cell or tissue is called metabolomics. The term 'metabolite(s)' is generally used for biomolecules having a molecular weight less than 1500 Da. These metabolites can be structural components of cells or mediators involved in intracellular signaling. Usually, metabolomics emphasizes the products and substrates of metabolism, containing biomolecules such as lipids, nucleotides, amino acids, carboxylic acids, and carbohydrates. The metabolome is less complex than the proteome and genome. The number of human genes, metabolites, and proteins (including posttranslational modifications) are estimated as 20 000–25 000, 2000–2500, and 250 000–1 000 000, respectively. Comparing with other 'omes', the metabolome tells us exactly what is happening in the organism and reflects the current status of the phenotype [99]. During cancer initiation and progression, alteration of cellular metabolism occurs, allowing cancer cells to avoid apoptosis, increase anabolic synthesis, and adapt to low oxygen and nutrient availability. Thus, the cancer's metabolic nature can assist in patient cancer status monitoring through lipidomics and metabolomics. Moreover, monitoring a patient's metabolic status may also be used to understand the mode of action of anticancer therapeutics [100]. Early detection strategies are required to ensure an increased overall survival rate among cancer cases. Cancer metabolomics helps in the early detection of lung cancer by describing metabolites which are related either directly or indirectly to tumor growth and its formation [101]. Metabolomics together with proteomics and genomics provide valuable information regarding the metabolic processes of cells that are responsible for tumor formation and its progression. Metabolomics also helps in the assessment of patient variability in the type and number of metabolites that are expressed in lung tumors. Based on metabolite absence or presence with respect to a particular condition, one can easily differentiate the stage, type, and drug response to treatment. The metabolic activity of a cell is actually the measurement of its survival capacity and thus is directly responsible for disease proliferation. Tumor cells adopt different tactics to sustain biosynthetic precursors, in particular for maintaining aerobic glycolysis at a faster rate [102]. The Warburg approach is used to describe the metabolic phenotype of tumors. It refers to the glycolysis at a very high rate followed by the production of lactic acid. A few studies have been carried out to determine the role of the glutamine pathway in cancer development and progression, which actually provides essential substances such as ATP and macromolecules for biosynthesis to sustain cellular proliferation [103].

This part of the chapter sheds light on the use of metabolomic techniques and biomarkers to differentiate between tumor type and stage. Furthermore, the role of metabolome is discussed in predicting disease progression and survival.

5.7.2 Metabolomic techniques used to analyze metabolites

Two different techniques are commonly used to examine metabolites in lung cancer, including nuclear magnetic resonance (NMR) and mass spectrometry (MS). These techniques are well-known for extracting metabolic information from blood, urine, sweat, sputum, and tumor samples as well as normal cells [104]. Normally, the results from MS and NMR are combined to completely analyze the related metabolites.

Particular alterations of metabolites in human beings can be examined using the following techniques: (i) obtaining metabolites from post-resection tumor samples, (ii) gaining metabolites from serum, urine, sweat and sputum samples, (iii) inserting patients resected tumor cells into animal models such as the mouse, or (iv) developing tumor cells resected *in vitro* along with metabolic extraction. Moreover, stable-isotope classification has been utilized to define pathways stimulated in diverse tumors. Some studies have reported the detection of labeled metabolites in different pathways, such as glycolysis, anaplerotic pyruvate carboxylation, and Krebs cycle. These are all considerably changed in lung cancer tumors [105, 106].

5.7.3 Lipidomics

Lipidomics, a branch of metabolomics, involves the systematic study of all lipids and their complete examination in the biological system. All biological membranes and the metabolites of organisms have lipids as basic components, as they play an important role in structure, cellular energy storage, and signaling [107]. The imbalance of lipids causes various diseases relevant to human lifestyle such as atherosclerosis, obesity [108], diabetes, Alzheimer's disease [109], and cancer [110]. Lipidomics is acknowledged as a research tool for lipids in lipid biochemistry, clinical biomarker discovery [110], disease diagnosis [111], and in understanding disease pathology [112].

Lipidomics not only gives an understanding of the particular purposes of lipid species in disease and health, but also classifies potential biomarkers for defensive or therapeutic programs for different human diseases. The use of lipidomics in the NSCLC biomarker offers a new prospect for exploring NSCLC related biochemical mechanisms [113]. Chen *et al* demonstrated that altered sphingolipid and phospholipid profiles in NSCLC might have significant biological effects and potential for biomarker growth [107].

5.7.4 Classification of diagnostic metabolic biomarkers

Lung cancer diagnostic markers are divided into the following four groups. (i) Metabolites relevant to energy such as citric acid and glucose. Glucose supplies energy for the development of lung cancer cells through the tricarboxylic acid cycle and glycolysis. Among the most studied pathways known for cancer cell multiplication is upregulation of the tricarboxylic acid cycle and glycolysis in tumor cells [114]. Glucose, D-isomer enhances lung cancer progression by stimulating proteins associated with glucose [115]. Acylcarnitines take part in the fatty acid oxidation in mitochondria, the powerhouse of the cell, producing energy for the cell and representing normal functioning of mitochondria. Lower acylcarnitine levels were found in the serum of newly diagnosed NSCLC cases [116]. (ii) Protein biosynthesis along with its building blocks (amino acids), such as alanine, threonine, and glutamic acid as molecular markers in disease diagnostics. The important sources of nitrogen for lung cancer cells are the amino acids. The source of carbon for anaplerosis of tricarboxylic acid cycle is glutamic acid. (iii) Metabolites which are associated with the synthesis of cell membrane, such as carnitine and choline have a significant role in Ca lung cell metabolism. Choline is most important metabolite helping in cell proliferation of cancer cells by providing initial substrates and materials for synthesis of the cell membrane along with other essential lipid materials. DNA methylation requires methyl which is also provided by choline and, as a result, methylation affects the expression of genes in normal cells and DNA repair [117]. The strength of all membrane glycerophospholipids and the important molecule in lipid biosynthesis is glycerol. A recent study showed that glycerol is dramatically amplified in lung cancer patients' serum [118]. Apart from this, for early detection of Ca lung, lactic acid is also identified as strong marker. It enhances cancer cell proliferation and metastasis by decreasing extracellular pH and inducing immunosuppression in native cells [119]. (iv) In lung cancer pathogenicity, gut microbiome dysbiosis has been identified as vital by means of the gut–lung axis [120]. Gut microbial metabolite benzaldehyde upregulation has been shown to distinguish the first stage cancer individuals from healthy ones with 100% sensitivity and 95% specificity [104].

5.7.5 Body fluids based metabolic biomarkers

As the lung is linked to the respiratory system, sputum samples, bronchoalveolar lavage fluid (BALF), and expiration concentrate have also been collected in studies along with other body fluids such as serum, blood, and urine, respectively.

Lung cancer and chronic obstructive pulmonary disease (COPD) are general lung diseases mostly caused by smoking. Therefore, it is necessary to differentiate between these pathological conditions, particularly to understand the primary stages of lung cancer. Novel monitoring and diagnostic tools are needed to identify lung carcinogenesis in order to decide proper treatment and drug dosage regimes. One study compared the diagnostic patterns with different nuclear magnetic resonance fingerprints in serum samples of 22 COPD and 77 lung cancer patients of I–IV tumor stages, and found it helped to differentiate the early stages of lung cancer from COPD. Moreover, an increase in leucine, mannose, *N*-acetylated glycoproteins, choline, lysine, and lipid levels along with a reduction in citrate, acetate, and methanol levels were detected in lung cancer cases when compared to COPD. It was reported that metabolite markers were useful in discriminating lung cancer stages: acetoacetate, isoleucine, and creatine plus two NMR signals of glycerol and *N*-acetylated glycoproteins [121].

LC/MS was also employed to examine serum metabolic molecules for lung cancer diagnosis. Serum metabolic features of lung cancer were studied using a non-targeted metabolomics strategy. About 23 Ca lung individuals with metabolic profiling and 23 healthy people were examined by employing ultrahigh performance liquid chromatography/quadrupole time-of flight mass spectrometry (UPLC/Q-TOF MS). Twenty-seven different metabolites were recognized; most of them were associated with malfunctioning of lipid metabolism comprising choline, free fatty acids, and others. It was reported that serum metabolic profiling by LC/MS can be an influential tool for lung cancer detection [122].

A study involving human urine screening highlighted an important variation of acylcarnitines and carnitine levels between healthy individuals and NSCLC patients. Another study reported that advanced acylcarnitines and carnitine profiling by MALDI-TOF can be used for NSCLC screening [123].

It is the need of the hour to discover diagnostic non-invasive biomarkers for better and early treatment. Creatine riboside was found to be the potential diagnostic lung cancer marker in all stages. It was proved to be important in early detection and linked to poor prognosis among stage I and II lung cancer cases. The two mentioned metabolites were considerably more developed in tumor cells than the neighboring non-tumor cells. Quantification of the aforementioned metabolites in urine samples by mass spectrometry offers a novel prospect for lung cancer detection followed by the recognition of new targets and therapeutic strategies. In addition to this, it provided the framework for analyzing the direct effect of these metabolites in lung tumorigenesis [124].

5.7.6 Alterations of metabolites in healthy individuals versus cancer patients

Different studies have reported variations in serum lipid and fatty acid levels between lung cancer cases and controls [125, 126]. Lung cancer cases usually have lower serum choline levels, because it is used for tumor proliferation, being a raw material for membrane phospholipids [127]. As membrane lipids, lysophosphatidylcholines can cause inflammation and are over-regulated in lung cancer cases

[122]. In contrast, a membrane sphingolipid sphingosine which is vital as apoptosis is found to be lower in lung cancer patients [128]. Furthermore, low density lipoproteins are examined in lung cancer patient's sera as they are a prerequisite for additional triglyceride proliferation, invasion, and metastasis [127, 129]. Other metabolite changes, including a reduction of 2,3,4,-trihydroxybutyric acid and prasterone sulfate and an increase in α-hydroxyisobutyric acid in lung cancer cases, making them beneficial lung cancer diagnostic markers [128].

A major aim of metabolomics research is to ascertain clinical biomarkers for the detection of lung cancer. Various studies have emphasized metabolite changes that can differentiate between cancer patients and healthy controls. Zhang *et al* demonstrated that lung cancer patient's serum samples displayed increased glutamine levels compared to controls. The amino acid glutamine may be transformed into glutamate, whose deamination goes towards the α-ketoglutarate formation, which is an intermediate of the tricarboxylic acid cycle. In addition to its conversion into glutamate it can be changed into aspartate, which makes malate, pyruvate, and axaloacetate by means of the tricarboxylic acid cycle. In this way, glutamine is important for the development and augmentation of cancer cells [129]. On the other hand, Puchades-Carrasco *et al* discovered a reduction in the levels of glutamine in sera from patients with lung cancer because glutamine is associated with the synthesis of amino acids and nucleotides [127]. A possible reason behind the inconsistent results is the differences in patients in terms of inclusion criteria, as Puchades *et al* used cases of all stages, while Zhang *et al* recruited only Ia and Ib stage patients [127, 129]. Therefore, the glutamine requirement increases with the advancement in disease, leading to its deficiency in the serum. Moreover, decreased serum levels of threonine and histidine were observed in lung tumors [101, 130].

5.7.7 Metabolite alterations in lung cancer stages and their significance as disease progression indicators and overall survival

Recently, some metabolites have been recognized in the bio-fluids and tumor tissues of cancer patients that are used for estimating lung cancer development and can be used to predict survival outcomes. Various serum metabolites were reported in early and advanced lung cancer. High levels of benzoic acid, lactic acid, and fumaric acid were observed in advanced-stage tumors showing disease metastasis [131]. As a support of triglycerides, glycerol is also amplified in advanced-stage lung cancer patients' sera, indicating either rearrangement of the cell membrane or lipid breakdown [121]. In contrast, decreased levels of L-glutamic and glyceric acid were observed in last stage tumors, which suggests that these might permeate from blood into lung tissues and then undergo metabolization [131]. Increased levels of lactate and ketone bodies (2-hydroxybutyrate, 3-hydroxybutyrate, acetone, and acetoacetate) were observed in early stage patients (the Warburg effect), which are general symbols of cancer metabolism. This decrease in the concentration of glucose along with increase in lactate is observed prominently in advanced-stage patients. Likewise, decreases in glutamine along with increases in *N*-acetyl-cysteine, serum leucine/isoleucine, and glutamate were observed in advance stage NSCLC cases [127].

Constant elevation in levels of *N*-acetyl cysteine, involved in antioxidant production, is over-regulated with the advancement of disease in NSCLC patients [127]. The upregulation of antioxidants contributes to lung cancer progression by p53 repression [132]. Glutamine has been widely studied in NSCLC and glutaminolysis was recognized as an important precursor for tumor proliferation, indicating its lower levels in the later stages of cancer [103]. Furthermore, other metabolites whose levels are upregulated in the progressive stages of lung cancer are phenylalanine and adipic acid. The changes in tumor cells' lipid metabolism cause high concentrations of adipic acid in advanced tumor stages. Phenylalanine is a precursor for tyrosine activation and neurotransmitters such as epinephrine and dopamine etc. Elevated serum levels of phenylalanine are due to the suppression of genes which are involved in NSCLC development [133]. A new metabolite, N^{12}-diacetylspermine, could prove a good biomarker for timely lung tumor detection. The literature has confirmed that Krebs cycle, glycolysis, membrane lipid degradation and biosynthesis, and nucleotide biosynthesis associated biomarkers are helpful in differentiating cancerous and non-cancerous tissues.

5.8 Immunotherapy markers

Immunotherapy has achieved remarkable outcomes for some cancer patients. However, there remains a clinical challenge for the selection of patients who are most likely to respond immunotherapy. One of the key modulators of tumor biology is the immune system, with its capability to inhibit or support tumor development, growth, invasion, and metastasis. Approaches intended to harness the immune system are the emphasis of numerous current promising therapeutic methods for cancer patients. For example, adoptive T cell therapy, which has produced promising remissions in people with advanced malignancies [134]. Moreover, some metastatic melanoma patients have shown long term survival benefits from therapeutic monoclonal antibodies which were designed to interrupt the inhibitory signals received by T cells through programmed cell death-1 (PD-1 or CD279) and cytotoxic T-lymphocyte-associated antigen 4 (CTLA-4 or CD152) [135]. However, all types of tumor do not respond to immunomodulatory approaches. This proves cancer heterogeneity and hypothesizes the existence of some other immune-regulatory mechanisms in patients. Therefore, one of the challenges faced by cancer immunotherapy today lies in understanding these resistance mechanisms to select the patients who are most likely to benefit [136].

Immune response is predicted by tumor–immune infiltrates called 'immune contexture' and stated as the composition, organization, mass, and active state of tumor-invading immune cells. In addition, these can either inhibit or promote tumorigenesis and can thus predict response and treatment outcomes [137]. Multiple immune-regulatory mechanisms can inhibit anti-tumor immune responses, for example the production of immunosuppressive mediators [138], resistance to immune effector pathways [86], inhibitory receptor overexpression, and recruitment of immune cells that have a suppressive role, such as myeloid-derived suppressor cells (MDSC) and T regulatory cells (Tregs) [139]. The management of these regulatory pathways in therapeutics may prolong cancer patients' survival and enhance anti-tumor immune responses. Currently monoclonal antibodies are mostly used in medical oncology because they can target immune check points [140].

5.8.1 Immunotherapy in NSCLC and SCLC

The latest innovations in immunotherapy have revolutionized medical practice in lung cancer therapy [141]. The United States Food and Drug Administration (FDA) have approved four checkpoint blockers, anti-PD-L1 antibodies atezolizumab and durvalumab and anti-PD-1 antibodies nivolumab and pembrolizumab, for the treatment of NSCLC since 2015 [142]. Regardless of the histological subtype, antibodies (anti-PD-1 and anti-PD-L1) give significant results in NSCLC patients whether pre-treated or not with increased overall survival [141]. Amazingly, patients with negative expression of anti-PD-L1 showed comparable consequences in OS to chemotherapy treated patients [143]. Although some NSCLC patients responded to anti-PD-L1 and anti-PD-1 immunotherapies, clinical trials showed only 15%–25% in NSCLC cases and the majority of them developed primary resistance [144]. Overall the mutation frequency is ten-fold higher in smokers compared to non-smoker lung cancer patients and this higher tumor mutational burden is considerably related to resilient medical benefits for patients treated with ICB therapy [145].

Clinical development of immuno-oncological agents for SCLC is at the early stages of development. Recent data from various phase I–III clinical trials show they have not progressed as for NSCLC. Although the progress in PFS observed in various clinical trials is promising, the clinical data are still sparse in this field [146]. The lower median survival time for SCLC patients with chemotherapy has moved researchers' attention towards immunotherapeutics [147].

5.8.2 PD-L1

In 2015, the trends of NSCLC treatment changed when two phase III trials, checkmate 057 and checkmate 017, were published. In checkmate 017, docetaxel or nivolumab was given randomly to locally advanced/metastatic NSCLC patients with disease progression. In the nivolumab-treated patients the median OS was about 9.2 months while it was 6 months in the docetaxel treated patients. The checkmate 057 trial recruited 582 NSCLC patients with the same study design as checkmate 017. In the nivolumab-treated group the median OS among 292 patients was 12.2 months while it was 9.4 months among the 290 patients in the docetaxel treated group. It was observed in both trials that nivolumab showed fewer adverse effects than docetaxel and was related to longer response rates, OS, and progression free survival in patients with PD-L1 expression on ⩾1%, 5%, and 10% of tumor cells. Both these clinical trials were practice-changing for NSCLC treatment by incorporating nivolumab as the second-line treatment standard of care [148, 149]. Mutual analysis of both studies verified that the OS rates of nivolumab were superior to docetaxel and revealed that it provides a favorable tolerability profile along with long term benefits [150]. The phase II/III KEYNOTE 010 clinical trial conducted on locally advanced or advanced NSCLC patients compared pembrolizumab and docetaxel as second-line treatment. Individuals possessing PD-L1 expression on more than 1% of tumor cells showed significant improvement in PFS, ORR, and OS with pembrolizumab [9]. Irrespective of the PD-L1 expression, individuals with metastatic NSCLC or previously treated locally advanced NSCLC showed significant prolonged OS with atezolizumab. Both atezolizumab and pembrolizumab had a more promising safety profile than docetaxel in phase II (POPLAR) and phase III (OAK) clinical trials and in KEYNOTE 010 [83, 151]. For first-line treatment, the KEYNOTE 024 clinical trial demonstrated that for advanced NSCLC with greater than 50% PD-L1 expression on tumor cells, pembrolizumab gives longer progression free survival and OS than chemotherapy [85]. One current clinical trial, KEYNOTE 042, is being carried out on individuals with PD-L1 expression ⩾1% and has shown that pembrolizumab was a better option compared to first-line chemotherapy with few side effects [152]. The KEYNOTE 189 trial was conducted on advanced non-squamous NSCLC with no mutations in ALK or EGFR genes. This trial verified that chemotherapy with pembrolizumab resulted in improved OS and PFS compared to first-line chemotherapy, regardless of PD-L1 expression [153]. In CkeckMate 026, PFS or OS was not improved in previously treated NSCLC cases with PD-L1 expression on ⩾50% of tumor cells or on at least 5% of tumor cells by nivolumab treatment [154]. With reference to published data on first-line treatments, for patients with no EGFR, ALK changes, and PD-L1 expression on at least 50% of tumor cells, pembrolizumab monotherapy should be the first choice of treatment. But for the remaining cases with low expression of PD-L1, chemotherapy combined with pembrolizumab or atezolizumab gave better results than chemotherapy alone.

In NSCLC patients, PD-L1 expression on tumor cells is a potential prognostic factor in immune checkpoint inhibitor therapy in respective clinical trials. However, the role of PDL-1 expression observed in qualification for immunotherapy among clinical trials is still contradictory due to the randomization differences of PD-L1 status on both immune and tumor cells [9].

5.8.3 Immune checkpoint inhibitors

Immune checkpoint inhibitors (ICIs) are being widely investigated in lung cancer. Immunotherapy as choice of treatment is not suitable for all individuals and also costs a huge amount. That is why it is important to personalize the use of immune check inhibitors. Factors responsible for the determination of response to ICIs are: the molecular tumor profile, tumor micro-environment, expression of immune checkpoint proteins such as PD-L1 or PD-1, and immune tumor infiltrates. Tumor shrinkage and prolonged survival can be achieved with selective inhibitors such as anti-ALK/ROS1 and anti-EGFR therapies. The effectiveness of ICIs can be increased by combining them with other anticancer therapies such as chemotherapy, radiation, or targeted therapy, or by collecting various immune checkpoint inhibitor strategies. Irrespective of the curative strategy, about half of lung cancer cases do not respond to immune checkpoint inhibitors. Sensitivity to immune check inhibitors depends on various factors such as tumor genetic history and immune regulator levels, such as PD-1 expression and PD-L1 expression. Increased response to immune checkpoint inhibitors was related to expression of their targets, such as PD-L1 and PD-1. Cases with PD-L1 negative tumors were clinically beneficial while PD-L1 patients could be non-responders. Tumor heterogeneity and the antibodies used to test PD-L1 expression were important factors. Irrespective of the drawbacks of PD-L1 immunohistochemistry, it is only one established biomarker used in daily clinics for the selection of individuals who will respond to first-line pembrolizumab monotherapy [85].

5.8.4 Circulating tumor DNA

Circulating tumor DNA (ctDNA) is now widely used in EGFR mutated NSCLC patients. A study reported increased overall survival and more clinical benefits that were related to low ctDNA concentration at first evaluation in NSCLC individuals treated with nivolumab. In addition, a low ctDNA level between first evaluation and diagnosis was also related to tumor response and PFS [155]. For the assessment of immunotherapy response in lung cancer patients, ctDNA level can be used in combination with medical imaging. A radiological response to immunotherapy is associated with an approximately >50% reduction in mutant ratio from the baseline [156]. In clinics the patients receiving ICIs have the feasibility of quantification of ctDNA due to the development of a targeted NGS panel in routine diagnostics.

5.8.5 Tumor mutational burden (TMB)

A potential biomarker which can respond to immunotherapy still needs to be explored. Since both PD-L1 negative and positive tumors give a response to their corresponding immune checkpoint blockers, PD-L1 expression is not considered as a predictive biomarker. Tumor mutational burden (TMB) in several tumor types including NSCLC is recommended as a predictive biomarker for immune checkpoint blocker treatments. A very high mutational rate was seen in genomic profiling of 110 SCLC samples [157]. About 22 910 mutations comprising 134 in exons were observed in the SCLC cell line, NCI-H209 correlated with tobacco smoking [158]. Approximately ninety five percent of these substitutions were single base and most of them are C→A mutations, dependent on polycyclic aromatic hydrocarbon exposure [159]. TMB in NSCLC was significantly correlated with total reported mutations, including those variants whose significance is not yet known along with functional variants. In SCLC pathogenicity, enhanced genomic instability by whole genomic functional loss of RB1 and p53 is inevitable [160]. SCLC represents one of the highest mutational loads comprising about 200 mutations per tumor. In a large phase III trial conducted on NSCLC, a greater mutational burden was observed in smokers with a better response to immunotherapy than never smokers [161]. A clinical trial, CheckMate 012, carried out on 75 advanced NSCLC patients suggested nivolumab and ipilimumab as first-line therapy. Longer progression free survival and a higher overall response rate was exhibited by a high TMB in tumor cells and in ctDNA than in patients with low TMB [162].

5.8.6 Immunotherapy side effects

Although immunotherapy is a very effective treatment providing resilient remission in some NSCLC patients, it can have various adverse effects due to overstimulation of the immune system. Usually chemotherapy is more toxic than monoclonal antibodies. However, some mild or severe immunotherapy associated side effects have been observed effecting the bronchi, large intestine mucosa, and the endocrine organs. Side effects of immunotherapy which could be severe include hepatitis, thyroiditis, and immune-related colitis, etc [163]. In some cases, immunotherapy was found to be involved in greater tumor progression. After the immunotherapy, the first imaging examination confirming hyper-progression is related to EGFR mutations, previous irradiation, older age, and higher metastatic load. Pseudo-progression is linked to enhanced infiltration of the tumor by immune cells and it should not be confused with hyper-progression [164]. A lot of aspects remain to be explored in cancer immunotherapy. The selection of patients for immunotherapy based on predictive factors is a major challenge for clinicians [165].

5.9 The emerging role of microRNAs

The family of small non-coding RNAs of about 21–25 nucleotides that can uphold mRNA breakdown by pairing to target messenger RNAs' complementary sites and can inhibit mRNA translation is called microRNA. MicroRNAs can alter gene expression by post-transcriptional modifications and are under investigation for their potential role in the pathogenesis, screening, and treatment of lung cancer. The literature shows the potential of microRNAs in the differentiation of lung cancer subtypes, with, for example, miR-21-5p and miR-375 were reported to be highly expressed in SCLC [166].

Advancement in liquid biopsies and body fluids have shown the potential of circulating miRNAs in disease diagnosis. A major advantage of targeting circulating miRNAs is their stability in body fluids without the effects of endogenous RNases. Furthermore, microRNAs overcome the tumor heterogeneity problem by collecting all pathological signals from different metastatic tumor sites [167]. A meta-analysis conducted in 2014 showed low expression of *let-7* microRNA in lung cancer patients as a predictor of poor prognosis [168]. In NSCLC poorer recurrence free survival is linked to miR-155 [169]. The patient response to chemotherapy, targeted therapy, and radiotherapy can also be modified by miRNAs [170]. The upregulation of miR-106b cisplatin activity was reported to be increased in a NSCLC cell line. This upregulated expression of miR-106b results in a decreased polycystin 2 (PKD2) level, followed by lowering of P-glycoprotein levels, affecting the efflux of various anticancer therapeutics [171]. On the other hand, upregulated miR-196 expression increases ERCC1, MDR1, and Bcl-2 levels, leading to cisplatin and drug efflux resistance [172].

In lung cancer radiotherapy, clinical applications of microRNAs have also been reported. Four microRNAs of plasma, including miR-613, miR-302e, miR-495-3p, and miR-98-5p, were identified as radiotherapy response predictors in NSCLC patients [173]. Cell-free DNA and miRNA is an upcoming technique for lung cancer, but it has certain limitations to be used in diagnostics, such as lack of reproducibility. Limited literature is available in this field and inconsistency among the already reported results can be attributed to variability in serum microRNA levels among patients. Variations in technical aspects, such as statistical methodologies, RNA purification methods, etc, may also contribute to inconsistent results [174]. Therefore, large-scale studies and clinical trials are recommended to explore the exact role and underlying mechanisms of various microRNAs in lung carcinogenesis.

5.10 Clinical trials with targetable oncogenic drivers

Clinical trials may be of various types such as diagnostic trials, in which new and improved tests are identified for diagnosing a particular disease. Other types of clinical trials include screening studies, prevention studies, treatment studies, etc.

Necitumumab is a recently developed novel monoclonal antibody which is effective in the treatment of metastatic squamous NSCLC by targeting epidermal growth factor receptor (EGFR) [22]. Durvalumab is a human immunoglobulin G1 kappa(Igg1k) monoclonal antibody and is an FDA-approved immunotherapy for cancer, which works by blocking the interaction of PD-L1 with the PD-1 and CD80 molecules. Most NSCLC advanced patients have faced disease progression despite the fact that they had completed a course of chemoradiotherapy. A phase III study (NCT02125461) compared durvalumab to a placebo as a consolidation therapy in stage III NSCLC patients who showed no disease progression after more than one cycle of platinum based chemoradiotherapy. Progression free survival was considerably greater with durvalumab than the placebo. The safety was the same between the groups, but the secondary end points favored durvalumab. Secondary end points included progression free survival, safety, response rate, response duration, time to distant metastasis, and time to death [175].

ALK rearrangement can act as a potent oncogenic driver in NSCLC patients as it occurs in 2%–7% of patients and is a newer molecular target. Crizotinib, which was synthesized as a cMET inhibitor, was found to be more effective in ALK rearranged NSCLC patients than chemotherapy. But patients developed recurrent disease advancement in the brain and resistance within a year. Hence, more effective and better therapeutic alternatives are needed. Ceritinib is a stronger anaplastic lymphoma kinase inhibitor than crizotinib and provides better results in crizotinib resistant NSCLC cases. In ASCEND-1, a phase I trial, ceritinib whole body activity was assessed in analplastic lymphoma kinase rearranged NSCLC in both analplastic lymphoma kinase inhibitor pre-treated and naïve individuals. This study concluded that ceritinib could be a good substitute for crizotinib in ALK rearranged NSCLC patients with brain metastasis. A phase II confirmation clinical trial is in progress on ceritinib performance in NSCLC individuals with analplastic lymphoma kinase rearrangement and brain metastasis [176]. Some of the ongoing clinical trials for lung cancer treatment which are registered with https://clinicaltrials.gov are listed in table 5.1.

Table 5.1. Ongoing clinical trials for lung cancer treatment.

Trial ID	Phase	Agents	Patient population	Study start date	Estimated completion date
NCT03191149	II	Osimertinib	NSCLC, recurrent EGFR exon20ins, Stage IIIb–IV	5 April 2018	31 July 2022
NCT03727724	II	Afatinib + cetuximab	Advanced EGFR exon20ins + NSCLC	4 December 2018	March 2021
NCT03505710	II	Trastuzumab deruxtecan (DS-8201a)	Metastatic NSCLC, HER2-mutated or overexpressing	21 May 2018	25 August 2020
NCT01542437	II	Afatinib	HER2 + NSCLC, progressive on chemotherapy	January 2012	June 2017
NCT02568267	II	Entrectinib	ALK, ROS1 gene fusions	19 November 2015	31 October 2020
NCT02771626	1/2	CB-839 + nivolumab	Melanoma, clear cell renal cell carcinoma, and NSCLC	August 2016	June 2019
NCT03215511	I/II	(LOXO-195)	Pre-treated with TRK inhibitor and NTRK fusion cancer	10 July 2017	December 2019
NCT02716116	1/2	TAK-788	Anti-tumor activity of oral EGFR/HER2 inhibitor TAK-788 in NSCLC	30 April 2016	28 January 2021
NCT02201992	III	Crizotinib	With stage IB–IIIA NSCLC (already gone through surgery) and ALK fusion mutations	18 August 2014	1 May 2022

NSCLC = non-small-cell lung carcinoma; EGFR = epidermal growth factor receptor; HER2 = human epidermal growth factor receptor 2; ALK = anaplastic lymphoma kinase; ROS = proto-oncogene 1, receptor tyrosine kinase; NTRK = neurotrophic-tropomyosin receptor kinase; TRK = tropomyosin receptor kinase; TAK-788 = tyrosine kinase inhibitor of HER2 and EGFR.

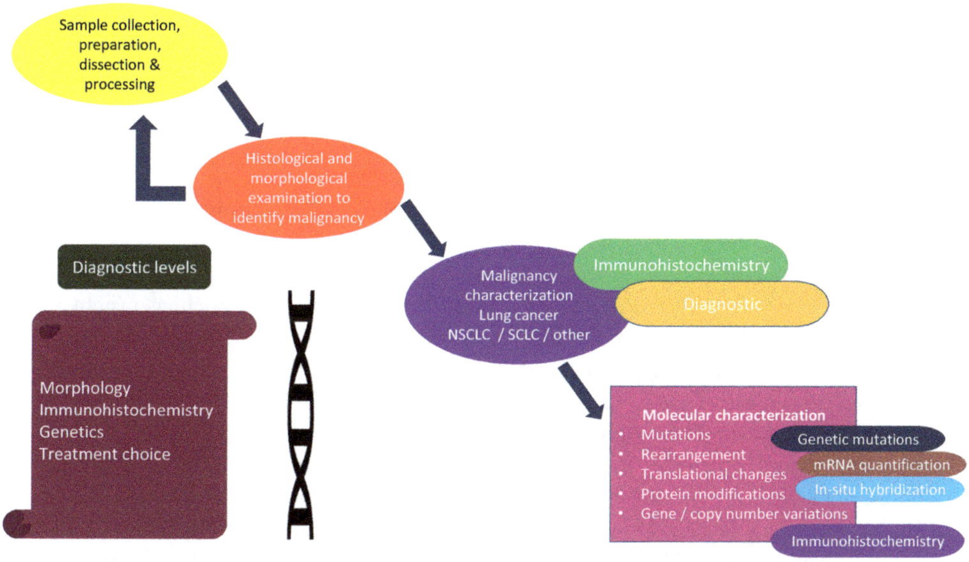

Figure 5.2. Overview of the pathological diagnostic algorithm in lung cancer.

5.11 Conclusion

The pathologists' role in guiding treatment strategies for lung cancer patients has been greatly changed in the last few years and is continuously evolving to understand and explore complex diagnostic and prognostic algorithms (figure 5.2). Pathologists' recommendations are gaining importance in lung cancer classification and will become more important in the future to interpret emerging molecular targets. Even with the advent of novel biomarkers, immunohistochemistry will remain part of lung cancer stratification. Morphology is the bedrock of lung cancer diagnosis. However, molecular biology and immunotherapy are continuously evolving fields to improve lung cancer diagnosis leading to better health outcomes.

Keeping in mind all the difficulties related to technical issues, new biomarkers for lung carcinoma are still being discovered. However, great knowledge is required to interpret the data obtained from screenings as the biological data are complex. One of the reasons may be that the diagnostic and prognostic biomarkers that are identified to be associated with lung cancer cannot be removed, as they may be playing important roles in some other pathway in the body that may disrupt their functioning. This means that the proper function of proteins needs to be studied before targeting them. Nonetheless the fact remains that most of these genes and proteins are potential potent therapeutic agents in cancer treatment strategies.

References

[1] Siegel R L, Miller K D and Jemal A 2016 Cancer statistics, 2016 *CA Cancer J. Clin.* **66** 7–30

[2] Miller K D, Siegel R L, Lin C C, Mariotto A B, Kramer J L, Rowland J H, Stein K D, Alteri R and Jemal A 2016 Cancer treatment and survivorship statistics, 2016 *CA Cancer J. Clin.* **66** 271–89

[3] Razi S S, John M M, Sainathan S and Stavropoulos C 2016 Sublobar resection is equivalent to lobectomy for T_{1a} non–small cell lung cancer in the elderly: a surveillance, epidemiology, and end results database analysis *J. Surg. Res.* **200** 683–9

[4] Shen J, Liu Y, Dai C, Chen B, Chen C, Rocco G, Brunelli A, Liu C-C, Petersen R H and He J 2016 A complicated clinical problem: surgical treatment decisions for patients with early-stage lung cancer *J. Thorac. Dis.* **8** E1787

[5] Tanaka F and Yoneda K 2016 Adjuvant therapy following surgery in non-small cell lung cancer (NSCLC) *Surg. Today* **46** 25–37

[6] Ettinger D S, Wood D E, Akerley W, Bazhenova L A, Borghaei H, Camidge D R, Cheney R T, Chirieac L R, D'Amico T A and Dilling T J 2016 NCCN guidelines insights: non-small cell lung cancer, version 4.2016 *J. Natl. Compr. Cancer Netw.* **14** 255–64

[7] Mascaux C, Tomasini P, Greillier L and Barlesi F 2017 Personalised medicine for nonsmall cell lung cancer *Eur. Respir. Rev.* **26** 170066

[8] Pfister D G, Johnson D H, Azzoli C G, Sause W, Smith T J, Baker S Jr, Olak J, Stover D, Strawn J R and Turrisi A T 2004 American Society of Clinical Oncology treatment of unresectable non-small-cell lung cancer guideline: update 2003 *J. Clin. Oncol.* **22** 330–53

[9] Herbst R S, Baas P, Kim D-W, Felip E, Pérez-Gracia J L, Han J-Y, Molina J, Kim J-H, Arvis C D and Ahn M-J 2016 Pembrolizumab versus docetaxel for previously treated, PD-L1-positive, advanced non-small-cell lung cancer (KEYNOTE-010): a randomised controlled trial *Lancet* **387** 1540–50

[10] Scagliotti G V, De Marinis F, Rinaldi M, Crino L, Gridelli C, Ricci S, Matano E, Boni C, Marangolo M and Failla G 2002 Phase III randomized trial comparing three platinum-based doublets in advanced non-small-cell lung cancer *J. Clin. Oncol.* **20** 4285–91

[11] Kelly K, Crowley J, Bunn P A Jr, Presant C A, Grevstad P K, Moinpour C M, Ramsey S D, Wozniak A J, Weiss G R and Moore D F 2001 Randomized phase III trial of paclitaxel plus carboplatin versus vinorelbine plus cisplatin in the treatment of patients with advanced non-small-cell lung cancer: a Southwest Oncology Group trial *J. Clin. Oncol.* **19** 3210–8

[12] Fossella F, Pereira J R, von Pawel J, Pluzanska A, Gorbounova V, Kaukel E, Mattson K V, Ramlau R, Szczesna A and Fidias P 2003 Randomized, multinational, phase III study of docetaxel plus platinum combinations versus vinorelbine plus cisplatin for advanced non-small-cell lung cancer: the TAX 326 study group *J. Clin. Oncol.* **21** 3016–24

[13] Schiller J H, Adak S, Feins R H, Keller S M, Fry W A, Livingston R B, Hammond M E M, Wolf B, Sabatini L and Jett J 2001 Lack of prognostic significance of p53 and K-ras mutations in primary resected non-small-cell lung cancer on E4592: a laboratory ancillary study on an Eastern Cooperative Oncology Group prospective randomized trial of post-operative adjuvant therapy *J. Clin. Oncol.* **19** 448–57

[14] Rizvi N A, Hellmann M D, Brahmer J R, Juergens R A, Borghaei H, Gettinger S, Chow L Q, Gerber D E, Laurie S A and Goldman J W 2016 Nivolumab in combination with platinum-based doublet chemotherapy for first-line treatment of advanced non-small-cell lung cancer *J. Clin. Oncol.* **34** 2969

[15] Scagliotti G V, Parikh P, Von Pawel J, Biesma B, Vansteenkiste J, Manegold C, Serwatowski P, Gatzemeier U, Digumarti R and Zukin M 2008 Phase III study comparing cisplatin plus gemcitabine with cisplatin plus pemetrexed in chemotherapy-naive patients with advanced-stage non-small-cell lung cancer *J. Clin. Oncol.* **26** 3543–51

[16] Treat J, Scagliotti G V, Peng G, Monberg M J, Obasaju C K and Socinski M A 2012 Comparison of pemetrexed plus cisplatin with other first-line doublets in advanced non-

small cell lung cancer (NSCLC): a combined analysis of three phase 3 trials *Lung Cancer* **76** 222–7

[17] Paz-Ares L, de Marinis F, Dediu M, Thomas M, Pujol J-L, Bidoli P, Molinier O, Sahoo T P, Laack E and Reck M 2012 Maintenance therapy with pemetrexed plus best supportive care versus placebo plus best supportive care after induction therapy with pemetrexed plus cisplatin for advanced non-squamous non-small-cell lung cancer (PARAMOUNT): a double-blind, phase 3, randomised controlled trial *Lancet Oncol.* **13** 247–55

[18] Scagliotti G, Hanna N, Fossella F, Sugarman K, Blatter J, Peterson P, Simms L and Shepherd F A 2009 The differential efficacy of pemetrexed according to NSCLC histology: a review of two phase III studies *Oncologist* **14** 253–63

[19] Johnson D H, Fehrenbacher L, Novotny W F, Herbst R S, Nemunaitis J J, Jablons D M, Langer C J, DeVore R F III, Gaudreault J and Damico L A 2004 Randomized phase II trial comparing bevacizumab plus carboplatin and paclitaxel with carboplatin and paclitaxel alone in previously untreated locally advanced or metastatic non-small-cell lung cancer *J. Clin. Oncol.* **22** 2184–91

[20] Sandler A, Gray R, Perry M C, Brahmer J, Schiller J H, Dowlati A, Lilenbaum R and Johnson D H 2006 Paclitaxel–carboplatin alone or with bevacizumab for non-small-cell lung cancer *New Engl. J. Med.* **355** 2542–50

[21] Paz-Ares L, Mezger J, Ciuleanu T E, Fischer J R, von Pawel J, Provencio M, Kazarnowicz A, Losonczy G, de Castro G Jr and Szczesna A 2015 Necitumumab plus pemetrexed and cisplatin as first-line therapy in patients with stage IV non-squamous non-small-cell lung cancer (INSPIRE): an open-label, randomised, controlled phase 3 study *Lancet Oncol.* **16** 328–37

[22] Thatcher N, Hirsch F R, Luft A V, Szczesna A, Ciuleanu T E, Dediu M, Ramlau R, Galiulin R K, Bálint B and Losonczy G 2015 Necitumumab plus gemcitabine and cisplatin versus gemcitabine and cisplatin alone as first-line therapy in patients with stage IV squamous non-small-cell lung cancer (SQUIRE): an open-label, randomised, controlled phase 3 trial *Lancet Oncol.* **16** 763–74

[23] Watanabe S, Yoshioka H, Sakai H, Hotta K, Takenoyama M, Yamada K, Sugawara S, Takiguchi Y, Hosomi Y and Tomii K 2019 Necitumumab plus gemcitabine and cisplatin versus gemcitabine and cisplatin alone as first-line treatment for stage IV squamous non-small cell lung cancer: a phase 1b and randomized, open-label, multicenter, phase 2 trial in Japan *Lung Cancer* **129** 55–62

[24] Lindeman N I, Cagle P T, Beasley M B, Chitale D A, Dacic S, Giaccone G, Jenkins R B, Kwiatkowski D J, Saldivar J-S and Squire J 2013 Molecular testing guideline for selection of lung cancer patients for EGFR and ALK tyrosine kinase inhibitors: guideline from the College of American Pathologists, International Association for the Study of Lung Cancer, and Association for Molecular Pathology *J. Mol. Diagn.* **15** 415–53

[25] Best D H and Swensen J J 2012 *Molecular Genetics and Personalized Medicine* (Berlin: Springer)

[26] Goodwin S, McPherson J D and McCombie W R 2016 Coming of age: ten years of next-generation sequencing technologies *Nat. Rev. Genet.* **17** 333

[27] Ambardar S, Gupta R, Trakroo D, Lal R and Vakhlu J 2016 High throughput sequencing: an overview of sequencing chemistry *Indian J. Microbiol.* **56** 394–404

[28] Bleidorn C 2017 Sequencing techniques *Phylogenomics* (Berlin: Springer), pp 43–60

[29] Kamps R, Brandão R, Bosch B, Paulussen A, Xanthoulea S, Blok M and Romano A 2017 Next-generation sequencing in oncology: genetic diagnosis, risk prediction and cancer classification *Int. J. Mol. Sci.* **18** 308

[30] Salto-Tellez M and Gonzalez de Castro D 2014 Next-generation sequencing: a change of paradigm in molecular diagnostic validation *J. Pathol.* **234** 5–10

[31] Pearce M, Nakorchevsky A, Nygren A and Irwin D 2014 Targeted mutation profiling of non-small cell lung cancer samples using the sequenom Lungcarta™ Panel* for clinical research *Sequenom* https://www.genehk.com/news/doc/LungCarta%20Application%20Note.pdf

[32] Rosell R, Carcereny E, Gervais R, Vergnenegre A, Massuti B, Felip E, Palmero R, Garcia-Gomez R, Pallares C and Sanchez J M 2012 Erlotinib versus standard chemotherapy as first-line treatment for European patients with advanced EGFR mutation-positive non-small-cell lung cancer (EURTAC): a multicentre, open-label, randomised phase 3 trial *Lancet Oncol.* **13** 239–46

[33] Shaw A T, Friboulet L, Leshchiner I, Gainor J F, Bergqvist S, Brooun A, Burke B J, Deng Y-L, Liu W and Dardaei L 2016 Resensitization to crizotinib by the lorlatinib ALK resistance mutation L1198F *New Engl. J. Med.* **374** 54–61

[34] Shaw A T and Engelman J A 2013 ALK in lung cancer: past, present, and future *J. Clin. Oncol.* **31** 1105

[35] Hutarew G, Hauser-Kronberger C, Strasser F, Llenos I C and Dietze O 2014 Immunohistochemistry as a screening tool for ALK rearrangement in NSCLC: evaluation of five different ALK antibody clones and ALK FISH *Histopathology* **65** 398–407

[36] Calvayrac O, Pradines A, Pons E, Mazieres J and Guibert N 2017 Molecular biomarkers for lung adenocarcinoma *Eur. Respir. J.* **49** 1601734

[37] Malik S S, Masood N, Asif M, Ahmed P, Shah Z U and Khan J S 2019 Expressional analysis of MLH1 and MSH2 in breast cancer *Curr. Probl. Cancer* **43** 97–105

[38] Lee S E, Lee B, Hong M, Song J-Y, Jung K, Lira M E, Mao M, Han J, Kim J and Choi Y-L 2015 Comprehensive analysis of RET and ROS1 rearrangement in lung adenocarcinoma *Mod. Pathol.* **28** 468

[39] Torre L A, Siegel R L, Ward E M and Jemal A 2016 Global cancer incidence and mortality rates and trends—an update *Cancer Epidemiol. Prev. Biomarkers* **25** 16–27

[40] Cheng L, Alexander R E, MacLennan G T, Cummings O W, Montironi R, Lopez-Beltran A, Cramer H M, Davidson D D and Zhang S 2012 Molecular pathology of lung cancer: key to personalized medicine *Mod. Pathol.* **25** 347

[41] Henson E S and Gibson S B 2006 Surviving cell death through epidermal growth factor (EGF) signal transduction pathways: implications for cancer therapy *Cell. Signal.* **18** 2089–97

[42] Lynch T J, Bell D W, Sordella R, Gurubhagavatula S, Okimoto R A, Brannigan B W, Harris P L, Haserlat S M, Supko J G and Haluska F G 2004 Activating mutations in the epidermal growth factor receptor underlying responsiveness of non-small-cell lung cancer to gefitinib *New Engl. J. Med.* **350** 2129–39

[43] Indovina P, Marcelli E, Maranta P and Tarro G 2011 Lung cancer proteomics: recent advances in biomarker discovery *Int. J. Proteomics* **2011** 726869

[44] Arrieta O, Cardona A F, Corrales L, Campos-Parra A D, Sánchez-Reyes R, Amieva-Rivera E, Rodríguez J, Vargas C, Carranza H and Otero J 2015 The impact of common and rare EGFR mutations in response to EGFR tyrosine kinase inhibitors and platinum-based chemotherapy in patients with non-small cell lung cancer *Lung Cancer* **87** 169–75

[45] Beau-Faller M, Prim N, Ruppert A-M, Nanni-Metellus I, Lacave R, Lacroix L, Escande F, Lizard S, Pretet J-L and Rouquette I 2013 Rare EGFR exon 18 and exon 20 mutations in non-small-cell lung cancer on 10 117 patients: a multicentre observational study by the French ERMETIC-IFCT network *Ann. Oncol.* **25** 126–31

[46] D'Arcangelo M and Hirsch F R 2014 Clinical and comparative utility of afatinib in non-small cell lung cancer *Biologics* **8** 183

[47] D'arcangelo M, D'incecco A and Cappuzzo F 2013 Rare mutations in non-small-cell lung cancer *Future Oncol.* **9** 699–711

[48] Gainor J F, Varghese A M, Ou S-H I, Kabraji S, Awad M M, Katayama R, Pawlak A, Mino-Kenudson M, Yeap B Y and Riely G J 2013 ALK rearrangements are mutually exclusive with mutations in EGFR or KRAS: an analysis of 1,683 patients with non–small cell lung cancer *Clin. Cancer Res.* **19** 4273–81

[49] Shi Y, Li J, Zhang S, Wang M, Yang S, Li N, Wu G, Liu W, Liao G and Cai K 2015 Molecular epidemiology of EGFR mutations in Asian patients with advanced non-small-cell lung cancer of adenocarcinoma histology—Mainland China subset analysis of the PIONEER study *PLoS One* **10** e0143515

[50] Rahman S, Kondo N, Yoneda K, Takuwa T, Hashimoto M, Orui H, Okumura Y, Tanaka F, Kumamoto K and Mostafa M G 2014 Frequency of epidermal growth factor receptor mutations in Bangladeshi patients with adenocarcinoma of the lung *Int. J. Clin. Oncol.* **19** 45–9

[51] Arrieta O, Cardona A F, Bramuglia G F, Gallo A, Campos-Parra A D, Serrano S, Castro M, Avilés A, Amorin E and Kirchuk R 2011 Genotyping non-small cell lung cancer (NSCLC) in Latin America *J. Thorac. Oncol.* **6** 1955–9

[52] Midha A, Dearden S and McCormack R 2015 EGFR mutation incidence in non-small-cell lung cancer of adenocarcinoma histology: a systematic review and global map by ethnicity (mutMapII) *Am. J. Cancer Res.* **5** 2892

[53] Jackman D M, Yeap B Y, Sequist L V, Lindeman N, Holmes A J, Joshi V A, Bell D W, Huberman M S, Halmos B and Rabin M S 2006 Exon 19 deletion mutations of epidermal growth factor receptor are associated with prolonged survival in non-small cell lung cancer patients treated with gefitinib or erlotinib *Clin. Cancer Res.* **12** 3908–14

[54] Karachaliou N, Molina-Vila M A and Rosell R 2015 *The Impact of Rare EGFR Mutations on the Treatment Response of Patients with Non-small Cell Lung Cancer* (London: Taylor and Francis)

[55] Choi Y L, Takeuchi K, Soda M, Inamura K, Togashi Y, Hatano S, Enomoto M, Hamada T, Haruta H and Watanabe H 2008 Identification of novel isoforms of the EML4-ALK transforming gene in non-small cell lung cancer *Cancer Res.* **68** 4971–6

[56] Takeuchi K, Choi Y L, Togashi Y, Soda M, Hatano S, Inamura K, Takada S, Ueno T, Yamashita Y and Satoh Y 2009 KIF5B-ALK, a novel fusion oncokinase identified by an immunohistochemistry-based diagnostic system for ALK-positive lung cancer *Clin. Cancer Res.* **15** 3143–9

[57] Gridelli C, Peters S, Sgambato A, Casaluce F, Adjei A A and Ciardiello F 2014 ALK inhibitors in the treatment of advanced NSCLC *Cancer Treat. Rev.* **40** 300–6

[58] Bergethon K, Shaw A T, Ou S-H I, Katayama R, Lovly C M, McDonald N T, Massion P P, Siwak-Tapp C, Gonzalez A and Fang R 2012 ROS1 rearrangements define a unique molecular class of lung cancers *J. Clin. Oncol.* **30** 863

[59] Kwak E L, Bang Y-J, Camidge D R, Shaw A T, Solomon B, Maki R G, Ou S-H I, Dezube B J, Jänne P A and Costa D B 2010 Anaplastic lymphoma kinase inhibition in non-small-cell lung cancer *New Engl. J. Med.* **363** 1693–703

[60] Ou S-H I, Kwak E L, Siwak-Tapp C, Dy J, Bergethon K, Clark J W, Camidge D R, Solomon B J, Maki R G and Bang Y-J 2011 Activity of crizotinib (PF02341066), a dual mesenchymal-epithelial transition (MET) and anaplastic lymphoma kinase (ALK) inhibitor, in a non-small cell lung cancer patient with de novo MET amplification *J. Thorac. Oncol.* **6** 942–6

[61] Solomon B J, Mok T, Kim D-W, Wu Y-L, Nakagawa K, Mekhail T, Felip E, Cappuzzo F, Paolini J and Usari T 2014 First-line crizotinib versus chemotherapy in ALK-positive lung cancer *New Engl. J. Med.* **371** 2167–77

[62] Camidge D R, Bang Y-J, Kwak E L, Iafrate A J, Varella-Garcia M, Fox S B, Riely G J, Solomon B, Ou S-H I and Kim D-W 2012 Activity and safety of crizotinib in patients with ALK-positive non-small-cell lung cancer: updated results from a phase 1 study *Lancet Oncol.* **13** 1011–9

[63] Riely G J, Kris M G, Rosenbaum D, Marks J, Li A, Chitale D A, Nafa K, Riedel E R, Hsu M and Pao W 2008 Frequency and distinctive spectrum of KRAS mutations in never smokers with lung adenocarcinoma *Clin. Cancer Res.* **14** 5731–4

[64] Fiala O, Pesek M, Finek J, Benesova L, Belsanova B and Minarik M 2013 The dominant role of G12C over other KRAS mutation types in the negative prediction of efficacy of epidermal growth factor receptor tyrosine kinase inhibitors in non-small cell lung cancer *Cancer Genet.* **206** 26–31

[65] Dearden S, Stevens J, Wu Y-L and Blowers D 2013 Mutation incidence and coincidence in non-small-cell lung cancer: meta-analyses by ethnicity and histology (mutMap) *Ann. Oncol.* **24** 2371–6

[66] Porta M, Crous-Bou M, Wark P A, Vineis P, Real F X, Malats N and Kampman E 2009 Cigarette smoking and K-ras mutations in pancreas, lung and colorectal adenocarcinomas: etiopathogenic similarities, differences and paradoxes *Mutat. Res./Rev. Mutat. Res.* **682** 83–93

[67] Ihle N T, Byers L A, Kim E S, Saintigny P, Lee J J, Blumenschein G R, Tsao A, Liu S, Larsen J E and Wang J 2012 Effect of KRAS oncogene substitutions on protein behavior: implications for signaling and clinical outcome *J. Natl. Cancer Inst.* **104** 228–39

[68] Cserepes M, Ostoros G, Lohinai Z, Raso E, Barbai T, Timar J, Rozsas A, Moldvay J, Kovalszky I and Fabian K 2014 Subtype-specific KRAS mutations in advanced lung adenocarcinoma: a retrospective study of patients treated with platinum-based chemotherapy *Eur. J. Cancer* **50** 1819–28

[69] Shepherd F A, Lacas B, Le Teuff G, Hainaut P, Jänne P A, Pignon J-P, Le Chevalier T, Seymour L, Douillard J-Y and Graziano S 2017 Pooled analysis of the prognostic and predictive effects of TP53 comutation status combined with KRAS or EGFR mutation in early-stage resected non-small-cell lung cancer in four trials of adjuvant chemotherapy *J. Clin. Oncol.* **35** 2018

[70] Broermann P, Junker K, Brandt B H, Heinecke A, Freitag L, Klinke F, Berdel W E and Thomas M 2002 Trimodality treatment in stage III nonsmall cell lung carcinoma: prognostic impact of K-ras mutations after neoadjuvant therapy *Cancer* **94** 2055–62

[71] Rodenhuis S, Boerrigter L, Top B, Slebos R, Mooi W J, van't Veer L and van Zandwijk N 1997 Mutational activation of the K-ras oncogene and the effect of chemotherapy in advanced adenocarcinoma of the lung: a prospective study *J. Clin. Oncol.* **15** 285–91

[72] Khambata-Ford S, Harbison C T, Hart L L, Awad M, Xu L-A, Horak C E, Dakhil S, Hermann R C, Lynch T J and Weber M R 2010 Analysis of potential predictive markers of cetuximab benefit in BMS099, a phase III study of cetuximab and first-line taxane/carboplatin in advanced non-small-cell lung cancer *J. Clin. Oncol.* **28** 918–27
[73] Garnett M J and Marais R 2004 Guilty as charged: B-RAF is a human oncogene *Cancer Cell* **6** 313–9
[74] Paik P K, Arcila M E, Fara M, Sima C S, Miller V A, Kris M G, Ladanyi M and Riely G J 2011 Clinical characteristics of patients with lung adenocarcinomas harboring BRAF mutations *J. Clin. Oncol.* **29** 2046
[75] Cardarella S, Ogino A, Nishino M, Butaney M, Shen J, Lydon C, Yeap B Y, Sholl L M, Johnson B E and Jänne P A 2013 Clinical, pathologic, and biologic features associated with BRAF mutations in non-small cell lung cancer *Clin. Cancer Res.* **19** 4532–40
[76] Hyman D M, Puzanov I, Subbiah V, Faris J E, Chau I, Blay J-Y, Wolf J, Raje N S, Diamond E L and Hollebecque A 2015 Vemurafenib in multiple nonmelanoma cancers with BRAF V600 mutations *New Engl. J. Med.* **373** 726–36
[77] Gautschi O, Milia J, Cabarrou B, Bluthgen M-V, Besse B, Smit E F, Wolf J, Peters S, Früh M and Koeberle D 2015 Targeted therapy for patients with BRAF-mutant lung cancer results from the European EURAF cohort *J. Thorac. Oncol.* **10** 1451–7
[78] Litvak A M, Paik P K, Woo K M, Sima C S, Hellmann M D, Arcila M E, Ladanyi M, Rudin C M, Kris M G and Riely G J 2014 Clinical characteristics and course of 63 patients with BRAF mutant lung cancers *J. Thorac. Oncol.* **9** 1669–74
[79] Wykes M N and Lewin S R 2018 Immune checkpoint blockade in infectious diseases *Nat. Rev. Immunol.* **18** 91
[80] Platten M, Wick W and Van den Eynde B J 2012 Tryptophan catabolism in cancer: beyond IDO and tryptophan depletion *Cancer Res.* **72** 5435–40
[81] Jiang W, Cai G, Hu P C and Wang Y 2018 Personalized medicine in non-small cell lung cancer: a review from a pharmacogenomics perspective *Acta Pharm. Sin.* B **8** 530–8
[82] Leventakos K and Mansfield A S 2016 Advances in the treatment of non-small cell lung cancer: focus on nivolumab, pembrolizumab, and atezolizumab *BioDrugs* **30** 397–405
[83] Rittmeyer A, Barlesi F, Waterkamp D, Park K, Ciardiello F, Von Pawel J, Gadgeel S M, Hida T, Kowalski D M and Dols M C 2017 Atezolizumab versus docetaxel in patients with previously treated non-small-cell lung cancer (OAK): a phase 3, open-label, multicentre randomised controlled trial *Lancet* **389** 255–65
[84] Rizvi N A, Mazières J, Planchard D, Stinchcombe T E, Dy G K, Antonia S J, Horn L, Lena H, Minenza E and Mennecier B 2015 Activity and safety of nivolumab, an anti-PD-1 immune checkpoint inhibitor, for patients with advanced, refractory squamous non-small-cell lung cancer (CheckMate 063): a phase 2, single-arm trial *Lancet Oncol.* **16** 257–65
[85] Reck M, Rodríguez-Abreu D, Robinson A G, Hui R, Csőszi T, Fülöp A, Gottfried M, Peled N, Tafreshi A and Cuffe S 2016 Pembrolizumab versus chemotherapy for PD-L1-positive non-small-cell lung cancer *New Engl. J. Med.* **375** 1823–33
[86] Zaretsky J M, Garcia-Diaz A, Shin D S, Escuin-Ordinas H, Hugo W, Hu-Lieskovan S, Torrejon D Y, Abril-Rodriguez G, Sandoval S and Barthly L 2016 Mutations associated with acquired resistance to PD-1 blockade in melanoma *New Engl. J. Med.* **375** 819–29
[87] Deyati A, Younesi E, Hofmann-Apitius M and Novac N 2013 Challenges and opportunities for oncology biomarker discovery *Drug Discov. Today* **18** 614–24

[88] Hu X, Bao J, Wang Z, Zhang Z, Gu P, Tao F, Cui D and Jiang W 2016 The plasma lncRNA acting as fingerprint in non-small-cell lung cancer *Tumor Biol.* **37** 3497–504
[89] Kang S-M, Sung H-J, Ahn J-M, Park J-Y, Lee S-Y, Park C-S and Cho J-Y 2011 The haptoglobin β chain as a supportive biomarker for human lung cancers *Mol. Biosyst.* **7** 1167–75
[90] Zhang G, Sun X, Lv H, Yang X and Kang X 2012 Serum amyloid A: a new potential serum marker correlated with the stage of breast cancer *Oncol. Lett.* **3** 940–4
[91] Cho W C S, Yip T, Cheng W and Au J S 2010 Serum amyloid A is elevated in the serum of lung cancer patients with poor prognosis *Br. J. Cancer* **102** 1731
[92] Varani J, Hattori Y, Chi Y, Schmidt T, Perone P, Zeigler M, Fader D and Johnson T 2000 Collagenolytic and gelatinolytic matrix metalloproteinases and their inhibitors in basal cell carcinoma of skin: comparison with normal skin *Br. J. Cancer* **82** 657
[93] Tian T, Hao J, Xu A, Hao J, Luo C, Liu C, Huang L, Xiao X and He D 2007 Determination of metastasis-associated proteins in non-small cell lung cancer by comparative proteomic analysis *Cancer Sci.* **98** 1265–74
[94] Luo C-H, Zhang P-F, Li M-Y, Chen Z-C and Liu Y-F 2013 Prognostic significance of annexin II expression in non-small cell lung cancer *Clin. Transl. Oncol.* **15** 938–46
[95] Gharib T G, Chen G, Wang H, Huang C-C, Prescott M S, Shedden K, Misek D E, Thomas D G, Giordano T J and Taylor J M 2002 Proteomic analysis of cytokeratin isoforms uncovers association with survival in lung adenocarcinoma *Neoplasia* **4** 440–8
[96] Xu A, Hao J, Zhang Z, Tian T, Jiang S, Hao J, Liu C, Huang L, Xiao X and He D 2010 14-kDa phosphohistidine phosphatase and its role in human lung cancer cell migration and invasion *Lung Cancer* **67** 48–56
[97] Maeda J, Hirano T, Ogiwara A, Akimoto S, Kawakami T, Fukui Y, Oka T, Gong Y, Guo R and Inada H 2008 Proteomic analysis of stage I primary lung adenocarcinoma aimed at individualisation of postoperative therapy *Br. J. Cancer* **98** 596
[98] Xu B J, Gonzalez A L, Kikuchi T, Yanagisawa K, Massion P P, Wu H, Mason S E, Olson S J, Shyr Y and Carbone D P 2008 MALDI-MS derived prognostic protein markers for resected non-small cell lung cancer *Proteomics–Clin. Appl.* **2** 1508–17
[99] Jelonek K and Widłak P 2018 Metabolome-based biomarkers: their potential role in the early detection of lung cancer *Contemp. Oncol.* **22** 135
[100] Armitage E G and Southam A D 2016 Monitoring cancer prognosis, diagnosis and treatment efficacy using metabolomics and lipidomics *Metabolomics* **12** 146
[101] Bamji-Stocke S, van Berkel V, Miller D M and Frieboes H B 2018 A review of metabolism-associated biomarkers in lung cancer diagnosis and treatment *Metabolomics* **14** 81
[102] Fan T W, Lane A N, Higashi R M, Farag M A, Gao H, Bousamra M and Miller D M 2009 Altered regulation of metabolic pathways in human lung cancer discerned by 13 C stable isotope-resolved metabolomics (SIRM) *Mol. Cancer* **8** 41
[103] Van Den Heuvel A P J, Jing J, Wooster R F and Bachman K E 2012 Analysis of glutamine dependency in non-small cell lung cancer: GLS1 splice variant GAC is essential for cancer cell growth *Cancer Biol. Ther.* **13** 1185–94
[104] Yu L, Li K and Zhang X 2017 Next-generation metabolomics in lung cancer diagnosis, treatment and precision medicine: mini review *Oncotarget* **8** 115774
[105] Bruntz R C, Lane A N, Higashi R M and Fan T W-M 2017 Exploring cancer metabolism using stable isotope-resolved metabolomics (SIRM) *J. Biol. Chem.* **292** 11601–9

[106] Fan T W, Lane A N and Higashi R M 2016 Stable isotope resolved metabolomics studies in *ex vivo* tissue slices *Bio Protoc.* **6** e1730

[107] Chen Y, Ma Z, Shen X, Li L, Zhong J, Min L S, Xu L, Li H, Zhang J and Dai L 2018 Serum lipidomics profiling to identify biomarkers for non-small cell lung cancer *BioMed. Res. Int.* **2018** 5276240

[108] Rauschert S, Uhl O, Koletzko B, Kirchberg F, Mori T A, Huang R-C, Beilin L J, Hellmuth C and Oddy W H 2016 Lipidomics reveals associations of phospholipids with obesity and insulin resistance in young adults *J. Clin. Endocrinol. Metab.* **101** 871–9

[109] Xiang Y, Lam S M and Shui G 2015 What can lipidomics tell us about the pathogenesis of Alzheimer disease? *Biol. Chem.* **396** 1281–91

[110] Perrotti F, Rosa C, Cicalini I, Sacchetta P, Del Boccio P, Genovesi D and Pieragostino D 2016 Advances in lipidomics for cancer biomarkers discovery *Int. J. Mol. Sci.* **17** 1992

[111] Zhao Y-Y, Cheng X-L and Lin R-C 2014 Lipidomics applications for discovering biomarkers of diseases in clinical chemistry *International Review of Cell and Molecular Biology* vol 313 (Amsterdam: Elsevier), pp 1–26

[112] Kasuga K, Suga T and Mano N 2015 Bioanalytical insights into mediator lipidomics *J. Pharm. Biomed. Anal.* **113** 151–62

[113] Zhao Y-Y, Miao H, Cheng X-L and Wei F 2015 Lipidomics: novel insight into the biochemical mechanism of lipid metabolism and dysregulation-associated disease *Chem. Biol. Interact.* **240** 220–38

[114] Wolf A, Agnihotri S, Micallef J, Mukherjee J, Sabha N, Cairns R, Hawkins C and Guha A 2011 Hexokinase 2 is a key mediator of aerobic glycolysis and promotes tumor growth in human glioblastoma multiforme *J. Exp. Med.* **208** 313–26

[115] Lee A S 2014 Glucose-regulated proteins in cancer: molecular mechanisms and therapeutic potential *Nat. Rev. Cancer* **14** 263

[116] Klupczynska A, Dereziński P, Garrett T J, Rubio V Y, Dyszkiewicz W, Kasprzyk M and Kokot Z J 2017 Study of early stage non-small-cell lung cancer using Orbitrap-based global serum metabolomics *J. Cancer Res. Clin. Oncol.* **143** 649–59

[117] Awwad H M, Geisel J and Obeid R 2012 The role of choline in prostate cancer *Clin. Biochem.* **45** 1548–53

[118] Louis E, Cantrelle F X, Mesotten L, Reekmans G, Bervoets L, Vanhove K, Thomeer M, Lippens G and Adriaensens P 2017 Metabolic phenotyping of human plasma by 1H-NMR at high and medium magnetic field strengths: a case study for lung cancer *Magn. Reson. Chem.* **55** 706–13

[119] Gillies R J and Gatenby R A 2015 Metabolism and its sequelae in cancer evolution and therapy *Cancer J.* **21** 88

[120] He Y, Wen Q, Yao F, Xu D, Huang Y and Wang J 2017 Gut–lung axis: the microbial contributions and clinical implications *Crit. Rev. Microbiol.* **43** 81–95

[121] Deja S, Porebska I, Kowal A, Zabek A, Barg W, Pawelczyk K, Stanimirova I, Daszykowski M, Korzeniewska A and Jankowska R 2014 Metabolomics provide new insights on lung cancer staging and discrimination from chronic obstructive pulmonary disease *J. Pharm. Biomed. Anal.* **100** 369–80

[122] Li Y, Song X, Zhao X, Zou L and Xu G 2014 Serum metabolic profiling study of lung cancer using ultra high performance liquid chromatography/quadrupole time-of-flight mass spectrometry *J. Chromatogr.* B **966** 147–53

[123] Wu Q, Wang Y, Gu X, Zhou J, Zhang H, Lv W, Chen Z and Yan C 2014 Urinary metabolomic study of non-small cell lung carcinoma based on ultra high performance liquid chromatography coupled with quadrupole time-of-flight mass spectrometry *J. Sep. Sci.* **37** 1728–35

[124] Mathé E A, Patterson A D, Haznadar M, Manna S K, Krausz K W, Bowman E D, Shields P G, Idle J R, Smith P B and Anami K 2014 Noninvasive urinary metabolomic profiling identifies diagnostic and prognostic markers in lung cancer *Cancer Res.* **74** 3259–70

[125] Reddy A V, Killampalli L K, Prakash A R, Naag S, Sreenath G and Biraggari S K 2016 Analysis of lipid profile in cancer patients, smokers, and nonsmokers *Dent. Res. J.* **13** 494

[126] Zhang F and Du G 2012 Dysregulated lipid metabolism in cancer *World J. Biol. Chem.* **3** 167

[127] Puchades-Carrasco L, Jantus-Lewintre E, Pérez-Rambla C, García-García F, Lucas R, Calabuig S, Blasco A, Dopazo J, Camps C and Pineda-Lucena A 2016 Serum metabolomic profiling facilitates the non-invasive identification of metabolic biomarkers associated with the onset and progression of non-small cell lung cancer *Oncotarget* **7** 12904

[128] Chen Y, Ma Z, Li A, Li H, Wang B, Zhong J, Min L and Dai L 2015 Metabolomic profiling of human serum in lung cancer patients using liquid chromatography/hybrid quadrupole time-of-flight mass spectrometry and gas chromatography/mass spectrometry *J. Cancer Res. Clin. Oncol.* **141** 705–18

[129] Zhang X, Zhu X, Wang C, Zhang H and Cai Z 2016 Non-targeted and targeted metabolomics approaches to diagnosing lung cancer and predicting patient prognosis *Oncotarget* **7** 63437

[130] Zhang W C, Shyh-Chang N, Yang H, Rai A, Umashankar S, Ma S, Soh B S, Sun L L, Tai B C and Nga M E 2012 Glycine decarboxylase activity drives non-small cell lung cancer tumor-initiating cells and tumorigenesis *Cell* **148** 259–72

[131] Hori S, Nishiumi S, Kobayashi K, Shinohara M, Hatakeyama Y, Kotani Y, Hatano N, Maniwa Y, Nishio W and Bamba T 2011 A metabolomic approach to lung cancer *Lung Cancer* **74** 284–92

[132] Sayin V I, Ibrahim M X, Larsson E, Nilsson J A, Lindahl P and Bergo M O 2014 Antioxidants accelerate lung cancer progression in mice *Sci. Transl. Med.* **6** 221ra215

[133] Long F, Su J-H, Liang B, Su L-L and Jiang S-J 2015 Identification of gene biomarkers for distinguishing small-cell lung cancer from non-small-cell lung cancer using a network-based approach *BioMed. Res. Int.* **2015**

[134] Kalos M and June C H 2013 Adoptive T cell transfer for cancer immunotherapy in the era of synthetic biology *Immunity* **39** 49–60

[135] Hamid O, Robert C, Daud A, Hodi F S, Hwu W-J, Kefford R, Wolchok J D, Hersey P, Joseph R W and Weber J S 2013 Safety and tumor responses with lambrolizumab (anti-PD-1) in melanoma *New Engl. J. Med.* **369** 134–44

[136] Beatty G L and Gladney W L 2015 Immune escape mechanisms as a guide for cancer immunotherapy *Clini. Cancer Res.* **21** 687–92

[137] Fridman W H, Zitvogel L, Sautès-Fridman C and Kroemer G 2017 The immune contexture in cancer prognosis and treatment *Nat. Rev. Clin. Oncol.* **14** 717

[138] Gotwals P, Cameron S, Cipolletta D, Cremasco V, Crystal A, Hewes B, Mueller B, Quaratino S, Sabatos-Peyton C and Petruzzelli L 2017 Prospects for combining targeted and conventional cancer therapy with immunotherapy *Nat. Rev. Cancer* **17** 286

[139] Bronte V, Brandau S, Chen S-H, Colombo M P, Frey A B, Greten T F, Mandruzzato S, Murray P J, Ochoa A and Ostrand-Rosenberg S 2016 Recommendations for myeloid-derived suppressor cell nomenclature and characterization standards *Nat. Commun.* **7** 12150

[140] Allard B, Aspeslagh S, Garaud S, Dupont F, Solinas C, Kok M, Routy B, Sotiriou C, Stagg J and Buisseret L 2018 Immuno-oncology-101: overview of major concepts and translational perspectives *Seminars in Cancer Biology* (Amsterdam: Elsevier), pp 1–11

[141] Pu X, Wu L, Su D, Mao W and Fang B 2018 Immunotherapy for non-small cell lung cancers: biomarkers for predicting responses and strategies to overcome resistance *BMC Cancer* **18** 1082

[142] Cho J H 2017 Immunotherapy for non-small-cell lung cancer: current status and future obstacles *Immune Netw.* **17** 378–91

[143] Rolfo C, Caglevic C, Santarpia M, Araujo A, Giovannetti E, Gallardo C D, Pauwels P and Mahave M 2017 Immunotherapy in NSCLC: a promising and revolutionary weapon *Immunotherapy* (Berlin: Springer), pp 97–125

[144] Franklin C, Livingstone E, Roesch A, Schilling B and Schadendorf D 2017 Immunotherapy in melanoma: recent advances and future directions *Eur. J. Surg. Oncol.* **43** 604–11

[145] Califano R, Kerr K, Morgan R D, Russo G L, Garassino M, Morgillo F and Rossi A 2016 Immune checkpoint blockade: a new era for non-small cell lung cancer *Curr. Oncol. Rep.* **18** 59

[146] Pujol J and Roch B 2018 Small cell lung cancer and immuno-oncologic agents: end of the cisplatin-etoposide era? *Rev. Mal. Respir.* **35** 846–51

[147] Gazdar A F, Bunn P A and Minna J D 2017 Small-cell lung cancer: what we know, what we need to know and the path forward *Nat. Rev. Cancer* **17** 725

[148] Brahmer J, Reckamp K L, Baas P, Crinò L, Eberhardt W E, Poddubskaya E, Antonia S, Pluzanski A, Vokes E E and Holgado E 2015 Nivolumab versus docetaxel in advanced squamous-cell non-small-cell lung cancer *New Engl. J. Med.* **373** 123–35

[149] Borghaei H, Paz-Ares L, Horn L, Spigel D R, Steins M, Ready N E, Chow L Q, Vokes E E, Felip E and Holgado E 2015 Nivolumab versus docetaxel in advanced nonsquamous non-small-cell lung cancer *New Engl. J. Med.* **373** 1627–39

[150] Horn L, Spigel D R, Vokes E E, Holgado E, Ready N, Steins M, Poddubskaya E, Borghaei H, Felip E and Paz-Ares L 2017 Nivolumab versus docetaxel in previously treated patients with advanced non-small-cell lung cancer: two-year outcomes from two randomized, open-label, phase III trials (CheckMate 017 and CheckMate 057) *J. Clin. Oncol.* **35** 3924

[151] Fehrenbacher L, Spira A, Ballinger M, Kowanetz M, Vansteenkiste J, Mazieres J, Park K, Smith D, Artal-Cortes A and Lewanski C 2016 Atezolizumab versus docetaxel for patients with previously treated non-small-cell lung cancer (POPLAR): a multicentre, open-label, phase 2 randomised controlled trial *Lancet* **387** 1837–46

[152] Lopes G, Wu Y-L, Kudaba I, Kowalski D, Cho B C, Castro G, Srimuninnimit V, Bondarenko I, Kubota K and Lubiniecki G M 2018 Pembrolizumab (pembro) versus platinum-based chemotherapy (chemo) as first-line therapy for advanced/metastatic NSCLC with a PD-L1 tumor proportion score (TPS) ⩾1%: open-label, phase 3 KEYNOTE-042 study *J. Clin. Oncol.* **36**(Suppl.) LBA4

[153] Gandhi L, Rodríguez-Abreu D, Gadgeel S, Esteban E, Felip E, De Angelis F, Domine M, Clingan P, Hochmair M J and Powell S F 2018 Pembrolizumab plus chemotherapy in metastatic non-small-cell lung cancer *New Engl. J. Med.* **378** 2078–92

[154] Carbone D P, Reck M, Paz-Ares L, Creelan B, Horn L, Steins M, Felip E, van den Heuvel M M, Ciuleanu T-E and Badin F 2017 First-line nivolumab in stage IV or recurrent non-small-cell lung cancer *New Engl. J. Med.* **376** 2415–26

[155] Giroux Leprieur E, Herbretau G, Dumenil C, Julie C, Giraud V, Labrune S, Dumoulin J, Tisserand J, Emile J-F and Blons H 2018 Circulating tumor DNA evaluated by next-generation sequencing is predictive of tumor response and prolonged clinical benefit with nivolumab in advanced non-small cell lung cancer *Oncoimmunology* **7** e1424675

[156] Goldberg S B, Narayan A, Kole A J, Decker R H, Teysir J, Carriero N J, Lee A, Nemati R, Nath S K and Mane S M 2018 Early assessment of lung cancer immunotherapy response via circulating tumor DNA *Clin. Cancer Res.* **24** 1872–80

[157] George J, Lim J S, Jang S J, Cun Y, Ozretić L, Kong G, Leenders F, Lu X, Fernández-Cuesta L and Bosco G 2015 Comprehensive genomic profiles of small cell lung cancer *Nature* **524** 47

[158] Pleasance E D, Stephens P J, O'Meara S, McBride D J, Meynert A, Jones D, Lin M-L, Beare D, Lau K W and Greenman C 2010 A small cell lung cancer genome reports complex tobacco exposure signatures *Nature* **463** 184

[159] Lawrence M S, Stojanov P, Polak P, Kryukov G V, Cibulskis K, Sivachenko A, Carter S L, Stewart C, Mermel C H and Roberts S A 2013 Mutational heterogeneity in cancer and the search for new cancer-associated genes *Nature* **499** 214

[160] Koeppel F, Blanchard S, Jovelet C, Genin B, Marcaillou C, Martin E, Rouleau E, Solary E, Soria J-C and André F 2017 Whole exome sequencing for determination of tumor mutation load in liquid biopsy from advanced cancer patients *PLoS One* **12** e0188174

[161] Pirker R 2018 Is smoking history the truly best biomarker for immune checkpoint inhibitor treatment in advanced non-small cell lung cancer? *BMJ* **3** e000421

[162] Hellmann M D, Ciuleanu T-E, Pluzanski A, Lee J S, Otterson G A, Audigier-Valette C, Minenza E, Linardou H, Burgers S and Salman P 2018 Nivolumab plus ipilimumab in lung cancer with a high tumor mutational burden *New Engl. J. Med.* **378** 2093–104

[163] Brahmer J R, Lacchetti C, Schneider B J, Atkins M B, Brassil K J, Caterino J M, Chau I, Ernstoff M S, Gardner J M and Ginex P 2018 Management of immune-related adverse events in patients treated with immune checkpoint inhibitor therapy: American Society of Clinical Oncology Clinical Practice Guideline *J. Clin. Oncol.* **36** 1714

[164] Fuentes-Antrás J, Provencio M and Díaz-Rubio E 2018 Hyperprogression as a distinct outcome after immunotherapy *Cancer Treat. Rev.* **70** 16–21

[165] Wojas-Krawczyk K, Kalinka E, Grenda A, Krawczyk P and Milanowski J 2019 Beyond PD-L1 markers for lung cancer immunotherapy *Int. J. Mol. Sci.* **20** 1915

[166] Demes M, Aszyk C, Bartsch H, Schirren J and Fisseler-Eckhoff A 2016 Differential miRNA-expression as an adjunctive diagnostic tool in neuroendocrine tumors of the lung *Cancers* **8** 38

[167] Han Y and Li H 2018 miRNAs as biomarkers and for the early detection of non-small cell lung cancer (NSCLC) *J. Thorac. Dis.* **10** 3119

[168] Xia Y, Zhu Y, Zhou X and Chen Y 2014 Low expression of let-7 predicts poor prognosis in patients with multiple cancers: a meta-analysis *Tumor Biol.* **35** 5143–8

[169] Yang M, Shen H, Qiu C, Ni Y, Wang L, Dong W, Liao Y and Du J 2013 High expression of miR-21 and miR-155 predicts recurrence and unfavourable survival in non-small cell lung cancer *Eur. J. Cancer* **49** 604–15

[170] Lu J, Zhan Y, Feng J, Luo J and Fan S 2018 MicroRNAs associated with therapy of non-small cell lung cancer *Int. J. Biol. Sci.* **14** 390

[171] Yu S, Qin X, Chen T, Zhou L, Xu X and Feng J 2017 MicroRNA-106b-5p regulates cisplatin chemosensitivity by targeting polycystic kidney disease-2 in non-small-cell lung cancer *Anti-Cancer Drugs* **28** 852–60

[172] Li J-H, Luo N, Zhong M-Z, Xiao Z-Q, Wang J-X, Yao X-Y, Peng Y and Cao J 2016 Inhibition of microRNA-196a might reverse cisplatin resistance of A549/DDP non-small-cell lung cancer cell line *Tumor Biol.* **37** 2387–94

[173] Chen X, Xu Y, Liao X, Liao R, Zhang L, Niu K, Li T, Li D, Chen Z and Duan Y 2016 Plasma miRNAs in predicting radiosensitivity in non-small cell lung cancer *Tumor Biol.* **37** 11927–36

[174] Larrea E, Sole C, Manterola L, Goicoechea I, Armesto M, Arestin M, Caffarel M, Araujo A, Araiz M and Fernandez-Mercado M 2016 New concepts in cancer biomarkers: circulating miRNAs in liquid biopsies *Int. J. Mol. Sci.* **17** 627

[175] Antonia S J, Villegas A, Daniel D, Vicente D, Murakami S, Hui R, Yokoi T, Chiappori A, Lee K H and De Wit M 2017 Durvalumab after chemoradiotherapy in stage III non–small-cell lung cancer *New Engl. J. Med.* **377** 1919–29

[176] Kim D-W, Mehra R, Tan D S, Felip E, Chow L Q, Camidge D R, Vansteenkiste J, Sharma S, De Pas T and Riely G J 2016 Activity and safety of ceritinib in patients with ALK-rearranged non-small-cell lung cancer (ASCEND-1): updated results from the multicentre, open-label, phase 1 trial *Lancet Oncol.* **17** 452–63

Chapter 6

Radiomics and lung cancer: promising news for early detection of nodules

Stefania Rizzo, Filippo Del Grande and Francesco Petrella

6.1 Introduction

In the new era of 'precision medicine', radiomics is an emerging translational field of research aiming to find associations between information extracted from clinical images and clinical data, with or without associated gene expression (the latter case is better referred to as 'radiogenomics').

Lung cancer is the leading cause of cancer-related death in the United States [1]. Because of the large number of lung cancer patients, diagnosis at an early, potentially curable, stage would lead to major benefits in terms of possible limited resections, a low rate of post-operative complications, longer overall survival, and, last but not least, higher adherence to proposed therapies.

Two main kind of nodules fall in the early diagnosis family: those detected as incidental findings during a chest CT exam performed for other reasons, and those detected within a screening program. In both scenarios the goal of imaging, corroborated by new tools, is to guarantee correct classification of the nodule as benign or malignant.

6.2 Interpretation of small lung nodules

6.2.1 Incidentally detected nodules

Pulmonary nodules are a frequently encountered incidental finding in CT, and the challenge for radiologists and clinicians is differentiating benign from malignant nodules. In current practice, pulmonary nodules identified by CT are managed according to widely accepted guidelines, such as those released by the Fleischner Society [2]. According to these guidelines, single solid nodules smaller than 6 mm do not require routine follow-up in patients at low risk; multiple solid noncalcified nodules smaller than 6 mm do not require routine follow-up; for pure ground-glass nodules smaller than 6 mm (i.e. 5 mm and smaller) in diameter no routine follow-up

doi:10.1088/978-0-7503-2540-0ch6

is recommended; and for solitary part-solid nodules smaller than 6 mm, no routine follow-up is recommended. In patients with multiple subsolid nodules smaller than 6 mm, one must consider infectious causes; however, in patients with multiple subsolid nodules with at least one nodule larger than 6 mm, that persists after 3–6 months of follow-up, then multiple primary adenocarcinoma has to be considered. According to these guidelines, nodule size and morphology remain the dominant factors to predict risk, but it is important to consider additional clinical risk factors, including smoking, exposure to other carcinogens, emphysema, fibrosis, upper lobe location, a family history of lung cancer, age, and sex. Low risk, which corresponds to an estimated risk of cancer of <5%, would be associated with young age, less smoking, smaller nodule size, regular margins, and location in an area other than the upper lobe; high-risk factors include older age, heavy smoking, larger nodule size, irregular or spiculated margins, and upper lobe location. Subjects with intermediate risk share both high- and low-risk characteristics.

It is of note that these guidelines are not intended for use in patients with known primary cancers, who are at risk of metastases, nor for use in immunocompromised patients, who are at risk of infection, nor for children and adults younger than 35 years. In these patients, treatment should be based on the specific clinical situation.

6.2.2 CT screening and Lung-RADS

The US National Lung Screening Trial (NLST) compared low-dose computed tomography (LDCT) to standard chest radiography across three annual screenings, demonstrating that the LDCT group presented a 20% relative reduction in lung cancer mortality compared to the chest radiography arm [3]. An important issue that arose from different lung cancer screening trials was the high detection of 4–12 mm diameter indeterminate pulmonary nodules. Indeed, among the indeterminate pulmonary nodules, only 3.6% were nascent cancers [4]. Overdiagnosis is harmful because it causes patient anxiety, and leads to unnecessary costs and morbidity for a condition that may pose no threat [5].

In 2014, the American College of Radiology (ACR) published the Lung-RADS Assessment Categories to standardize the CT lung screening reporting and management recommendations and to facilitate outcome monitoring [6]. Lung-RADS contains five categories to differentiate high-risk from low-risk nodules, based on size, solidity, and location using nodule type, nodule size, and growth as criteria. For nodule type, solid is differentiated from subsolid nodule composition with the latter having a relatively higher malignancy risk [7]. Nodule size is determined using manual diameter measurements and volumetry measurements, and growth is defined as an increase of at least 1.5 mm in diameter or 2 mm^3. A negative screening result corresponds to category 1 (negative) or 2 (benign appearance), whereas a positive screening corresponds to category 3 (probably benign) or 4 (suspicious). The last category is further divided into category 4A and 4B based on the probability of malignancy (5%–15% or greater than 15%), indicating that additional diagnostic testing (4A) and/or tissue sampling (4B) is recommended. Category 4X is a special category for lesions that demonstrate additional features or imaging findings that increase the suspicion of malignancy. It is well known that both visual assessment of nodule type and manual diameter measurements suffer from substantial observer variability [8–10].

Although Lung-RADS was not used in the National Lung Cancer Screening Trial, for prospective structured reporting, it has been evaluated in a large retrospective study, demonstrating a decrease in false positive results from 26.6% to 12.8% [11], thus producing a significant reduction in overdiagnosis and overtreatment.

6.3 Computer-aided detection/diagnosis (CAD)

Computer-aided detection/diagnosis systems have been investigated to detect pulmonary nodules and to classify malignant and benign nodules [12–15]. Kawata *et al* proposed quantitative surface characterization to classify malignant and benign pulmonary nodules [16]. McNitt-Gray *et al* proposed a pattern classification approach to characterize PNs, which used quantitative features including attenuation (intensity), size, shape, and texture [17]. Another group proposed an automatic scheme to segment pulmonary nodules using a dynamic programming technique and to determine malignant nodules using linear discriminant analysis classification [18].

Suzuki *et al* developed a massive training artificial neural network to filter out benign appearances in CT images [14]. Han *et al* investigated texture feature analysis to differentiate malignant and benign nodules [19]. The early successes of the CAD systems demonstrated that quantitative medical image analysis has the potential to improve the performance of detecting cancer, and such systems may allow the radiologist to be more confident in making hypotheses and diagnoses.

6.4 Radiomics

6.4.1 What radiomics is

The suffix 'omics' in clinical medicine research denotes the concept of examining large volumes of complex data to identify precise characteristics or outcomes.

Radiomics is an approach to extract quantitative features from the standard-of-care medical images, to generate high dimensional mineable data, and to associate them with selected outcomes. Radiomics has been applied to many different tumors to find associations with prognosis and response to therapies [20–23], as well as with genetic alterations [9, 24, 25].

The radiomics process can be divided into distinct steps with definable inputs and outputs, such as: image acquisition and reconstruction; segmentation; feature extraction and qualification; and analysis and model building [8]. For each of the above-mentioned steps, there are still unresolved issues, such as: to what extent acquisition and reconstruction parameters may have an impact on the features [26, 27]; what kind of segmentation is more precise among manual, semi-automatic, and automatic; what features are really stable and reproducible; how overfitting can be avoided; and what type of statistical analysis is more appropriate for model building [8, 28].

In the setting of lung nodules, radiomics is aimed at deriving quantitative imaging features that can non-invasively predict the nature of the nodule and its behavior. Since pulmonary nodules are usually detected and followed up by CT, problems related to the variability in acquisition and reconstruction do exist, but are limited to a small number of variables.

The high contrast resolution between pulmonary nodules and lung parenchyma makes them ideal candidates for volumetric segmentation. Radiomic features may include semantic qualitative features, such as shape, margins, density [24], and agnostic quantitative features mathematically extracted by different software [29]. The quantitative features may have different levels of complexity, such as describing lesion shape, intensity, texture, and wavelet. More specifically, first-order statistics features describe the distribution of individual voxel values without concern for spatial relationships. These are generally histogram-based methods and reduce a region of interest to single values for mean, median, maximum, minimum, and uniformity or randomness (entropy) of the intensities on the image, as well as the skewness (asymmetry) and kurtosis (flatness) of the histogram of values [8]. Shape features describe the shape and geometric properties of the analyzed volume, such as maximum diameter or the diameters along the three orthogonal directions, maximum surface, tumor compactness, and sphericity.

Second-order statistics features generally describe the so-called textural features, indicating the statistical relationships between voxels with similar (or dissimilar) values and take into account the spatial arrangement of the values [30]. Examples of these features belong to the category of the gray level co-occurrence matrix (GLCM) and gray level run length matrix (GLRLM). Higher order statistics features are generated by statistical methods after imposing filter grids on the image to extract repetitive or non-repetitive patterns, such as fractal analyses, Minkowski functionals, wavelets, and Laplacian transforms of Gaussian bandpass filters. As a result, extraction of textural features may generate hundreds of variables, some of which may be redundant and require co-variance evaluation [8, 31, 32].

Once features have been extracted, the next process in radiomics is establishing relationships between patterns of features and clinical variables, also known as data mining. This can vary from straightforward statistical analyses based on *a priori* hypotheses, to machine learning methods. Machine learning is a field of computer science which combines the study of pattern recognition and computational learning theory to construct algorithms that can learn from data and make predictions on outcomes as well as uncover hidden insights. Random forests is an example of a machine learning algorithm which works by constructing a collection of decision trees [33].

6.4.2 Radiomics models and lung nodules

Nodule size is a known prognostic factor (the larger it is, the worst the prognosis), as demonstrated by the above-mentioned guidelines for management of incidentally detected nodules according to size, and by the indications of different strategies for follow-up of nodules with different sizes. Radiomic features related to nodule size can be more accurate than the mere manual caliper measurements.

Choi *et al* developed a model of only two radiomic features: the bounding box anterior–posterior dimension and the standard deviation of inverse difference moment, related to the nodule size and to the local homogeneity, respectively. They compared the performance of this model to the Lung-RADS classification accuracy, demonstrating that Lung-RADS misclassified 19 cases because it was mainly based on PN size, whereas their model correctly classified ten of these cases by combining a size feature and a texture feature. Moreover, the prediction improvement of their model comparing to Lung-RADS was statistically significant (McNemar's test $P = 0.026$) [34].

With the aim of elaborating a radiomics signature to predict the emergence of cancer from low-dose computed tomography, Hawkins *et al* used the public data from the National Lung Screening Trial (ACRIN 6684) [4]. The authors assembled two cohorts of 104 and 92 patients with screen-detected lung cancer; then matched these cohorts with two different cohorts of 208 and 196 screening subjects with benign pulmonary nodules. Their best model, elaborated in a random forest classifier, included 23 features and was able to predict nodules that would become cancerous in 1 and 2 years, with accuracies of 80% and 79%. They also demonstrated that radiomics outperformed the Lung-RADS and volume-only approaches [4].

Mao *et al* extracted 385 radiomics features and included 11 of them in a radiomics model to predict malignant differentiation, of 81.0% and 92.2%, respectively, with a demonstrated accuracy superior to Lung-RADS (89.8% versus 76.5%) [35].

Paul *et al* used a transfer learning approach to differentiate lung cancer nodules versus positive controls among subsets of participants from the National Lung Screening Trial (NLST) [36]. The authors used three different pretrained convolutional neural networks (CNNs) for extracting deep features and used five different classifiers. Selected deep features were combined with radiomics features. Combinations of features from pretrained, CNNs trained on NLST data, and classical radiomics were used to build classifiers. The best accuracy (76.79%) was then obtained using feature combinations; an area under the receiver operating characteristic curve of 0.87 was obtained using a CNN trained on an augmented NLST data cohort [36].

A study by Ma *et al* illustrated the potentially vast number of radiomic textural features that can be extracted from pulmonary nodules [37]. The authors assessed 127 indeterminate pulmonary nodules and identified 583 features of nodule intensity, shape, and heterogeneity. By analyzing these features, they achieved 82.7% accuracy in classification of malignant primary lung nodules and benign nodules [33, 37].

Radiomic analysis has also been shown to have a role in evaluating subsolid nodules. Studies have identified textural features that are able to differentiate transient inflammatory nodules from malignant part-solid nodules, and differentiate indolent adenocarcinoma *in situ* from invasive adenocarcinoma. Lee *et al* assessed textural features of 86 part-solid nodules, demonstrating that low mean attenuation and higher positive skewness of attenuation were significant discriminators of transient from persistent part-solid nodules. When texture analysis was used in combination with clinical and CT features, differentiating power increased significantly when compared to clinical and CT features alone; the AUC rising from 79% to 92.9% [38]. In another study of 86 part-solid ground-glass nodules Chae *et al* successfully differentiated preinvasive lesions from invasive lung adenocarcinoma using a combination of texture based features with higher kurtosis and smaller mass being particularly good differentiators [39].

6.5 Conclusion

In conclusion, pulmonary nodules, either detected incidentally or during low-dose CT for cancer screening, provide diagnostic challenges. Radiomics, as a tool able to provide quantitative information from diagnostic images, has the potential to help in more accurate differentiation of benign and malignant nodules, in addition to helping in prognostication.

Although more studies are needed to validate the robustness of quantitative radiomics features, to harmonize image acquisition parameters and feature extraction, it is very likely that in the near future radiomics signatures will replace pre-existing classifications, such as Lung-RADS, in order to improve the accuracy of lung nodule characterization.

References

[1] Siegel R L, Miller K D and Jemal A 2019 Cancer statistics, 2019 *CA Cancer J. Clin.* **69** 7–34

[2] MacMahon H *et al* 2017 Guidelines for management of incidental pulmonary nodules detected on CT images: from the Fleischner Society 2017 *Radiology* **284** 228–43

[3] Aberle D R *et al* 2011 Reduced lung cancer mortality with low-dose computed tomographic screening *N. Engl. J. Med.* **365** 395–409

[4] Hawkins S *et al* 2016 Predicting malignant nodules from screening CT scans *J. Thorac. Oncol.* **11** 2120–8

[5] Patz E F Jr *et al* 2014 Overdiagnosis in low-dose computed tomography screening for lung cancer *JAMA Intern. Med.* **174** 269–74

[6] American College of Radiology 2019 Lung-RADS assessment categories, version 1.1 (2019 release) *Lung CT Screening Reporting and Data System (Lung-RADS™)* https://acr.org/Clinical-Resources/Reporting-and-Data-Systems/Lung-Rads (Accessed: 7 August 2019)

[7] Henschke C I, Yankelevitz D F, Mirtcheva R, McGuinness G, McCauley D and Miettinen O S 2002 CT screening for lung cancer: frequency and significance of part-solid and nonsolid nodules *Am. J. Roentgenol.* **178** 1053–7

[8] Rizzo S, Botta F, Raimondi S, Origgi D, Fanciullo C, Morganti A G and Bellomi M 2018 Radiomics: the facts and the challenges of image analysis *Eur. Radiol. Exp.* **2** 36

[9] Gillies R J, Kinahan P E and Hricak H 2016 Radiomics: images are more than pictures, they are data *Radiology* **278** 563–77

[10] Bellomi M, Rizzo S, Travaini L L, Bazzi L, Trifirò G, Zampino M G, Radice D and Paganelli G 2007 Role of multidetector CT and FDG-PET/CT in the diagnosis of local and distant recurrence of resected rectal cancer *Radiol. Med.* **112** 681–90

[11] Pinsky P F *et al* 2015 Performance of Lung-RADS in the National Lung Screening Trial: a retrospective assessment *Ann. Intern. Med.* **62** 485–91

[12] Armato S G, Giger M L, Moran C J, Blackburn J T, Doi K and MacMahon H 1999 Computerized detection of pulmonary nodules on CT scans *Radiographics* **19** 1303–11

[13] Doi K 2005 Current status and future potential of computer-aided diagnosis in medical imaging *Br. J. Radiol.* **78** s3–19

[14] Suzuki K 2012 A review of computer-aided diagnosis in thoracic and colonic imaging *Quant. Imaging Med. Surg.* **2** 163–76

[15] El-Baz A *et al* 2013 Computer-aided diagnosis systems for lung cancer: challenges and methodologies *Int. J. Biomed. Imaging* **2013** 942353

[16] Kawata Y *et al* 1998 Quantitative surface characterization of pulmonary nodules based on thin-section CT images *IEEE Trans. Nucl. Sci.* **45** 2132–8

[17] McNitt-Gray M F, Hart E M, Wyckoff N, Sayre J W, Goldin J G and Aberle D R 1999 A pattern classification approach to characterizing solitary pulmonary nodules imaged on high resolution CT: preliminary results *Med. Phys.* **26** 880–8

[18] Aoyama M, Li Q, Katsuragawa S, Li F, Sone S and Doi K 2003 Computerized scheme for determination of the likelihood measure of malignancy for pulmonary nodules on low-dose CT images *Med. Phys.* **30** 387–94

[19] Han F *et al* 2015 Texture feature analysis for computer-aided diagnosis on pulmonary nodules *J. Digit. Imaging* **28** 99–115

[20] Rizzo S *et al* 2018 Radiomics of high-grade serous ovarian cancer: association between quantitative CT features, residual tumour and disease progression within 12 months *Eur. Radiol.* **28** 4849–59

[21] Karlo C A *et al* 2013 Radiogenomics of clear cell renal cell carcinoma: associations between CT imaging features and mutations *Radiology* **270** 464–71

[22] Segal E *et al* 2007 Decoding global gene expression programs in liver cancer by noninvasive imaging *Nat. Biotechnol.* **25** 675–80

[23] Kuo M D, Gollub J, Sirlin C B, Ooi C and Chen X 2007 Radiogenomic analysis to identify imaging phenotypes associated with drug response gene expression programs in hepatocellular carcinoma *J. Vasc. Interv. Radiol.* **18** 821–31

[24] Rizzo S *et al* 2016 CT radiogenomic characterization of EGFR, K-RAS, and ALK mutations in non-small cell lung cancer *Eur. Radiol.* **26** 32–42

[25] Aurilio G *et al* 2013 Discordant hormone receptor and human epidermal growth factor receptor 2 status in bone metastases compared to primary breast cancer *Acta Oncol.* **52** 1649–56

[26] Rizzo S, Kalra M K, Schmidt B, Raupach R, Maher M M, Blake M A and Saini S 2005 CT images of abdomen and pelvis: effect of nonlinear three-dimensional optimized reconstruction algorithm on image quality and lesion characteristics *Radiology* **237** 309–15

[27] Dalal T, Kalra M K, Rizzo S, Schmidt B, Suess C, Flohr T, Blake M A and Saini S 2005 Metallic prosthesis: technique to avoid increase in CT radiation dose with automatic tube current modulation in a phantom and patients *Radiology* **236** 671–5

[28] Aerts H J W L *et al* 2014 Decoding tumour phenotype by noninvasive imaging using a quantitative radiomics approach *Nat. Commun.* **5** 4006

[29] Larue R T H M *et al* 2017 Influence of gray level discretization on radiomic feature stability for different CT scanners, tube currents and slice thicknesses: a comprehensive phantom study *Acta Oncol.* **56** 1544–53

[30] Balagurunathan Y *et al* 2014 Test–retest reproducibility analysis of lung CT image features *J. Digit. Imaging* **27** 805–23

[31] De Jong E E C *et al* 2018 Applicability of a prognostic CT-based radiomic signature model trained on stage I–III non-small cell lung cancer in stage IV non-small cell lung cancer *Lung Cancer* **124** 6–11

[32] Rizzo S *et al* 2019 Genomics of non-small cell lung cancer (NSCLC): association between CT-based imaging features and EGFR and K-RAS mutations in 122 patients—an external validation *Eur. J. Radiol.* **110** 148–55

[33] Wilson R and Devaraj A 2017 Radiomics of pulmonary nodules and lung cancer *Transl. Lung Cancer Res.* **6** 86–91

[34] Choi W *et al* 2018 Radiomics analysis of pulmonary nodules in low-dose CT for early detection of lung cancer *Med. Phys.* **45** 1537–49

[35] Mao L, Chen H, Liang M, Li K, Gao J, Qin P, Ding X, Li X and Liu X 2019 Quantitative radiomic model for predicting malignancy of small solid pulmonary nodules detected by low-dose CT screening *Quant. Imaging Med. Surg.* **9** 263–72

[36] Paul R, Hawkins S H, Schabath M B, Gillies R J, Hall L O and Goldgof D B 2018 Predicting malignant nodules by fusing deep features with classical radiomics features *J. Med. Imaging* **5** 011021

[37] Ma J *et al* 2016 Automatic lung nodule classification with radiomics approach *Proc. SPIE* **9879**

[38] Lee S H *et al* 2014 Usefulness of texture analysis in differentiating transient from persistent partsolid nodules (PSNs): a retrospective study *PLoS One* **9** e85167

[39] Chae H D *et al* 2014 Computerized texture analysis of persistent part-solid ground-glass nodules: differentiation of preinvasive lesions from invasive pulmonary adenocarcinomas *Radiology* **273** 285–93

Chapter 7

Photodynamic diagnosis and treatment of lung cancer

Anine Crous and Heidi Abrahamse

7.1 Introduction

Cancer is ultimately a genetic DNA disease. Changes in chromosomal sequences lead to altered gene expression, protein composition, and function of enzymes, resulting in enhanced cell growth, motility, and related clinical signs. Every cancer is distinct, and knowing the mutations is essential in selecting the right therapy [115]. This applies in particular to lung cancer, the most severe cancer disease, and a significant contributor to cancer deaths [16]. Lung cancer is caused by respiratory epithelium cells that have undergone genetic mutation. Small cell lung cancer (SCLC) and non-small cell lung cancer (NSCLC) are two common types of lung cancer. Patients with lung cancer have a life expectancy of 5 years, which decreases with variables such as metastasis [27]. Better testing, early diagnosis, and suitable and new medications can help with the prognosis. Screening is provided to individuals with enhanced danger of lung cancer, including x-ray imaging, sputum cytology, and tissue biopsy, where lung cancer is staged after diagnosis. The staging of lung cancer includes CT, MRI, and PET tests, which help to determine suitable therapy schedules [94]. Chemotherapy, radiation therapy, surgery, targeted drug therapy, and immunotherapy are the current options for lung cancer. However, these types of therapies can trigger distinct side effects and appear to have reached a therapeutic plateau based on chemotherapy regimens. Effective, better tolerated medicines are therefore required to deal with this problem and hopefully resolve it [47].

Specifically, one therapy provides a multi-modal strategy that can be used both as a diagnostic instrument and as an alternative for therapy. This treatment uses a photochemotherapeutic agent or photosensitizer (PS) that can be used for photodynamic diagnosis (PDD) and photodynamic therapy (PDT).

doi:10.1088/978-0-7503-2540-0ch7

PSs are molecules that undergo photochemical reactions to emit fluorescence in response to specific light irradiation. This effect is used in the production of reactive oxygen species (ROS) such as singlet oxygen ($^1O_2$) by PDT and is a current treatment for cancer. PDT has several advantages over conventional cancer treatments, as it is relatively non-invasive and less toxic [85]. In 1990, Kennedy *et al* registered the first PDT case, with δ-aminolaevulinic acid (ALA) provided to individuals with basal cell carcinoma [60]. The use of PDT in cancer therapy is usually palliative and typically for developed stage cancers, where it was also seen that PDT's distinctive processes of tumour cell and microenvironment destruction could be used to solve cancer drug resistance [114].

Its fluorescent nature can also be used for cancer imaging in relation to the use of PSs for PDT. PDD has a variety of important characteristics, including diagnosis, therapy guidelines, monitoring, treatment assessment, and mechanical study. The uniqueness of PDT, in that the same molecule can work both as a medicinal agent and as a contrasting imaging agent, has resulted in an increase in PS fluorescence application for surgical guides and other processes [21].

PDD and PDT have been used for several carcinomas, including actinic keratosis, Bowen's and basal cell carcinoma, liver and lung disease, gastrointestinal malignancy, intrathoracic malignancy, and many other carcinomas [79]. Since the advent of PDT and PDD more than half a century ago, distinct alternatives have been tested for higher clinical results, including the inclusion of photochemical wavelengths, developments in laser generation, improved drug delivery technologies, and, of course, distinctive and improved PS chemicals [52].

7.2 Cancer

Cancer is a major public health crisis worldwide. GLOBOCAN recorded 18.1 million new cancer cases and 9.6 million cancer deaths in 2018 [16]. This burden is expected to rise worldwide due to demographic growth and aging, particularly in less developed countries where around 82% of the world's population lives. Implementing lifestyle behaviours known to increase the risk of cancer, such as smoking, poor diet, physical inactivity, and reproductive changes, has further increased the risk of cancer in less developed nations [119]. With cancer having such an enormous impact on humanity, not only physically but also financially, addressing the the causes, diagnosis, and treatment of cancer has fostered the need for developments in the field of research.

One of the cancer research objectives is to understand the biological cancer model, where studies have defined malignancy as a cell disease defined by somatic cell genomic disorder. Hereditary and epigenetic influences affect the development of cell genomics leading to heterogeneity, providing a rich background for further development in a cancer cell's molecular biology [9]. Cancer's biochemical mechanism allows uncontrolled cell growth and invasion-led genetic mutation. Hence, the arrest of normal cellular procedures where uncontrolled neoplastic formation occurs can result in mortality. Carcinogenesis is a multi-stage process that incorporates the accumulation of mutagenic characteristics that promote metastatic ability with each

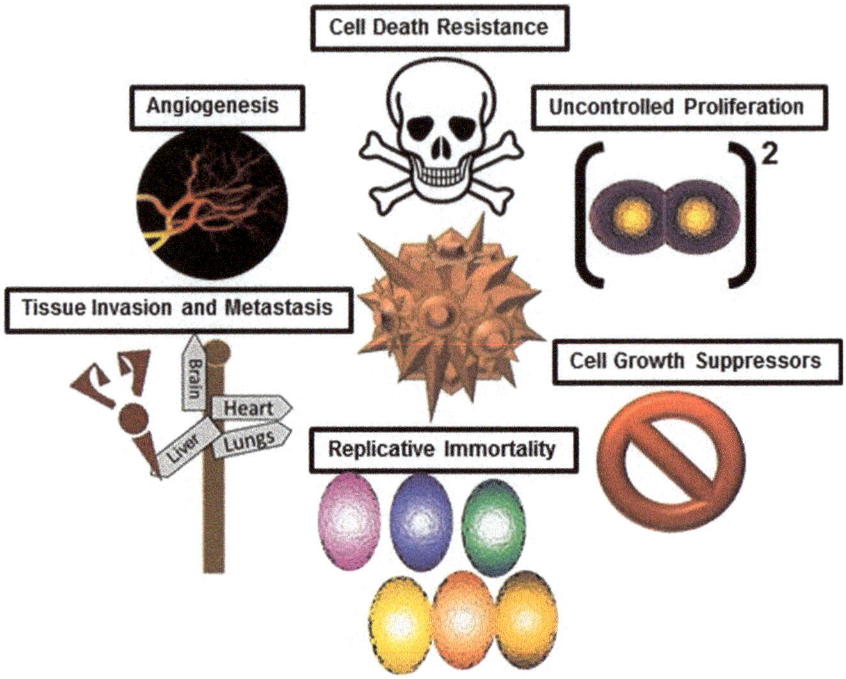

Figure 7.1. Cancer cell characteristics acquired through mutagenesis.

mutagenic advantage including oncogene activation, tumour suppressor gene suppression, and altered genes for DNA repair. The characteristics acquired (figure 7.1) throughout this multi-stage process enable resistance to cell death, uncontrolled proliferation, cell growth suppressors, replicative immortality, invasion and metastasis of tissues, and angiogenesis [7, 99].

7.2.1 Lung cancer

Despite current developments in pulmonary cancer aetiology, diagnosis, and treatment, pulmonary cancer remains the most frequently found cancer globally (11.6% of complete instances) and the major cause of cancer mortality (18.4% of complete cancer fatalities) in both women and men [16]. Current statistics show that the cancer incidence rate will double from 2012 to 2035, when most of the diagnoses will be made in older adults in less developed regions most at risk. This anticipated rise in cancer instances will have significant financial and social effects worldwide, presenting significant and distinctive difficulties to healthcare systems in all regions of the globe, in particular in those with limited resources and weaker health systems [91].

Lung carcinoma is a neoplastic cell that shows uninhibited development of altered pulmonary cells produced in the lung tissue aerial sections. The transformed cells quickly diffuse the tumour structure. As tumour development advances, the various mutated cells begin to undermine the vital capacity of the lungs, preventing oxygen supply to the circulatory system [83].

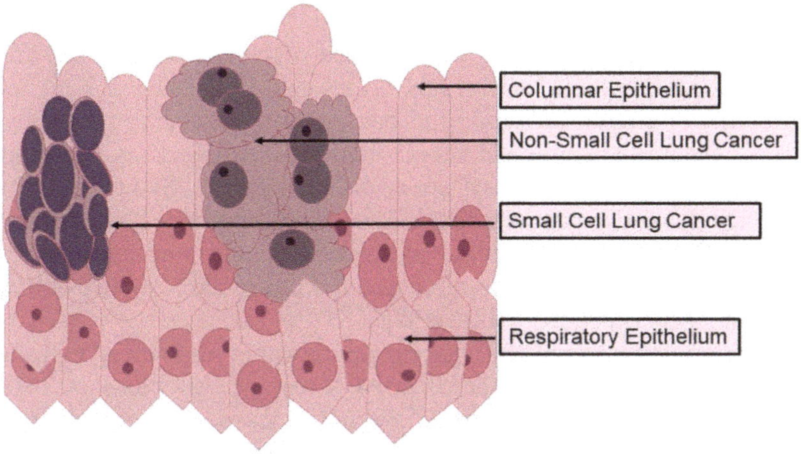

Figure 7.2. The two main types of lung cancer, small cell lung cancer and non-small cell lung cancer.

Lung cancer is categorised into two groups. SCLC is characterized by its neuroendocrine appearance and includes 15% of instances of pulmonary disease. The remaining 85% of instances are caused by NSCLC (figure 7.2). Subtypes include: adenocarcinoma (38.5%), squamous cell carcinoma (20%), and large cell carcinoma (2.9%) [72]. If they are determined to have restricted pulmonary carcinoma, 52% of patients have an estimated 5-year life expectancy. At the moment of treatment, more than 52% of people with metastatic illness have a 5-year survival level of 3.6% [27].

The administrative circuits in lung carcinoma that maintain normal cell development and homeostasis are faulty. From a typical lung cell to a malignant phenotype, a multistep shift is followed, with a sequence of hereditary and epigenetic changes, causing a powerful damaging growth. Malignant progression results in a continuous development of hereditary and epigenetic variants and multiplication of disease, invasion of tissue, metastasis, and safety from conventional treatment choices [73]. Reducing malignancy through early detection and treatment depends on the classification and recognition of these genetic changes. Data on tumour characteristics and hereditary properties will promote the prognostic result and the selection of an ideal therapy [111].

Smoking, second-hand smoking, and radon are cancer-causing variables that contribute to lung carcinoma. For example, asbestos, arsenic and arsenic mixtures, and beryllium and beryllium oxide, are work-related exposures. Inhalation of synthetic compounds including cadmium, silica, vinyl chloride, nickel mixtures, chromium mixtures, coal products, mustard gas, diesel fumes, and chloromethyl esters, and extended exposure to air contamination, including outflows of polycyclic aromatic hydrocarbons, are fully recognised as threat variables for lung disease. Lung illness may also be inherent, where family heritage of lung carcinoma increases the probability of pulmonary cancer due to inherited genetic abnormalities that can be activated upon exposure to cancer-causing agents [134].

7.2.2 Diagnosis and staging of lung cancer

The procedures used to determine the presence of cancer include the following: history, physical examination, routine laboratory evaluations, chest x-ray, chest CT scan with contrast material infusion, and biopsy where cancer is staged by extent. Lung cancer is generally assumed in people with an unusual radiograph of the chest or symptoms induced by local or systemic tumour impacts. Symptoms of primary lung cancer include, but are not restricted to, vomiting, dyspnoea, chest pain, weight loss, and exhaustion [44]. The technique of diagnosing lung cancer relies on the form of pulmonary cancer, the primary tumour size and place, the existence of metastasis, and the patient's general clinical status [98].

Pulmonary nodule management choices include watchful waiting with follow-up CT imaging, PET imaging, or further invasive screening depending on malignancy probability. Longer distances between follow-up CT scans are suggested for patients with a small projected danger of malignancy in an incidentally identified solitary pulmonary nodule. For individuals at elevated danger of malignancy or patients with nodules of at least 8 mm, either incidentally, with test detection or with symptoms, a diagnostic biopsy is required to determine the cause of the solitary pulmonary nodule [84]. Only low-dose helical CT testing has been shown to change survival in patients deemed to be at elevated risk of developing pulmonary cancer. Lung cancer screening studies with chest x-rays and sputum cytology have failed to show that screening reduces the mortality levels of lung cancer [29].

Staging is one of the most significant prognostic indicators for lung cancer. The tumour, node, metastasis (TNM) scheduling scheme, operated by the American Joint Committee on Cancer (AJCC) and the International Union Against Cancer (UICC), is the most widely used cancer staging scheme [51]. The lung cancer classification of TNM defines the magnitude of the disease in terms of main tumour magnitude, place, and magnitude (T descriptor), the existence and place of lymph cell participation (N descriptor), and the existence or lack of remote metastatic illness (M descriptor) [39]. TNM staging in conjunction with the updated pulmonary cancer classification scheme by the International Association for the Study of Lung Cancer (IASLC), involves main tumour volume and local invasion (T1-4), whether it involves ipsilateral hilar (N1) and mediastinal lymph nodes (N2), contralateral hilar or mediastinal nodes (N3), or supraclavicular nodes (N3); and whether intrathoracic nodes are engaged [75].

Proper lung cancer staging using TNM plays a significant role in choosing the best therapy options. Staging includes two clinical and pathological elements, wherein cTNM includes clinical assessment and computed tomography (CT) offering original assessment of illness magnitude, and pathological staging (pTNM) utilizes clinical staging (cTNM) and extra pathological data acquired through surgical processes including mediastinal lymph node examination and/or mediastinoscopy [66]. The degree of consensus between the two specifies the result of the therapy diagnosis and prognosis. For example, an inaccurate or inadequate ranking of cTNM can contribute to the wrong choice among possible therapy alternatives for both curative and palliative treatment. While patients with NSCLC phase IA, IB, IIA, and IIB may benefit from curative surgical resection, this operation rarely benefits patients with phase IIIA, IIIB, and IV disease. In individuals with SCLC, with the exception of rare limited-stage surgically operable disease, the aim of staging is to determine whether therapy is for a restricted disease with chemotherapy and radiation or for comprehensive disease with chemotherapy alone [89].

7.2.3 Conventional treatments used in lung cancer

Research on presumed lung cancer patients focuses on confirming the diagnosis and determining the magnitude of the disease. Patient treatment choices are determined by the patient's histology, phase, and overall wellness and comorbidity [14].

The pathological material must be reviewed by an experienced lung cancer pathologist before a person starts therapy for lung cancer. This is critical because SCLC can be mistaken on microscopic examination for NSCLC, which reacts well to chemotherapy and is usually not surgically handled. Immunohistochemistry and electron microscopy are invaluable diagnostic and sub-classification methods, but most lung tumours can be categorized according to light microscopic requirements [14, 134].

The present approach to treating SCLC is combination chemotherapy. Platinum including combined regimens are inferior in restricted stage-SCLC to non-platinum regimens and potentially as first- and second-line medications in comprehensive stage-SCLC. Adding ifosfamide to regimens comprising platinum may enhance the result but at the cost of enhanced toxicity. Inferior survival results from suboptimal doses of chemotherapy. Early increased, accelerated, and high-dose chemotherapy has resulted in inconsistent outcomes and is not regarded a normal choice outside clinical trials. A variety of new drugs, for example gemcitabine, irinotecan, and topotecan, have produced successful outcomes when used in combined regimens. However, more research is needed to assess them properly [53].

Radiation therapy plays a significant role in the radical management of SCLC together with chemotherapy. The findings available to date have not yet answered questions about optimum radiotherapy timing, schedule, and dose. Despite the recognized SCLC chemosensitivity (reaction rates of 70%–80% with full reactions of up to 50% with combined treatment in patients with restricted illness), most people die from recurrent cancer [53, 110].

Radiation therapy is an important part of the management of all stages of SCLC, in the curative as well as in the palliative setting [38]. SCLC is extremely radiosensitive and thoracic radiation therapy enhances the survival of limited disease and extensive disease tumour patients [137]. Early concurrent radiochemotherapy may not be suitable for all patients. In patients with large tumour volumes or poor performance status, early radiotherapy may increase acute and late toxicities. In these cases, a deferred start to radiotherapy or even sequential treatment are the preferred options. Bulky tumours may require large treatment volumes; these can be reduced if initial chemotherapy shrinks the tumour, potentially reducing toxicity to the lungs and oesophagus [38]. Prophylactic cranial radiation avoids recurrence of the central nervous system and may enhance the long-term survival of individuals with excellent performance status who have responded to chemotherapy and offer symptomatic metastatic disease palliation [113]. Intrathoracic diseases such as tumour mass obstruction, pain, or haemoptysis can often be handled in the palliative environment with radiotherapy. It is also possible to treat symptoms triggered by extra thoracic metastases with radiotherapy. Interdisciplinary cooperation is vital in order to promote appropriate therapy for all elements of care [38].

For NSCLC, depending on the staging of lung cancer, patients are eligible for certain treatments ranging from surgery to radiation to chemotherapy as well as targeted therapy. In NSCLC, with the exception of most localized cancers, the findings for conventional therapy are poor. All newly diagnosed NSCLC patients are prospective applicants for new types of therapy evaluation research [134].

Surgery plays a major role in NSCLC diagnosis, staging, and definite management. Resection is the main method of therapy for phase I and II NSCLC and a significant element of the stage IIIA disease multimodality strategy. Standard resections include tumour extraction of the lobe and systematic assessment of ipsilateral hilar and mediastinal lymph nodes. The changing surgical therapy objectives for early phase disease are intended to decrease morbidity and death through less invasive methods including video-assisted thoracoscopic surgery and robotic methods, and possibly decrease the amount of lung removed for select patients with well-staged small peripheral tumours. For individuals with locally developed diseases, continuing study focuses on the proper identification of patients who will profit most from the addition of surgery to a multimodality system and the safe integration of resection with chemotherapy and radiotherapy [69], where chemo and radiation therapy can generate a curve in a tiny number of patients and in most patients can provide palliation [73]. The incidence of brain metastases may be reduced by prophylactic cranial irradiation, but there is no proof of survival benefits and the impact of prophylactic cranial irradiation on quality of life is not understood [4].

About 40% of recently diagnosed people with pulmonary disease are in phase IV. Treating these patients is aimed at improving survival and reducing adverse events associated with disease. Cytotoxic combination chemotherapy for phase IV NSCLC is the first-line therapy that could be affected by histology, age versus comorbidity, and performance status [96], where the treatment for patients with a good performance status is a regimen of a platinum (cisplatin or carboplatin) plus paclitaxel, gemcitabine, docetaxel, vinorelbine, irinotecan, or pemetrexed [78]. Patients with a median performance status are treated with one chemo agent excluding platinum [42], where adverse side effects will prompt a change in the agent used. Treatment will also be stopped if the tumour is enlarged, or if the tumour is not shrinking after four rounds of chemo [92, 107]. Patients with a poor performance status do not benefit from chemotherapy, where they run a risk of adverse side effects that will result in a poor quality of life and basic supportive care is the only option [134].

Radiotherapy utilizes high-energy beams to disrupt and destroy DNA in cancer cells. This treatment may assist in regulating or remove tumours at particular body locations. Radiation therapy may benefit patients with NSCLC located in the chest and who are not applicants for surgical resection. Radiotherapy can also be a component of palliative care for people with NSCLC who do not react to surgery or chemotherapy [5]. Stereotactic body radiation therapy is a technique that uses advanced placement of radiation to treat patients with early-stage NSCLC with a single small lung nodule without metastasis, and offers a greater than two year survival rate [43]. Inoperable NSCLC is locally controlled [33] and the patient survival rate amounts to three years for 55.8% of patients [118], with lower rates of treatment related morbidity in outcomes approaching surgical resection [70, 87].

Molecular-targeted therapies are currently in use or under construction to bypass the side effects caused by standard treatments. Current molecularly targeted therapies efficiently target particular biomarkers that are frequently over-expressed in lung cancers and may result in enhanced tumourigenicity [106]. A range of molecularly targeted therapies concentrate on different tyrosine kinase receptors (TKRs) engaged in cell growth and survival. TKRs are frequently mutated in NSCLC, resulting in TKR signalling amplification and activation of upstream and alternative signalling mechanisms that often overlap with prevalent downstream signalling effectors that cause tumorigenesis [26]. Different RTKs, such as epidermal growth factor receptor (EGFR), hepatocyte growth factor receptor (HGFR/c-Met), and anaplastic lymphoma kinase (ALK), have been aimed at therapeutic development, as they are often discovered to be mutated in individuals with NSCLC [30]. Many of the current molecular therapies targeting TKRs use tyrosine kinase inhibitors (TKIs) that bind to TKRs and inhibit their corresponding signalling cascades, thereby inhibiting signalling processes that would otherwise cause cell growth and proliferation [30]. However, extended TKI therapy often leads to the growth of acquired drug resistance that reduces the duration of their clinical advantage. A prospective reason for gained TKI resistance may be the accumulation of RTK mutations, epithelial–mesenchymal transformation (EMT), and the activation of alternative signalling mechanisms [112].

7.3 Photodynamic diagnosis

7.3.1 Photodynamic diagnosis

The application of PDD requires a PS that can be excited by a laser or light source in the visible blue to blue–violet spectrum, where after optical imaging red fluorescence can be detected (figure 7.3(a)). There is a large Stokes shift between the emission and excitation wavelengths of porphyrins, where these PSs are diagnosed by exciting the 400 nm Soret band. Conventional medical imaging devices such as laparoscopes, endoscopes, cystoscopes, and neurochirurgical microscopes can generally be adjusted to fluorescence testing by using suitable light sources with relatively minor alteration of the imaging instrument [21]. This clinical translation suitability has enabled the use of PDD to selectively identify cancerous lesions in a wide spectrum of anatomical locations, including the cervix [41, 68], lung [56], head and neck, [74] and bladder [11]. In contrast to other diagnostic methods such as PET, MRI, CT, etc, that can be used in comparable capabilities as diagnostic imaging modalities, it is essential to remember that PDD is essentially a surface detection method. While the above-mentioned volume-sensitive methods provide structural information that

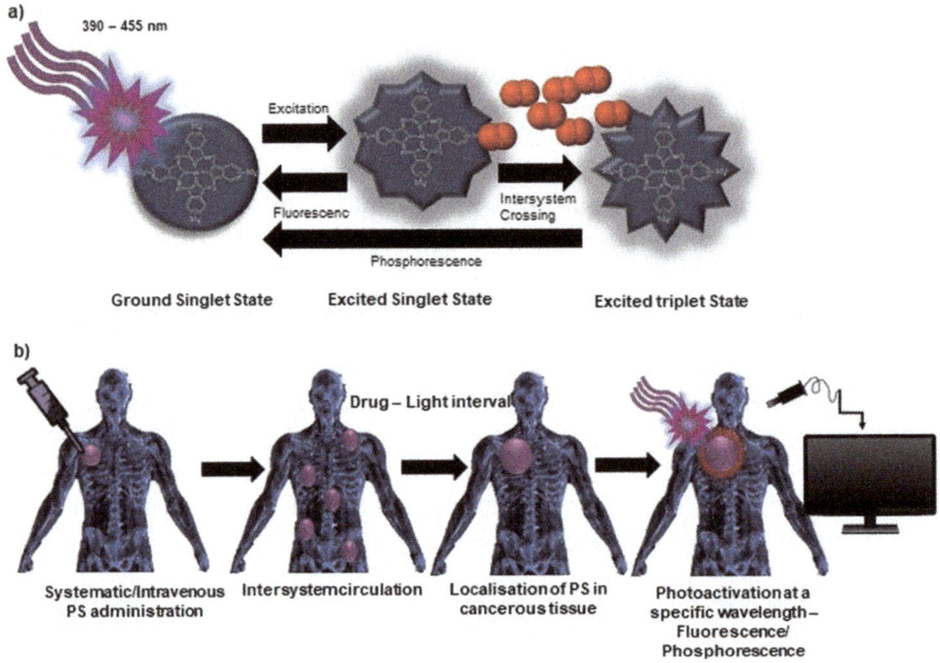

Figure 7.3. (a) A schematic representation of PDD where a PS is photo-activated using blue/violet light from its ground singlet state to its excited triplet state resulting in fluorescence and phosphorescence. (b) A schematic representation of PDD administration, localisation, and imaging.

is not obtained with fluorescence imaging, the sensitivity of identification decreases as the size of unresected disease decreases during the resection phase. On the other hand, the imaging sensitivity of fluorescence is not affected [21].

PDD involves the administration of a drug that is retained selectively by a tumour. When exposed to laser light at a wavelength that induces photo-excitation, the tumour fluoresces to distinguish the tumour from normal tissue [85]. Optical excitation of a PS can result both in an anticancer effect, but also in fluorescence emitted as a result of relaxing the excited single-state PS back to the ground state. Therefore, in addition to being clinical agents for PDT, PSs can be effectively used as the imaging agents that fluoresce after excitation in the visible region with the appropriate wavelength (figure 7.3(b)), although with a lower quantum yield than the conventional fluorescent dyes that are not also curative agents. Because PSs tend to collect preferentially in neoplastic tissues, this strategy allows early visualization of malignant tumours that are not visible to the human eye and thus improves the prognosis in patients [82]. The ability to properly recognize tumour margins is a main component in optimizing surgical procedures and constitutes an important subset of this fluorescence imaging method's implementation. Generally, the ability to attain cancer-free margins around cancer excision determines significantly whether the illness will recur [17, 21]. PSs' intrinsic ability to selectively identify disease and their use as an instrument for treatment optimization has resulted in important changes in the quality of life of people with various cancers [21].

Complementary innovations in imaging technology have resulted in a revolution over the past two decades, and fluorescence imaging now benefits a range of biomedical applications. Specifically, advances in fluorophore chemistry and imaging machinery and the finding of specific biomarkers have now made intraoperative fluorescence a highly specific technique of identification in real time [136]. In particular, the increased tissue density and limited autofluorescence of near-infrared (NIR) fluorescence imaging enhances the computational capacity of this component over visible-light fluorescence screening. Continuous advances in fluorophores with enhanced features, screening equipment, and targeting approaches resulted in clinical testing of the first NIR intraoperative cancer therapy in the mid-2010s. The foundation for the advancement this technique remains to be fostered by the interdisciplinary collaboration of pharmacists, scientists, engineers, and doctors [136].

7.3.2 Photosensitizers used in PDD

Scherer produced the initial fluorescent PS haematoporphyrin (HP) from a precipitate of dried blood warmed with sulphuric acid and rinsed of iron in 1841 [105]. The first written report stating that HP collects preferably in cancerous tumours is ascribed to Policard, who described the 1924 discovery of red HP fluorescence where UV-light from a Wood's lamp was used to illuminate rat sarcoma [93]. Another study found that certain investigated porphyrin species produced concentrated red fluorescence in tumours after ultraviolet stimulation but not in ordinary tissues [34]. This interesting finding laid the foundation for the Rassmussan-Taxdal *et al* clinical PDD research that intravenously introduced HP hydrochloride to patients before benign and malignant lesions were excised. The red fluorescence emission was noticeable in a larger percentage of malignant tumours compared to benign tumours, and the concentration increased with an increased quantity of HP, and solid tumours could be identified even through intact skin [97].

Due to their dependence on the crude type of HP, these first PS fluorescence experiments had minimal capacity for clinical translation, which needed large doses to generate a detectable fluorescence signal. Researchers were unable to identify HP fluorescence in human clinical trials with head and neck malignancies, probably owing to the much-reduced amount of HP used compared to prior animal studies. Additional chemical analysis of HP disclosed that the material was a combination of porphyrin compounds with variable absorption and fluorescent characteristics. This observation resulted in a sequence of extra purification measures on crude HP resulting in the HP derivative drug (HPD) with greater affinity for tumour location and greater phototoxicity [61]. HPD-based fluorescence screening was assessed for several clinical applications over the following decades, including the detection of cervical cancer [63], pulmonary cancer through fluorescence bronchoscopy [56], head and neck tumours [74], and the identification of multiple malignancies in the bladder [11]. The issue of drug impurity was obviously a limiting factor in its capacity to correctly and reliably define the limits of diseased tissue for diagnosis or surgical advice, in relation to the known side effects of HPD, including extended cutaneous toxicity. It was not until Kennedy and Pottier launched a fresh photosensitizing approach, i.e. increased endogenous protoporphyrin IX (PpIX) production through the *in situ* synthesis of ALA, a non-photoactivatable precursor, into PpIX, a naturally occurring photosensitizing species via the cellular haem biosynthesis pathway in the tumour, that PDD would achieve more extensive and effective applications [60]. With several stronger absorption bands, including one at 635 nm, PpIX heavily absorbs light at 409 nm and generates distinctive dual-peak red fluorescence at 635 nm and 700 nm. Longer PS wavelength activation is preferred for PDT procedures to obtain greater tissue penetration with decreased dispersion and absorption. Therefore, therapeutic light activation with illumination at 635 nm is usually performed for ALA-induced PpIX [101]. However, for PDD, stimulating the PS with red light is often not feasible as the Stokes-shifted spectral limit of the fluorescence emission has significant overlap with the excitation peak and is difficult to differentiate. In addition, an emission filter to block illumination light is intentionally not used in many PDD implementations in order to retain the ability to visualize the healthy tissue landscape surrounding the more intense malignant fluorescent regions. For these reasons, PpIX's 409 nm excitation, which is close to the 405 nm emission of frequently accessible blue–violet laser diodes, is often used for fluorescence emission generation. This also applies to other PSs, which are usually excited at 400 nm wavelengths for imaging applications, but also have powerful 600 nm absorption bands that are beneficial for PDT therapy [21].

Developments in fluorophores with improved characteristics led to the development of the detection of NIR fluorophore disease where excitation and resonance range fluorophores in the NIR range (700–900 nm) are most noticeable owing to their increased depth-penetration range compared to fluorophores emitting surface radiation of lower ranges. *In vivo*, background fluorescence and dispersion from water and chromophores are minimized within the wavelength range of NIR [35]. Fluorophores that can target cancer were widely investigated in preclinical designs, but have only been tested in clinical settings for the past three years. One of the first selected NIR fluorophores to enter clinical trials was cetuximab-800CW [102]. These agents' industrial growth for clinical implementation has synergized with simultaneous advances in instrumentation and software for identification.

The heptamethine cyanine fluorophore indocyanine green (ICG) is the first and only NIR fluorescent clinically approved fluorophore [35]. The readily accessible equipment for use in ICG identification is adapted to the features displayed by ICG in plasma with a maximum excitation wavelength of 807 nm and a maximum emission wavelength of 822 nm [104]. IGC is hydrophobic and is therefore often linked to plasma enzymes that limit ICG to the intravascular area and make it particularly suitable for angiography implementations [28]. ICG has also demonstrated enhanced detection, sensitivity, and specificity in identification of sentinel lymph nodes [46] and has shown intraoperative identification of metastatic cancer of the liver [90]. ICG is known for its passive extravasation into tumour tissue due to the EPR effect, which has been noted using ICG in detecting cancers of the ovaries

[121], pancreas [48], and peritoneal metastasis [76]. The PDT effects of ICG have been explored in melanoma [122], colon cancer [116], and hepatocellular carcinoma [109].

Methylene blue is a diagnostically authorized dye with fluorescent visible and NIR characteristics and a distinctive bio-distribution model used for tumour diagnosis. Methylene blue is frequently included as a blue dye to define sentinel lymph nodes in combination with radio colloids [24]. It shows far-red fluorescence with a maximum emission of 688 nm at low concentrations. Several cancers have been identified including neuroendocrine insulinomas [132], fibrous pancreatic tumours [128], paragangliomas [120], and parathyroid adenomas [127]. Methylene blue also has photodynamic characteristics, with elevated effectiveness when light excites the production of triplet oxygen species [117].

7.3.3 Photodynamic diagnosis and lung cancer

The concept of PS fluorescence imaging for cancer tissue detection can also be expanded in any situation where the PS can be introduced to the tissue of interest and the fluorescence emission of the tissue can be obtained by a testing tool. Since various drug delivery mechanisms can be used to access distinct anatomical locations and developments in fibre optic fluorescence microscopy, the use of submillimetre diameter samples can be guided across small inner luminous areas [95].

In the 1960s it was shown how the diagnosis of lung cancer was improved by the development of the fibre optic bronchoscope, which was further revolutionized by the fluorescence bronchoscope for PDD in the 1970s, where clinical implementation of endoscopic PDD found that HPD and photo-irradiation could be used to identify early bronchogenic carcinoma and small lung cancer tumours [45]. Further early studies included the use of Porfimer sodium (Photofrin I/II) where the efficacy of PDD and PDT were evaluated. This clinical application was tested on patients with early squamous carcinoma, however, unspecific localisation of the PS was found in healthy tissue [81]. In another study HPD or Photofrin II was used for the localisation of early bronchogenic carcinoma, and carcinoma *in situ* was detected with low-dose Photofrin II with no apparent skin phototoxicity [71]. However, these Photofrin compounds had low tumour selectivity and fluorescence quantum yield and very complex devices were necessary for their detection. A more sensitive compound was tested using ALA, while a technique of inhalation of the drug was used for early detection of lung neoplasia, and the results indicated continual PPIX synthesis and confirmed the interpretation of fluorescence images with subsequent analysis of biopsies, also no adverse clinical effects were noted [8].

Following the enhancement of imaging technologies and advancements of PSs, researchers developed a PDD technique using the second-generation PS, mono-L-aspartyl chlorine e6 (Talaporfin sodium, Laserphyrin, NPe6), which has a major absorption band at 664 nm and has lower photosensitivity than Photofrin, and was approved for use in the diagnosis/treatment of centrally located early lung cancer by the Japanese government [124]. The researchers used an autofluorescence diagnostic system called SAFE-300 and a diode laser. The results indicated that they were able to clearly detect red fluorescence from the tumour by the PDD system using SAFE-3000 and, therefore, to accurately determine the tumour extent [125].

Up-to-date PDT with a 664 nm wavelength diode laser (PD laser, Panasonic Healthcare, Tokyo, Japan) using Talaporfin sodium (Laserphyrin, Meiji Seika Pharma, Tokyo, Japan; L-PDT) as the PS is approved for the treatment of both early and advanced stage lung cancers and can be also used for photodynamic diagnosis [82]. A simultaneous method video endoscope system allows for a dynamic colour reproduction and a more accurate observation. Some simultaneous method magnifying video endoscopes with a high-quality colour CCD chip allow the visualization of red fluorescent light emitted by photosensitized tissues when excited by light from a shortwave purple diode laser (wavelength 405 nm). This confirms that PDD can be performed endoscopically. A novel high-resolution magnifying video endoscope system, whereby both PDT and PDD can be performed, was successfully developed (XG-0001, Fujifilm, Tokyo, Japan). The XG-0001 is a magnifying video endoscope based on the commercially available EG-590ZW (Fujifilm), the magnification rate of which is up to 135 times, visualized on a 19 inch high-definition colour monitor. It has a spectral image processing function known as flexible spectral imaging colour enhancement (FICE) which is regarded as image enhanced endoscopy. XG-0001 allows easy intra-procedural viewing of PS accumulation in the tumour before initial laser irradiation or prior to additional laser irradiation, with a high-resolution magnifying endoscopic observation [82].

7.4 Photodynamic therapy

7.4.1 Photodynamic therapy

PDT encompasses the administration of a tumour-localizing photosensitizing agent that may involve metabolic formulation (i.e. a prodrug), preceded by stimulation of the agent by light of a specific wavelength. This treatment results in a series of photochemical and photobiological procedures that lead tumour tissues to suffer irreversible photodamage [32]. The present PDT revolution began in 1960 with experiments at the Mayo Clinic by Lipson and Schwartz, who identified that the injection of crude HP preparations prompted the fluorescence visualization of neoplastic caries during surgery. Schwartz treated HP with acetic acid and sulphuric acid and acquired a porphyrin combination he called 'HP derivative' (HPD), used by Lipson *et al* [41]. HPD includes a number of porphyrins, monomers, dimers, and oligomers [80]. HPD was partially purified to form Photofrin with the removal of the less active porphyrin monomers [31], which is also the PS most commonly used in clinical PDT. Photofrin's long-lasting skin phototoxicity launched several innovative PSs in clinical trials [40]. Photofrin absorbs only about 640 nm light, while light at longer wavelengths penetrates further into the tissue, however, most current sensitizers have a greater absorption range of 650–850 nm.

The PS is typically administered intravenously or topically in clinical environments, accompanied by illumination using a light delivery system appropriate for the treatment of the anatomical location. The time limit between PS administration

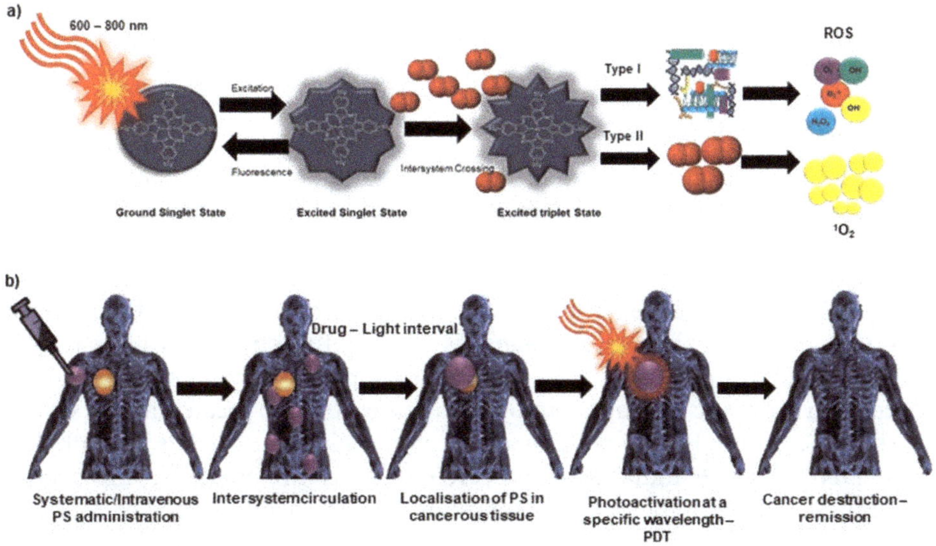

Figure 7.4. (a) A schematic representation of PDT where a PS is photo-activated, using red light, from its ground singlet state to its excited triplet state, that reacts with biomolecules and oxygen resulting in $^1O_2$ and ROS formation leading to cancer toxicity and cell death. (b) A schematic representation of PS administration, localisation, and PDT.

and the beginning of illumination with currently used PSs, often referred to as the drug–light interval (figure 7.4(b)), differs between 5 min to 24 h or more based on the particular PS and the target disease. Usually, the valuable spectrum of wavelengths for curative activation of PS is 600–800 nm, in order to avoid disruption by intracellular chromophores within the body, while maintaining the energy required to generate cytotoxic species such as $^1O_2$ [21].

In PDT, three basic components work simultaneously: molecular oxygen, a light source, and a PS. None of these are toxic individually [2]. Molecular oxygen (O_2) is the terminal electron acceptor of the aerobic respiration chain performed by the mitochondrial electron transport (MET) chain. Oxygen acts as an electron acceptor in the MET [126]. During PDT, a photochemical reaction uses free O_2, generating a highly reactive product called $^1O_2$ and ROS that can cause significant toxicity by apoptosis or necrosis leading to cancer cell death (figure 7.4(a)). Ground state/molecular oxygen has two unpaired electrons in the outermost antibonding orbitals residing separately. There are three possible states for O_2 depending on the electron configuration; the ground oxygen state is called a $^3O_2$ triplet state. $^1O_2$ is produced by inverting the spin of one of the outermost electrons during photo-oxygenation. Highly reactive, this type of oxygen is the predominant cytotoxic agent produced during PDT [10, 20, 77].

Due to the oxygen–hydrogen (O–H) energy stretching in water molecules, the lifetime of single oxygen in an aqueous environment is about 2 ms. The stretching and vibrational movements of water molecules dissipate the energy as heat. Because of the rapid reaction of $^1O_2$, its oxidative damage is reserved to a cell membrane diameter and confined to hydrophobic regions due to the nature of the hydrophobic PSs [77].

7.4.2 Photosensitizers used in PDT

A PS or photosensitizing agent is a chemical substance that can be stimulated with a particular wavelength linked to the absorption peak of the administered compound by monochromatic light and then pass energy to a chosen reactant. This is usually molecular oxygen that is transformed into ROS or (extremely unstable) single-state oxygen in the cancer tissue. This reacts quickly with any nearby biomolecules, leading to cytotoxicity through mechanisms of oxidative stress that ultimately kill the cancer cells [15, 67]. PDT PSs are primarily porphyrin or porphyrin-related products with aromatic hydrophobic ring structures and are located in one or more cell membrane. Many PSs do not penetrate cell nuclei, and PDT has a small ability to cause DNA damage, mutations, and carcinogenesis. Preferentially, PSs accumulates in cancer cells to mitochondrial membranes, endoplasmic reticulum, and Golgi complexes. $^1O_2$ species and other ROS generated in the membranes by PDT trigger photo-oxidant harm to proteins and lipids within a few nanometres of the PSs' binding locations. PDT causes rapid apoptosis, inflammatory reaction, tumour-specific and/or non-specific immune response, and damages the tumour bed's microvasculature. The impact on the vasculature is the most significant cause of its therapeutic effect with some PSs [124]. The PSs commonly used in cancer are based on the haemoglobin-based tetra pyrrole backbone that simulates protoporphyrin. Haemoglobin spectral absorbance ranges from 478–672 nm. This range transmits red light to visible blue, indicating that the PS structure has an impact on the bands of absorption. Beneficial PSs are anticipated to have a powerful absorbance maximum in the deep-red to near-infrared spectral region varying from 600 to 800 nm, enabling tissue absorption as density tends to increase with wavelength. However, due to their lower frequency, longer wavelengths are avoided as too little energy is provided for sufficient oxygen excitation. Preferably, a PS ought to have appropriate photophysical properties: a high-quantum yield of triplet formation ($\Phi T \geqslant 0.5$); a high $^1O_2$ quantum yield ($\Phi\Delta \geqslant 0.5$); a relatively long triplet-state lifetime (τT, μs range); and a high triplet-state energy ($\geqslant$94 kJ mol^{-1}). Other desired characteristics of PSs include: low dark toxicity in the absence of light and negligible cytotoxicity; preferential accumulation over healthy tissue in diseased/target tissue; rapid post-procedure clearance from the body to reduce side effects; high chemical stability; and single, well-characterised compounds, with a known and constant composition. The PS should be biologically accessible, as efficient PSs tend to be comparatively hydrophobic substances that diffuse rapidly into tumour cells and find themselves in intracellular membrane structures such as mitochondria and endoplasmic reticulum. This should generate a significant inflammatory reaction via apoptosis which has an immunogenic impact on cancerous cells [1, 15].

Tetra pyrroles have very good photophysical properties. They have long triplet lives and high quantity outputs. Due to the low energy gap between the triplets of most tetra pyrroles and molecular oxygen, the $^1O_2$ quantity yields are also high [49].

In haem (porphyrins), chlorophyll, and bacteriochlorophyll, naturally occurring tetra pyrrole structures are found. Phthalocyanines are synthetically synthesized tetra pyrroles. The Q-band moves to longer wavelengths and increases in size as the double bonds of the pyrrole ring start in porphyrins and go to chlorines and bacteriochlorin (figure 7.5) [54].

HPD and a purified form of HPD, Photofrin II, were the first-generation PSs used in early clinical trials [133]. HPD, used in a variety of cancers, has been shown to be minimally effective due to limitations including structural complexity, leading to unspecific tissue selectivity as well as unstable photochemical damage, and a short wavelength of activation preventing sufficient tissue penetration, resulting in photosensitive toxicity, thus promoting the development of second-generation PSs [65]. Second-generation PSs have been improved by changing their composition and structure, increasing the photosensitivity, spectrum of absorption, and selectivity of tissue. Second-generation PSs are built around the structure of porphyrin. Benzoporphyrins, purpurins, texaphyrins, phthalocyanines, naphthalocyanines, and PpIX are some of the second-generation PSs [12].

Improving chemically pure PSs of the first-generation with favourable photochemical and pharmacological properties leads to the synthesis of PSs based on chlorine [88]. Chlorine (e6) is derived from natural chlorophyll with a 650 and 700 nm absorption spectrum. Significant clinical chlorin PSs include: m-tetrahydroxyphenylchlorin (Temoporfin or Foscan) [130], benzoporphyrin derivative (Verteporfin) [22], and Radachlorin (now Bremachlorin) [13]. The aspartyl derivatives of chlorin-e6, monoaspartyl chlorin-e6 (MACE), and diaspartyl chlorin-e6 (DACE), have been reported as effective PSs *in vitro* compared to Photofrin II [100].

It was suggested that bacteriochlorin derivatives meet the characteristics of an ideal PS [25]. It has been shown that a bacteriochlorin-based PS has characteristics of a strong absorption band with a long wavelength of 732 nm, a high yield of $^1O_2$, low dark toxicity, and significant cytotoxicity when activated by light *in vitro* and

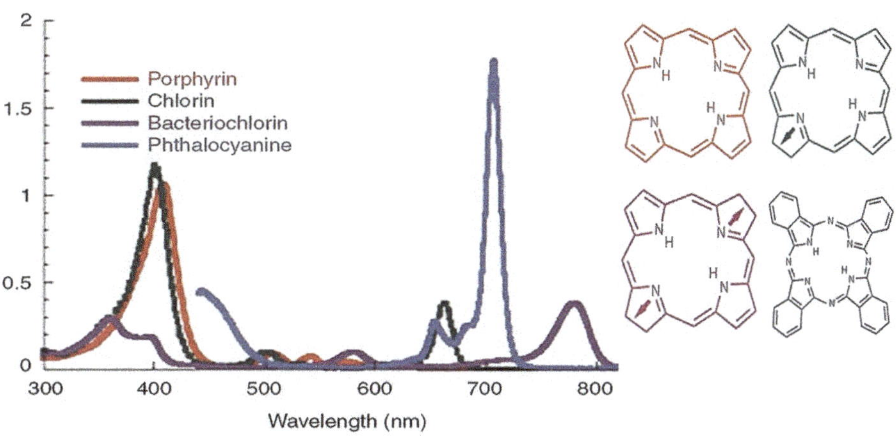

Figure 7.5. Tetrapyrrolic absorption spectra showing porphyrins, chlorins, bacteriochlorin, and phthalocyanines.

in vivo [135]. In clinical trials, the lead-containing bacteriophaeophorbide derivative and its new water-soluble derivative known as TOOKAD were tested as well as the new bacteriochlorin derivative known as LUZ11 [6, 103].

Phthalocyanines (PCs) are synthesized PSs. The most common method of synthesizing PCs is the reaction of o-cyanobenzamide to form tetrabenzoporphyrazine/phthalocyanine with phthalimide. By coordinating metal ions within their nitrogen core, their physical properties are easily altered. They have increased yields and spectroscopic properties compared to porphyrins. Typically, PCs with low energy Q-bands are much more intense between 650–750 nm [108]. PCs have a drawback that involves the lack of tumour cell specificity. However, this has led to experiments that have made the PS more specific by conjugating PCs with gold dispersed nanoparticles (Au-NPs) in an emulsion. In comparing PC alone to Au-NP conjugated PC, the findings showed a significant response to tumour tissue [19].

7.4.3 Photodynamic therapy and lung cancer

In 1980, in a patient with a weak cardiopulmonary status in which surgery was not feasible, the first endoscopic PDT operation for human lung disease was conducted. This was a developed squamous cell carcinoma that blocked the right main bronchus, and PDT led to the bronchus opening. The second instance in March 1980 was an early phase squamous cell carcinoma of the upper right bronchus [55]. The patient was a 74 year old man who refused surgical intervention, and this became the first case in history where PDT for early-stage lung cancer was performed. A full recovery was achieved and the patient stayed free of disease for >5 years [58].

It is essential to decrease the magnitude of lung resection in lung cancer patients with poor pulmonary function. Clinicians started using PDT before operations in 1985 [59]. In October 1994, the Japanese government endorsed PDT with Photofrin. In 1995 Photofrin was adopted in the United States for oesophageal cancer by the Food and Drugs Administration (FDA) and published in 1998 for the treatment of early NSCLC [32].

Okunaka *et al* noted that laser endoscopic surgery, in particular the efficacy of PDT using Photofrin as a PS, has now attained a status as an efficient lung cancer treatment method. Twenty-six people with lung cancer received preoperative PDT to either reduce the resection magnitude or increase operability. After the intravenous injection of Photofrin, PDT using a bronchoscope was conducted with topical anaesthesia. Two to nine weeks after the original PDT, the operation was conducted. The original objective of PDT was accomplished in 22 of the 26 individuals studied, i.e. to either decrease the magnitude of resection or transform inoperable disease to operable status. With the implementation of preoperative PDT, the survival level of T3 (primary bronchus infection) instances handled by operation alone improved considerably from 50.9% to 60.0%. This notable outcome meant that this choice of PDT as a preoperative laser irradiation could add to sophisticated lung malignancy management [86].

Photofrin is currently authorized for use in obstructive pulmonary cancer globally [129]. Skin photosensitivity, which can last as long as 4–6 weeks, is the main side effect of Photofrin itself. In cancer cells, photofrin remains longer than in ordinary cells, giving some selectivity of tissue. When the cancer cells are subjected to 630 nm red light, Photofrin absorbs the light and forms toxic radicals in the presence of oxygen [37]. Other trials using Photofrin demonstrated that in a small retrospective study the PS was well accepted and efficient as part of a multi-modal NSCLC endobronchial therapy. In combination with high-dose brachytherapy (HDR), PDT accomplished extended control of local tumours. PDT following HDR may attain long-term tumour control relative to other modalities or therapy alone [131]. Studies have also shown that postoperative PDT patients have an enhanced mean survival time relative to conventional postoperative care patients [23]. In another study, mesothelioma patients with radical pleurectomy accompanied by postoperative PDT showed exceptionally lengthy survival despite recurrences and no enhanced progression-free survival, most probably due to lung conservation and/or the impact of PDT [36]. PDT using Photofrin was an excellent option for palliative chemotherapy or radiation therapy in unresectable lung cancer as it reached a general reaction of nearly 87% and enhanced the quality of life for patients as a stand-alone treatment. With several instances of complete remission, it even showed curative possibilities [18].

Laserphyrin, which was clinically licensed by the Japanese government in 2003, is another PS used for lung cancer. NPe6 (Talaporfin sodium, Laserphyrin, Meiji Seika, Tokyo, Japan) is a second-generation, water-soluble photosensitizer with 799.69 molecular weight and an annulus of chlorine. Its maximum absorption peak is at 407 nm and a second peak is at 664 nm [125]. Laserphyrin has a strong tumour affinity and is stimulated by noticeable red light with a longer wavelength of 664 nm, making it possible to penetrate deeper and better into living tissues [57].

Usuda *et al* evaluated the PDT impact of NPe6 used for bronchogenic carcinomas in central airways >1.0 cm in diameter, concluding that NPe6-PDT has a powerful antitumor effect against centrally situated early pulmonary tumours >1.0 cm in diameter that have penetrated beyond the bronchial cartilage, thus allowing the remaining cancer lesions to be destroyed after the mass decrease of large nodular cancers. Therefore, the PDT rules for lung cancer should be amended with regard to tumour size, as the use of NPe6-PDT will allow clinical clues for PDT to be extended [123]. In the latest research by Kimura *et al* where they used PDT and chemotherapy to treat early phase lung cancer with airway stenosis, they discovered that PDT therapy was efficient in treating patients with advanced airway stenosis lung cancer. All individuals experienced enhanced symptoms and quality of life as soon as a week after therapy with PDT. Moreover, the significant increase in bronchial lumen openings and the avoidance of obstructive pneumonia suggested an objective reaction. In addition, the combination of PDT with conventional therapy techniques seems safe, even in patients with problems such as interstitial lung disease, without increased toxicity [62].

Radachlorin is a second-generation PS, also recognized in the EU as Bremachlorin, and it was created and clinically endorsed in Russia in 2009. This

PS has been researched for use in cutaneous basal cell carcinoma as a topical administrative medication. The drug's photo-activation involves 3 W 662 ± 3 nm with semiconductor lasers [64]. A pilot study examined its palliative effectiveness and safety as a multi-modal therapy for advanced phase lung cancer with main airway obstruction. Using the water-soluble chlorine E6 complex, the drug was administered intravenously, followed by light activation using a bronchoscopic fibre optic. With significantly improved lung capacity and function, all patients showed improvement in their symptoms. One year after PDT, survival for PDT-treated individuals was considerably enhanced relative to the one-year survival level for NSCLC-treated patients with systemic chemotherapy alone [50]. Radachlorin has been used as a neoadjuvant therapy in previous research in an effort to reduce tumours and enhance the chances of effective surgery. Chemotherapy and preoperative PDT significantly increased the number of patients eligible for radical resection compared to neoadjuvant chemotherapy alone [3].

Overall, Photofrin-PDT is efficient as a palliative therapy for lung cancer, but is linked with extended photosensitivity of the skin. In addition, with bigger lesions, it demonstrates less efficiency. On the other hand, newer PSs such as Talaporfin with greater bands of absorption at longer wavelengths demonstrate enhanced efficacy, making them appropriate for instances where Photofrin fails. An additional benefit of these second-generation PSs is the reduced half-life resulting in smaller phases of photosensitivity and fewer instances of associated adverse effects. These findings show that PDT can be readily introduced in conventional treatment schemes, either pre- or post-operative, to enhance treatment results.

7.5 Conclusion

Lung cancer continues to be a common cause of death associated with cancer. It grows over a time period in which early diagnosis by standard therapies can contribute to elimination. Existing diagnostic imaging methods are PET, MRI, CT, and x-rays, which provide structural information of the lung cancer tumour, where recognition sensitivity decreases during the resection phase as the size of the unresected disease decreases. Chemotherapy, radiation therapy, surgery, focused drug therapy, and immunotherapy are traditional lung cancer treatments. Most of these treatments, however, pose a danger of adverse side effects resulting in a poor standard of living.

It has become apparent that cancer imaging can play a crucial role in optimizing and improving cancer therapy's effect. Over the years, cancer imaging has been at the centre of the quest for effective drugs, taking advantage of the technical changes in different imaging modalities. It is evident that PSs can be applied with fluorescent tumour surgery for diagnostic reasons to create concise resection margins. This affects the prognosis and quality of life of the patient. PDD also demonstrates an improvement in the efficacy of PDT in PS dose administration and laser irradiation.

At present, PDT is increasingly being used alone or as an auxiliary treatment to cure thoracic malignancies. Exerted effects include apoptosis and necrosis, tumour vasculature harm, and inflammatory reactions. With repeated procedures, it does not lose effectiveness and allows combination therapy.

Given these benefits and important advances in optical technology that allowed deeper lying tumours to be penetrated by light, an absence of phase III clinical trials has limited the healthcare industry's utilization of PDT as a frontline cancer treatment. This can be attributed to current PDT problems involving poor tumour selectivity in malignant metastatic tumours in pulmonary cancer therapy. However, research needs to be carried out to show the potential advantages of PDT and the need to boost clinical study financing and uptake using next-generation PSs that offer sophisticated focused delivery and enhanced photodynamic dose, coupled with contemporary light distribution techniques.

Acknowledgements

The authors would like to thank the South African Research Chairs Initiative and National Research Foundation of the Department of Science and Technology (SARChI—NRF—DST) (grant number: 98337), the University of Johannesburg, and the National Laser Centre (NLC) for their financial grant support.

References

[1] Abrahamse H and Hamblin M R 2016 New photosensitizers for photodynamic therapy *Biochem. J.* **473** 347–64

[2] Agostinis P *et al* 2011 Photodynamic therapy of cancer: an update *CA Cancer J. Clin.* **61** 250–81

[3] Akopov A, Rusanov A, Gerasin A, Kazakov N, Urtenova M and Chistyakov I 2014 Preoperative endobronchial photodynamic therapy improves resectability in initially irresectable (inoperable) locally advanced non small cell lung cancer *Photodiagnosis Photodyn. Ther.* **11** 259–64

[4] Al Feghali K A, Ballout R A, Khamis A M, Akl E A and Geara F B 2018 Prophylactic cranial irradiation in patients with non-small-cell lung cancer: a systematic review and meta-analysis of randomized controlled trials *Front. Oncol.* **8** 115

[5] Amini A, Yeh N, Gaspar L E, Kavanagh B and Karam S D 2014 Stereotactic body radiation therapy (SBRT) for lung cancer patients previously treated with conventional radiotherapy: a review *Radiat. Oncol.* **9** 210

[6] Azzouzi A R, Lebdai S, Benzaghou F and Stief C 2015 Vascular-targeted photodynamic therapy with TOOKAD(R) soluble in localized prostate cancer: standardization of the procedure *World J. Urol.* **33** 937–44

[7] Basu A K 2018 DNA damage, mutagenesis and cancer *Int. J. Mol. Sci.* **19** 970

[8] Baumgartner R, Huber R M, Schulz H, Stepp H, Rick K, Gamarra F, Leberig A and Roth C 1996 Inhalation of 5-aminolevulinic acid: a new technique for fluorescence detection of early stage lung cancer *J. Photochem. Photobiol.* B **36** 169–74

[9] Ben-David U, Beroukhim R and Golub T R 2019 Genomic evolution of cancer models: perils and opportunities *Nat. Rev. Cancer* **19** 97–109

[10] Benov L 2015 Photodynamic therapy: current status and future directions *Med. Princ. Pract.* **24** 14–28

[11] Benson R C Jr, Farrow G M, Kinsey J H, Cortese D A, Zincke H and Utz D C 1982 Detection and localization of *in situ* carcinoma of the bladder with hematoporphyrin derivative *Mayo Clin. Proc.* **57** 548–55

[12] Berg K *et al* 2005 Porphyrin-related photosensitizers for cancer imaging and therapeutic applications *J. Microsc.* **218** 133–47

[13] Biswas R, Moon J H and Ahn J C 2014 Chlorin e6 derivative radachlorin mainly accumulates in mitochondria, lysosome and endoplasmic reticulum and shows high affinity toward tumors in nude mice in photodynamic therapy *Photochem. Photobiol.* **90** 1108–18

[14] Board PDQATE 2002 *PDQ Cancer Information Summaries* (Bethesda, MD: National Cancer Institute)

[15] Bown S G 2013 Photodynamic therapy for photochemists *Philos. Trans. Series* A **371** 20120371

[16] Bray F, Ferlay J, Soerjomataram I, Siegel R L, Torre L A and Jemal A 2018 Global cancer statistics 2018: GLOBOCAN estimates of incidence and mortality worldwide for 36 cancers in 185 countries *CA Cancer J. Clin.* **68** 394–424

[17] Bu L, Shen B and Cheng Z 2014 Fluorescent imaging of cancerous tissues for targeted surgery *Adv. Drug Deliv. Rev.* **76** 21–38

[18] Cai X J, Li W M, Zhang L Y, Wang X W, Luo R C and Li L B 2013 Photodynamic therapy for intractable bronchial lung cancer *Photodiagnosis Photodyn. Ther.* **10** 672–6

[19] Camerin M, Magaraggia M, Soncin M, Jori G, Moreno M, Chambrier I, Cook M J and Russell D A 2010 The *in vivo* efficacy of phthalocyanine-nanoparticle conjugates for the photodynamic therapy of amelanotic melanoma *Eur. J. Cancer* **46** 1910–8

[20] Castano A P, Demidova T N and Hamblin M R 2004 Mechanisms in photodynamic therapy: part one-photosensitizers, photochemistry and cellular localization *Photodiagnosis Photodyn. Ther.* **1** 279–93

[21] Celli J P, Spring B Q, Rizvi I, Evans C L, Samkoe K S, Verma S, Pogue B W and Hasan T 2010 Imaging and photodynamic therapy: mechanisms, monitoring, and optimization *Chem. Rev.* **110** 2795–838

[22] Chan W M, Lim T H, Pece A, Silva R and Yoshimura N 2010 Verteporfin PDT for non-standard indications—a review of current literature *Graefes Arch. Clin. Exp. Ophthalmol.* **248** 613–26

[23] Chen K C, Hsieh Y S, Tseng Y F, Shieh M J, Chen J S, Lai H S and Lee J M 2015 Pleural photodynamic therapy and surgery in lung cancer and thymoma patients with pleural spread *PLoS One* **10** e0133230

[24] Cousins A, Thompson S K, Wedding A B and Thierry B 2014 Clinical relevance of novel imaging technologies for sentinel lymph node identification and staging *Biotechnol. Adv.* **32** 269–79

[25] Dabrowski J M, Arnaut L G, Pereira M M, Urbanska K, Simoes S, Stochel G and Cortes L 2012 Combined effects of singlet oxygen and hydroxyl radical in photodynamic therapy with photostable bacteriochlorins: evidence from intracellular fluorescence and increased photodynamic efficacy *in vitro Free Radic. Biol. Med.* **52** 1188–200

[26] Daga A, Ansari A, Patel S, Mirza S, Rawal R and Umrania V 2015 Current drugs and drug targets in non-small cell lung cancer: limitations and opportunities *Asian Pac. J. Cancer Prev.* **16** 4147–56

[27] Dela Cruz C S, Tanoue L T and Matthay R A 2011 Lung cancer: epidemiology, etiology, and prevention *Clin. Chest Med.* **32** 605–44

[28] Desmettre T, Devoisselle J M and Mordon S 2000 Fluorescence properties and metabolic features of indocyanine green (ICG) as related to angiography *Surv. Ophthalmol.* **45** 15–27

[29] Detterbeck F C, Mazzone P J, Naidich D P and Bach P B 2013 Screening for lung cancer: diagnosis and management of lung cancer *Chest* **143** e78S–92S

[30] Domvri K *et al* 2013 Molecular targeted drugs and biomarkers in NSCLC, the evolving role of individualized therapy *J. Cancer* **4** 736–54

[31] Dougherty T J 1996 A brief history of clinical photodynamic therapy development at Roswell Park Cancer Institute *J. Clin. Laser Med. Surg.* **14** 219–21

[32] Dougherty T J, Gomer C J, Henderson B W, Jori G, Kessel D, Korbelik M, Moan J and Peng Q 1998 Photodynamic therapy *J. Natl. Cancer Inst.* **90** 889–905

[33] Fakiris A J, McGarry R C, Yiannoutsos C T, Papiez L, Williams M, Henderson M A and Timmerman R 2009 Stereotactic body radiation therapy for early-stage non-small-cell lung carcinoma: four-year results of a prospective phase II study *Int. J. Radiat. Oncol. Biol. Phys.* **75** 677–82

[34] Figge F H, Weiland G S and Manganiello L O 1948 Cancer detection and therapy; affinity of neoplastic, embryonic, and traumatized tissues for porphyrins and metalloporphyrins *Proc. Soc. Exp. Biol. Med.* **68** 640

[35] Frangioni J V 2003 *In vivo* near-infrared fluorescence imaging *Curr. Opin. Chem. Biol.* **7** 626–34

[36] Friedberg J S, Culligan M J, Mick R, Stevenson J, Hahn S M, Sterman D, Punekar S, Glatstein E and Cengel K 2012 Radical pleurectomy and intraoperative photodynamic therapy for malignant pleural mesothelioma *Ann. Thorac. Surg.* **93** 1658–67

[37] Furuse K *et al* 1993 A prospective phase II study on photodynamic therapy with photofrin II for centrally located early-stage lung cancer. The Japan Lung Cancer Photodynamic Therapy Study Group *J. Clin. Oncol.* **11** 1852–7

[38] Glatzer M, Schmid S, Radovic M, Früh M and Putora P M 2017 The role of radiation therapy in the management of small cell lung cancer *Breathe* **13** e87–94

[39] Goldstraw P, Crowley J, Chansky K, Giroux D J, Groome P A, Rami-Porta R, Postmus P E, Rusch V and Sobin L 2007 The IASLC Lung Cancer Staging Project: proposals for the revision of the TNM stage groupings in the forthcoming (seventh) edition of the TNM classification of malignant tumours *J. Thorac. Oncol.* **2** 706–14

[40] Gomer C J 1991 Preclinical examination of first and second generation photosensitizers used in photodynamic therapy *Photochem. Photobiol.* **54** 1093–107

[41] Gray M J, Lipson R, Maeck J V, Parker L and Romeyn D 1967 Use of hematoporphyrin derivative in detection and management of cervical cancer *Am. J. Obstet. Gynecol.* **99** 766–71

[42] Gridelli C, Ardizzoni A, Le Chevalier T, Manegold C, Perrone F, Thatcher N, van Zandwijk N, Di Maio M, Martelli O and De Marinis F 2004 Treatment of advanced non-small-cell lung cancer patients with ECOG performance status 2: results of an European Experts Panel *Ann. Oncol.* **15** 419–26

[43] Grutters J P, Kessels A G, Pijls-Johannesma M, De Ruysscher D, Joore M A and Lambin P 2010 Comparison of the effectiveness of radiotherapy with photons, protons and carbon-ions for non-small cell lung cancer: a meta-analysis *Radiother. Oncol.* **95** 32–40

[44] Hamilton W, Peters T J, Round A and Sharp D 2005 What are the clinical features of lung cancer before the diagnosis is made? A population based case-control study *Thorax* **60** 1059–65

[45] Hayata Y, Kato H and Konaka C 1982 Fiberoptic bronchoscopic laser photoradiation for tumor localization in lung cancer *Chest* **82** 10–4

[46] How J, Gotlieb W H, Press J Z, Abitbol J, Pelmus M, Ferenczy A, Probst S, Gotlieb R, Brin S and Lau S 2015 Comparing indocyanine green, technetium, and blue dye for sentinel lymph node mapping in endometrial cancer *Gynecol. Oncol.* **137** 436–42

[47] Huang C-Y, Ju D-T, Chang C-F, Muralidhar Reddy P and Velmurugan B K 2017 A review on the effects of current chemotherapy drugs and natural agents in treating non-small cell lung cancer *BioMedicine* **7** 23

[48] Hutteman M, van der Vorst J R, Mieog J S, Bonsing B A, Hartgrink H H, Kuppen P J, Lowik C W, Frangioni J V, van de Velde C J and Vahrmeijer A L 2011 Near-infrared fluorescence imaging in patients undergoing pancreaticoduodenectomy *Eur. Surg. Res.* **47** 90–7

[49] Imran M, Ramzan M, Qureshi A K, Khan M A and Tariq M 2018 Emerging applications of porphyrins and metalloporphyrins in biomedicine and diagnostic magnetic resonance imaging *Biosensors* **8** 95

[50] Ji W, Yoo J W, Bae E K, Lee J H and Choi C M 2013 The effect of Radachlorin(R) PDT in advanced NSCLC: a pilot study *Photodiagnosis Photodyn. Ther.* **10** 120–6

[51] Jin Y, Chen M and Yu X 2016 Comparison of the 7(th) and proposed 8(th) editions of the AJCC/UICC TNM staging system for non-small cell lung cancer undergoing radical surgery *Sci. Rep.* **6** 33587

[52] Juarranz A, Jaen P, Sanz-Rodriguez F, Cuevas J and Gonzalez S 2008 Photodynamic therapy of cancer. Basic principles and applications *Clin. Transl. Oncol.* **10** 148–54

[53] Karim S M and Zekri J 2012 Chemotherapy for small cell lung cancer: a comprehensive review *Oncol. Rev.* **6** e4

[54] Kashef N, Huang Y Y and Hamblin M R 2017 Advances in antimicrobial photodynamic inactivation at the nanoscale *Nanophotonics* **6** 853–79

[55] Kato H *et al* 1984 Clinical measurement of tumor fluorescence using a new diagnostic system with hematoporphyrin derivative, laser photoradiation, and a spectroscope *Lasers Surg. Med.* **4** 49–58

[56] Kato H and Cortese D A 1985 Early detection of lung cancer by means of hematoporphyrin derivative fluorescence and laser photoradiation *Clin. Chest Med.* **6** 237–53

[57] Kato H *et al* 2003 Phase II clinical study of photodynamic therapy using mono-L-aspartyl chlorin e6 and diode laser for early superficial squamous cell carcinoma of the lung *Lung Cancer* **42** 103–11

[58] Kato H, Konaka C, Kawate N, Shinohara H, Kinoshita K, Noguchi M, Ootomo S and Hayata Y 1986 Five-year disease-free survival of a lung cancer patient treated only by photodynamic therapy *Chest* **90** 768–70

[59] Kato H *et al* 1985 Preoperative laser photodynamic therapy in combination with operation in lung cancer *J. Thorac. Cardiovasc. Surg.* **90** 420–9

[60] Kennedy J C, Pottier R H and Pross D C 1990 Photodynamic therapy with endogenous protoporphyrin IX: basic principles and present clinical experience *J. Photochem. Photobiol. B Biol.* **6** 143–8

[61] Kessel D and Cheng M L 1985 Biological and biophysical properties of the tumor-localizing component of hematoporphyrin derivative *Cancer Res.* **45** 3053–7

[62] Kimura M, Miyajima K, Kojika M, Kono T and Kato H 2015 Photodynamic therapy (PDT) with chemotherapy for advanced lung cancer with airway stenosis *Int. J. Mol. Sci.* **16** 25466–75

[63] Kinsey J H, Cortese D A and Sanderson D R 1978 Detection of hematoporphyrin fluorescence during fiberoptic bronchoscopy to localize early bronchogenic carcinoma *Mayo Clin. Proc.* **53** 594–600

[64] Kochneva E V, Filonenko E V, Vakulovskaya E G, Scherbakova E G, Seliverstov O V, Markichev N A and Reshetnickov A V 2010 Photosensitizer Radachlorin(R): skin cancer PDT phase II clinical trials *Photodiagnosis Photodyn. Ther.* **7** 258–67

[65] Kou J, Dou D and Yang L 2017 Porphyrin photosensitizers in photodynamic therapy and its applications *Oncotarget* **8** 81591–603

[66] Koukis I, Gkiozos I, Ntanos I, Kainis E and Syrigos K N 2013 Clinical and surgical-pathological staging in early non-small cell lung cancer *Oncol. Rev.* **7** e7

[67] Kurutas E B 2016 The importance of antioxidants which play the role in cellular response against oxidative/nitrosative stress: current state *Nutr. J.* **15** 71

[68] Kyriazis G A, Balin H and Lipson R L 1973 Hematoporphyrin-derivative-fluorescence test colposcopy and colpophotography in the diagnosis of atypical metaplasia, dysplasia, and carcinoma *in situ* of the cervix uteri *Am. J. Obstet. Gynecol.* **117** 375–80

[69] Lackey A and Donington J S 2013 Surgical management of lung cancer *Semin. Intervent. Radiol.* **30** 133–40

[70] Lagerwaard F J, Verstegen N E, Haasbeek C J, Slotman B J, Paul M A, Smit E F and Senan S 2012 Outcomes of stereotactic ablative radiotherapy in patients with potentially operable stage I non-small cell lung cancer *Int. J. Radiat. Oncol. Biol. Phys.* **83** 348–53

[71] Lam S, Palcic B, McLean D, Hung J, Korbelik M and Profio E 1990 Detection of early lung cancer using low dose photofrin II *Chest* **97** 333–7

[72] Langer C J, Besse B, Gualberto A, Brambilla E and Soria J C 2010 The evolving role of histology in the management of advanced non-small-cell lung cancer *J. Clin. Oncol.* **28** 5311–20

[73] Lemjabbar-Alaoui H, Hassan O U, Yang Y-W and Buchanan P 2015 Lung cancer: biology and treatment options *Biochim. Biophys. Acta* **1856** 189–210

[74] Leonard J R and Beck W L 1971 Hematoporphyrin fluorescence: an aid in diagnosis of malignant neoplasms *Laryngoscope* **81** 365–72

[75] Liam C K, Andarini S, Lee P, Ho J C, Chau N Q and Tscheikuna J 2015 Lung cancer staging now and in the future *Respirology* **20** 526–34

[76] Liberale G, Vankerckhove S, Caldon M G, Ahmed B, Moreau M, Nakadi I E, Larsimont D, Donckier V and Bourgeois P 2016 Fluorescence imaging after indocyanine green injection for detection of peritoneal metastases in patients undergoing cytoreductive surgery for peritoneal carcinomatosis from colorectal cancer: a pilot study *Ann. Surg.* **264** 1110–5

[77] Macdonald I J and Dougherty T J 2001 Basic principles of photodynamic therapy *J. Porphyr. Phthalocya.* **05** 105–29

[78] Masters G A *et al* 2015 Systemic therapy for stage IV non-small-cell lung cancer: American Society of Clinical Oncology Clinical Practice Guideline update *J. Clin. Oncol.* **33** 3488–515

[79] Matoba Y, Banno K, Kisu I and Aoki D 2018 Clinical application of photodynamic diagnosis and photodynamic therapy for gynecologic malignant diseases: a review *Photodiagnosis Photodyn. Ther.* **24** 52–7

[80] Moan J 1986 Porphyrin photosensitization and phototherapy *Photochem. Photobiol.* **43** 681–90

[81] Monnier P, Savary M, Fontolliet C, Wagnieres G, Chatelain A, Cornaz P, Depeursinge C and Van Den Bergh H 1990 Photodetection and photodynamic therapy of 'early' squamous cell carcinomas of the pharynx, oesophagus and tracheo-bronchial tree *Lasers Med. Sci.* **5** 149–69

[82] Nakamura T and Oinuma T 2014 Usefulness of photodynamic diagnosis and therapy using talaporfin sodium for an advanced-aged patient with inoperable gastric cancer (a secondary publication) *Laser Ther.* **23** 201–10

[83] Nall R 2018 What to know about lung cancer *Medical News Today*

[84] Nasim F and Ost D E 2019 Management of the solitary pulmonary nodule *Curr. Opin. Pulm. Med.* **25** 344–53

[85] Nishie H, Kataoka H, Yano S, Kikuchi J-I, Hayashi N, Narumi A, Nomoto A, Kubota E and Joh T 2016 A next-generation bifunctional photosensitizer with improved water-solubility for photodynamic therapy and diagnosis *Oncotarget* **7** 74259–68

[86] Okunaka T, Hiyoshi T, Furukawa K, Yamamoto H, Tsuchida T, Usuda J, Kumasaka H, Ishida J, Konaka C and Kato H 1999 Lung cancers treated with photodynamic therapy and surgery *Diagn. Ther. Endosc.* **5** 155–60

[87] Onishi H *et al* 2011 Stereotactic body radiotherapy (SBRT) for operable stage I non-small-cell lung cancer: can SBRT be comparable to surgery? *Int. J. Radiat. Oncol. Biol. Phys.* **81** 1352–8

[88] Pandey R K, Bellnier D A, Smith K M and Dougherty T J 1991 Chlorin and porphyrin derivatives as potential photosensitizers in photodynamic therapy *Photochem. Photobiol.* **53** 65–72

[89] Paoletti L, Pastis N J, Denlinger C E and Silvestri G A 2011 A decade of advances in treatment of early-stage lung cancer *Clin. Chest Med.* **32** 827–38

[90] Peloso A *et al* 2013 Combined use of intraoperative ultrasound and indocyanine green fluorescence imaging to detect liver metastases from colorectal cancer *HPB* **15** 928–34

[91] Pilleron S, Sarfati D, Janssen-Heijnen M, Vignat J, Ferlay J, Bray F and Soerjomataram I 2019 Global cancer incidence in older adults, 2012 and 2035: a population-based study *Int. J. Cancer* **144** 49–58

[92] Pisters K M *et al* 2007 Cancer Care Ontario and American Society of Clinical Oncology adjuvant chemotherapy and adjuvant radiation therapy for stages I–IIIA resectable non small-cell lung cancer guideline *J. Clin. Oncol.* **25** 5506–18

[93] Policard A 1924 Etude sur les aspects offerts par des tumeurs experimentales examines a la lumiere de Wood *C. R. Soc. Biol.* **91** 1423–4

[94] Purandare N C and Rangarajan V 2015 Imaging of lung cancer: implications on staging and management *Indian J. Radiol. Imaging* **25** 109–20

[95] Rai P, Mallidi S, Zheng X, Rahmanzadeh R, Mir Y, Elrington S, Khurshid A and Hasan T 2010 Development and applications of photo-triggered theranostic agents *Adv. Drug Deliv. Rev.* **62** 1094–124

[96] Ramalingam S and Belani C 2008 Systemic chemotherapy for advanced non-small cell lung cancer: recent advances and future directions *Oncologist* **13** 5–13

[97] Rassmussen-Taxdal D S, Ward G E and Figge F H 1955 Fluorescence of human lymphatic and cancer tissues following high doses of intravenous hematoporphyrin *Cancer* **8** 78–81

[98] Rivera M P, Mehta A C and Wahidi M M 2013 Establishing the diagnosis of lung cancer: diagnosis and management of lung cancer *Chest* **143** e142S–65S

[99] Rivlin N, Brosh R, Oren M and Rotter V 2011 Mutations in the p53 tumor suppressor gene: important milestones at the various steps of tumorigenesis *Genes Cancer* **2** 466–74

[100] Roberts W G, Shiau F Y, Nelson J S, Smith K M and Berns M W 1988 *In vitro* characterization of monoaspartyl chlorin e6 and diaspartyl chlorin e6 for photodynamic therapy *J. Natl. Cancer Inst.* **80** 330–6

[101] Rollakanti K R, Kanick S C, Davis S C, Pogue B W and Maytin E V 2013 Techniques for fluorescence detection of protoporphyrin IX in skin cancers associated with photodynamic therapy *Photonics Lasers Med.* **2** 287–303

[102] Rosenthal E L *et al* 2015 Safety and tumor specificity of cetuximab-IRDye800 for surgical navigation in head and neck cancer *Clin. Cancer Res.* **21** 3658–66

[103] Saavedra R, Rocha L B, Dabrowski J M and Arnaut L G 2014 Modulation of biodistribution, pharmacokinetics, and photosensitivity with the delivery vehicle of a bacteriochlorin photosensitizer for photodynamic therapy *ChemMedChem* **9** 390–8

[104] Schaafsma B E, Mieog J S, Hutteman M, van der Vorst J R, Kuppen P J, Lowik C W, Frangioni J V, van de Velde C J and Vahrmeijer A L 2011 The clinical use of indocyanine green as a near-infrared fluorescent contrast agent for image-guided oncologic surgery *J. Surg. Oncol.* **104** 323–32

[105] Scherer J 1841 Untersuchungen Liebigs *Ann. Chem. Pharm.* **40** 1–64

[106] Schrank Z, Chhabra G, Lin L, Iderzorig T, Osude C, Khan N, Kuckovic A, Singh S, Miller R J and Puri N 2018 Current molecular-targeted therapies in NSCLC and their mechanism of resistance *Cancers* **10** 224

[107] Scott W J, Howington J, Feigenberg S, Movsas B and Pisters K 2007 Treatment of non-small cell lung cancer stage I and stage II: ACCP evidence-based clinical practice guidelines *Chest* **132** 234S–42S

[108] Swavey S and Tran M 2013 Porphyrin and Phthalocyanine Photosensitizers as PDT agents: a new modality for the treatment of melanoma *Recent Advances in the Biology, Therapy and Management of Melanoma* ed L M Davids (Rijeka: InTech) pp 253–82

[109] Shirata C *et al* 2017 Near-infrared photothermal/photodynamic therapy with indocyanine green induces apoptosis of hepatocellular carcinoma cells through oxidative stress *Sci. Rep.* **7** 13958

[110] Skarlos D V *et al* 1994 Randomized comparison of etoposide-cisplatin vs etoposide-carboplatin and irradiation in small-cell lung cancer. A Hellenic Co-operative Oncology Group study *Ann. Oncol.* **5** 601–7

[111] Sokolenko A P and Imyanitov E N 2018 Molecular diagnostics in clinical oncology *Front. Mol. Biosci.* **5** 76

[112] Soucheray M *et al* 2015 Intratumoral heterogeneity in EGFR-mutant NSCLC results in divergent resistance mechanisms in response to EGFR tyrosine kinase inhibition *Cancer Res.* **75** 4372–83

[113] Spencer K, Parrish R, Barton R and Henry A 2018 Palliative radiotherapy *Br. Med. J.* **360** k821

[114] Spring B Q, Rizvi I, Xu N and Hasan T 2015 The role of photodynamic therapy in overcoming cancer drug resistance *Photochem. Photobiol. Sci.* **14** 1476–91

[115] Jahn S C and Starostik P 2017 Clinical lung cancer mutation detection *Prevention, Diagnosis, and Treatment of Lung Cancer* (Rijeka: InTech) p 83

[116] Tamai K *et al* 2018 Photodynamic therapy using indocyanine green loaded on super carbonate apatite as minimally invasive cancer treatment *Mol. Cancer Ther.* **17** 1613–22

[117] Tardivo J P, Del Giglio A, de Oliveira C S, Gabrielli D S, Junqueira H C, Tada D B, Severino D, de Fatima Turchiello R and Baptista M S 2005 Methylene blue in photodynamic therapy: from basic mechanisms to clinical applications *Photodiagnosis Photodyn. Ther.* **2** 175–91

[118] Timmerman R *et al* 2010 Stereotactic body radiation therapy for inoperable early stage lung cancer *JAMA* **303** 1070–6

[119] Torre L A, Bray F, Siegel R L, Ferlay J, Lortet-Tieulent J and Jemal A 2015 Global cancer statistics, 2012 *CA Cancer J. Clin.* **65** 87–108

[120] Tummers Q R, Boonstra M C, Frangioni J V, van de Velde C J, Vahrmeijer A L and Bonsing B A 2015 Intraoperative near-infrared fluorescence imaging of a paraganglioma using methylene blue: a case report *Int. J. Surg. Case Rep.* **6c** 150–3

[121] Tummers Q R, Hoogstins C E, Peters A A, de Kroon C D, Trimbos J B, van de Velde C J, Frangioni J V, Vahrmeijer A L and Gaarenstroom K N 2015 The value of intraoperative near-infrared fluorescence imaging based on enhanced permeability and retention of indocyanine green: feasibility and false-positives in ovarian cancer *PLoS One* **10** e0129766

[122] Urbanska K, Romanowska-Dixon B, Matuszak Z, Oszajca J, Nowak-Sliwinska P and Stochel G 2002 Indocyanine green as a prospective sensitizer for photodynamic therapy of melanomas *Acta Biochim. Pol.* **49** 387–91

[123] Usuda J *et al* 2010 Outcome of photodynamic therapy using NPe6 for bronchogenic carcinomas in central airways >1.0 cm in diameter *Clin. Cancer Res.* **16** 2198–204

[124] Usuda J *et al* 2006 Photodynamic therapy (PDT) for lung cancers *J. Thorac. Oncol.* **1** 489–93

[125] Usuda J *et al* 2007 Photodynamic therapy for lung cancers based on novel photodynamic diagnosis using talaporfin sodium (NPe6) and autofluorescence bronchoscopy *Lung Cancer* **58** 317–23

[126] van Boxel G, Doherty W and Parmar M 2012 Cellular oxygen utilization in health and sepsis *BJA Educ.* **12** 207–12

[127] van der Vorst J R *et al* 2014 Intraoperative near-infrared fluorescence imaging of parathyroid adenomas with use of low-dose methylene blue *Head Neck* **36** 853–8

[128] van der Vorst J R, Vahrmeijer A L, Hutteman M, Bosse T, Smit V T, van de Velde C J, Frangioni J V and Bonsing B A 2012 Near-infrared fluorescence imaging of a solitary fibrous tumor of the pancreas using methylene blue *World J. Gastrointest. Surg.* **4** 180–4

[129] van Straten D, Mashayekhi V, de Bruijn H S, Oliveira S and Robinson D J 2017 Oncologic photodynamic therapy: basic principles, current clinical status and future directions *Cancers* **9** E19

[130] Wagner A *et al* 2015 Temoporfin improves efficacy of photodynamic therapy in advanced biliary tract carcinoma: a multicenter prospective phase II study *Hepatology* **62** 1456–65

[131] Weinberg B D, Allison R R, Sibata C, Parent T and Downie G 2010 Results of combined photodynamic therapy (PDT) and high dose rate brachytherapy (HDR) in treatment of obstructive endobronchial non-small cell lung cancer (NSCLC) *Photodiagnosis Photodyn. Ther.* **7** 50–8

[132] Winer J H, Choi H S, Gibbs-Strauss S L, Ashitate Y, Colson Y L and Frangioni J V 2010 Intraoperative localization of insulinoma and normal pancreas using invisible near-infrared fluorescent light *Ann. Surg. Oncol.* **17** 1094–100

[133] Yoon I, Li J Z and Shim Y K 2013 Advance in photosensitizers and light delivery for photodynamic therapy *Clin. Endosc.* **46** 7–23

[134] Zappa C and Mousa S A 2016 Non-small cell lung cancer: current treatment and future advances *Transl. Lung Cancer Res.* **5** 288–300

[135] Zhang L J, O'Shea D, Zhang C Y, Yan Y J, Wang L and Chen Z L 2015 Evaluation of a bacteriochlorin-based photosensitizer's anti-tumor effect *in vitro* and *in vivo J. Cancer Res. Clin. Oncol.* **141** 1921–30

[136] Zhang R R, Schroeder A B, Grudzinski J J, Rosenthal E L, Warram J M, Pinchuk A N, Eliceiri K W, Kuo J S and Weichert J P 2017 Beyond the margins: real-time detection of cancer using targeted fluorophores *Nat. Rev. Clin. Oncol.* **14** 347–64

[137] Zhu H, Zhou Z, Wang Y, Bi N, Feng Q, Li J, Lv J, Chen D, Shi Y and Wang L 2011 Thoracic radiation therapy improves the overall survival of patients with extensive-stage small cell lung cancer with distant metastasis *Cancer* **117** 5423–31

Chapter 8

Cold atmospheric plasma and iron oxide based magnetic nanoparticles for synergetic lung cancer therapy

Hongli Yu, Wentong Li and Weifen Zhang

Lung cancer is one of the most common malignancies. Despite the progress made in the past few decades, further research is needed to improve lung cancer treatment. Nanomedicine offers an unprecedented live cell pathway and is committed to the highest level of cancer detection and treatment. In particular, nano-based drug delivery devices allow the effective and sustained delivery of therapeutic agents to solid tumors, which has completely changed the treatment of cancer. Iron oxide based magnetic nanoparticles, with their biocompatibility, high supermagnetism, and excellent efficacy, are opening up a wide field of possible applications in modern cancer therapy. Likewise, cold atmospheric plasma (CAP), with various reactive species including reactive oxygen species (ROS), reactive nitrogen species (RNS), and UV photons, is an emerging biomedical technique that shows great potential for cancer treatment, making them a promising anti-cancer agent. Recent scientific studies have shown that there is a potential synergy between these two aspects. The induction of apoptosis/necrosis may be caused by multiple probable mechanisms of their cytotoxic effects. The synergetic effect of the integration of CAP and iron oxide based magnetic nanoparticles could be tantamount to maximized targeted efficacy in the treatment of lung cancer.

8.1 Introduction

Lung cancer is the most prevalent malignancy leading to cancer-related death in both men and women [1]. Globally, 1 378 400 people die of lung cancer every year and the overall 5-year survival rate is 15% [2, 3]. Historically, lung cancer has been divided based on histology into two major forms: non-small cell lung cancer and small cell lung cancer [4]. About 85% of lung cancers are non-small cell lung cancer (NSCLC) with small cell lung cancer (SCLC) making up the remaining 15% [5].

doi:10.1088/978-0-7503-2540-0ch8

Most NSCLC patients present with metastatic diseases, characterized by local and distant spread of cancer cells to lymph nodes, lungs, and other organs [4]. The current treatment of NSCLC mainly includes surgery, chemotherapy, and radiotherapy, of which chemotherapy is the mainstay. In the past few decades, several small molecule inhibitors have been introduced clinically, which has significantly improved the overall prognosis of NSCLC [6, 7]. However, many patients still suffer from poor response to drug therapy, and the overall survival rate for lung cancer remains discouragingly low. Therefore, precision medicine aiming to provide personalized targeted treatment is becoming an attractive strategy to improve the drug efficacy against lung cancer [8, 9].

8.2 Therapeutic effect of cold atmospheric plasma in lung cancer

8.2.1 Cold atmospheric plasma device structure, methods, and carrier gas types

Cold atmospheric plasma (CAP), considered the fourth fundamental state of matter, is an ionized gas that is composed of positive and negative charged ions, electrons, photons, and neutrals particles (radicals as well as excited atoms and molecules) [10]. The heavy particle temperature of CAP is less than 40 °C [11]. The therapeutic effect is reported by the most important composition of the CAP containing free radicals, include singlet oxygen ($^1O_2$), superoxide (O^{2-}), ozone (O^3), hydroxyl radicals (•OH), nitrogen radicals (N^2•), nitric oxide (•NO), nitrogen dioxide (•NO_2), peroxynitrite ($ONOO^-$), hydrogen peroxide (H_2O_2), organic radicals, electrons, energetic ions, and charged particles (RO•, RO_2•) [12]. This complicated chemistry leads to a myriad of interactions between the CAP and biological systems including cells and tissues [13].

Two main methods have been widely used to generate CAP, namely direct (plasma jet) and indirect dielectric barrier discharges (DBDs), although the majority of studies have used plasma jets rather than DBD (72.1% and 27.8%, respectively) [14]. A plasma jet was used at George Washington University with a configuration of a central powered electrode 1 mm in diameter and a grounded outer electrode wrapped around the outside of a 4.5 mm diameter quartz tube (figure 8.1(a)). The electrodes were connected to a secondary high voltage transformer (voltage up to 8 kV, frequency 25 kHz). Industrial grade helium (He) was used as the carrier gas at a flow rate of 4 L min^{-1} [15]. Helium alone was the most used carrier gas (35.8%), followed by air (26.3%), and argon (22.1%) [14]. Figure 8.1(b) shows the plasma jet for both *in vitro* experiments.

Barrier discharges (BDs) produce highly non-equilibrium plasmas in a controllable way at atmospheric pressure, and at moderate gas temperature. They provide the effective generation of atoms, radicals, and excited species by energetic electrons [16]. A DBD device can generate the plasma directly in air [17, 18]. However, DBD devices tend to generate a short but wide plasma.

8.2.2 The mechanism of cold atmospheric plasma treatment of lung cancer

In addition to traditional chemotherapy and radiotherapy, CAP is an emerging biomedical technique for selective cancer treatment [19]. Many publications have

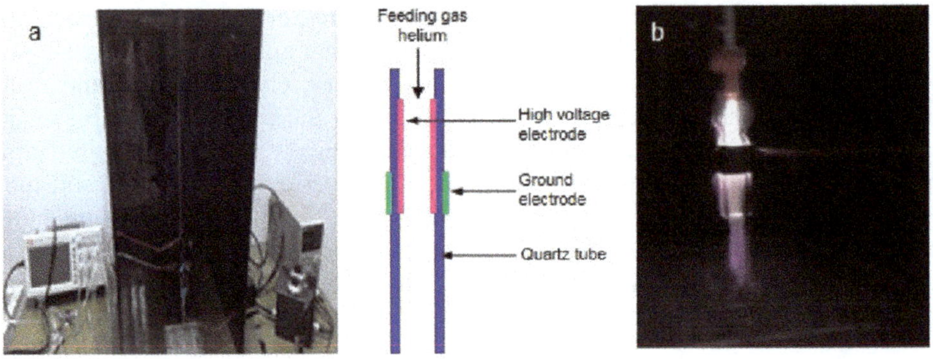

Figure 8.1. The plasma device. (a) Homemade CAP system and schematic diagram. (b) Treatment of tumor cells *in vitro* with CAP.

discussed that CAP has been extensively studied in the treatment of cancer, leaving normal cells relatively unharmed [20]. Some studies have demonstrated that CAP leads to cancer cell death through apoptosis [21]. In addition, there is evidence that CAP can prevent the development of resistant cells, which is the main problem of current treatments [22, 23].

The unique properties of CAP have enabled recent biomedical applications including wound healing, sterilization, blood coagulation, tooth bleaching, skin regeneration, and cancer therapy [24]. To date, the remarkable anti-cancer capacity of CAP has been demonstrated with dozens of cancer cell lines *in vivo* [25]. Our previous research revealed that CAP could effectively induce A549 cancer cell proliferation and apoptosis *in vitro* via the inhibition of the EGFR-RAS/ERK and EGFR-PI3K/AKT signaling pathways [26].

It was suggested that CAP treatment seems to induce malignant cells to generate RONS that may be involved in a bystander effect-like process of self-perpetuation of apoptosis induction [27]. Precancerous cells could be induced to die by apoptosis using a combination of transformed cell-derived RONS and signaling components either released by surrounding non-transformed cells or from RONS released by the transformed cells themselves. The former mechanism is the classical intercellular induction of apoptosis and the latter is an autocrine, RONS-mediated apoptotic self-destruction. Through the detection of intracellular reactive oxygen species, we found that the amount of reactive oxygen species in A549 cells was significantly increased after CAP treatment [26].

Additionally, extreme amounts of reactive species may lead to severe damage to DNA, proteins, mitochondria, and the cytoplasmic membrane, and a weakened intracellular antioxidant system [25]. Because the mechanism of CAP in the treatment of tumors is complex, the exact mechanism still needs to be further defined.

8.2.3 The impact of cold atmospheric plasma on EMT

Epithelial mesenchymal transition (EMT), a cellular mechanism that is known to contribute to normal embryonic development, can be co-opted by cancer cells during metastatic progression [28]. In particular, during EMT, epithelial cells lose cell–cell adherence complexes, resulting in increased migratory and invasive properties [29]. Cancer cells that have undergone EMT start to express mesenchymal markers, such as N-cadherin and Vimentin, displaying increased invasiveness, stem-like features, and resistance to apoptosis during tumor cell progression. In addition, epithelial cells lose indicators of differentiation, such as E-cadherin, and this leads to metastasis [30]. Our previous studies demonstrated that CAP treatment can reverse EMT in solid tumor cells by reducing the secretion of a number of proteins, resulting in the upregulation of epithelial markers such as E-cadherin. The inhibition of the PI3K/AKT pathway and the reversal of EMT prevented tumor cell growth in solid tumors [26]. Some studies have shown that phorbol ester, which initiates EMT, is regulated by the ROS signal derived from histone H3 acetylation and NADPH oxidase (NOX)2 [31], suggesting that CAP regulates the EMT process by producing ROS.

8.3 The therapeutic effect of magnetic iron oxide nanoparticles in lung cancer

8.3.1 Advantages of magnetic iron oxide nanoparticles in the treatment of lung cancer

Magnetic nanoparticles possessing unique properties such as high coercivity, low Curie temperature, and most importantly supermagnetism have been intensively investigated for various biomedical applications, in particular iron oxide based nanoparticles [32, 33].

In recent times, magnetic iron oxide nanoparticles have attracted the attention of the scientific community as an ideal candidate for carriers of drug or gene delivery, the hypothermal treatment of tumors, magnetic resonance contrast agents, and iron agents [34], due to their good chemical stability, magnetic responsiveness, and biocompatibility [35]. Our results demonstrate that iron oxide magnetic nanoparticles have a certain therapeutic effect on non-small cell lung cancer *in vitro* and *in vivo* [26]. Mohd *et al* found that bare iron oxide nanoparticles were significantly cytotoxic to human cancer cells (A549) but not to the normal human lung fibroblast cells. In other words, the nanoparticles selectively kill cancerous cells [34]. These findings are parallel to the observations of other researchers [36].

8.3.2 The mechanism of magnetic iron oxide nanoparticle treatment of lung cancer

In recent years, magnetic iron oxide nanoparticles have been used in different fields, in particular in biomedicine for diagnosis and therapy, with 'theranostic' effects. Several studies have reported the potential toxicity of iron oxide nanoparticles in different models, in particular in cells. In our study, we observed a significant increase in ROS levels by iron oxide nanoparticles in lung cancer cells [26]. Our observations and conclusions on ROS production are well supported by a couple of previous studies.

Khan *et al* also observed a significant increase in ROS levels in lung cancer cells treated with iron oxide nanoparticles. In addition, they also noted that ROS production is associated with autophagy and mitochondrial damage [34]. In short, their results indicate that iron oxide nanoparticles induce ROS and autophagy leading to final cell death. These toxic consequences may be due to mitochondrial damage caused by iron oxide nanoparticles. Similarly, another study by Wu *et al* showed the same results, but in colorectal cancer cells [37].

In addition, iron oxide nanoparticles exhibit toxicity dependent on oxidative stress. ROS generation induced by nanoparticles causes damage to DNA, protein, and organelles, including mitochondria [38]. Damaged mitochondria can induce endogenous and exogenous apoptotic pathways [39]. Excessive free radical production causes a decrease in mitochondrial membrane potential and leads to mitochondrial membrane damage, ultimately causing necrotic cell death [40, 41].

8.3.3 Magnetic iron oxide nanoparticles for the detection of lung cancer in magnetic resonance imaging

The traditional imaging mode magnetic resonance imaging (MRI) is considered to be one of the most useful and non-invasive diagnostic techniques, because it has excellent soft tissue contrast, high spatial resolution, and does not use radioisotopes or x-rays [42].

Among the variety used contrast agents, magnetic iron oxide nanoparticles have been investigated for their effectiveness as an MRI T_2-negative contrast agent because of their biocompatibility, nontoxicity, low particle dimensions, large surface area, and particular magnetic properties [43, 44]. In addition, magnetic iron oxide can shorten the T_2 relaxation time and attenuate the T_2-weighted signal. This type of contrast agent has a small particle size, strong penetrability, and, under the same conditions, the relaxation rate is 7–10 times that of Gd^{3+} in clinical cancer utility [45]. MRI can non-invasively obtain cross-sectional images of tissues or organs with high resolution, and MRI-guided targeted chemotherapy is expected to be used for the treatment of cancer [46].

Therefore, magnetic iron oxide, as a contrast agent, can be used for the imaging of tumor cells and molecule levels, improving the sensitivity of MRI techniques.

8.4 Synergistic therapeutic effects of cold atmospheric plasma and magnetic iron oxide nanoparticles in lung cancer

8.4.1 Limitations of cold atmospheric plasma

CAP shows its promising potential to be an anti-cancer tool with the aid of these selective, highly reactive species, targeting tumor cells selectively without conferring any detrimental effects on the surrounding normal tissue [11]. However, there are many key questions that have not been answered or even mentioned in this field.

First, active particles often need to penetrate to a certain depth to reach the target in the clinical application of plasma. To improve the effect of plasma may be difficult, and we are unlikely to make a breakthrough by plasma technology alone. Therefore, we need to consider combination therapy. Second, this study mainly focused on the description of the anti-cancer effect of CAP *in vitro* and *in vivo* [47].

The understanding of anti-cancer mechanisms is very limited. To become a mature anti-cancer therapy with a solid theoretical basis, we need to determine the basic mechanism.

Of course, the main challenge in using CAP as a treatment method is the lack of detailed clinical tests and its long-term negative effects from its interaction with the body. Successful clinical trials should be conducted to obtain reliable therapeutic effects [48].

In summary, satisfactory answers to these questions will help CAP to become a practical anti-cancer tool.

8.4.2 Cold atmospheric plasma science and nanotechnology

Currently, CAP is a recently emerged biomedical technique for selective cancer treatment, as shown by substantial research studies [49]. In a parallel way, nanotechnology, due to its advanced imaging applications and extensive engineering capabilities, has dramatically influenced drug delivery research to improve the therapeutic performance capabilities of drugs, along with its capacity for early detection of cancer [50]. In addition, compared to orthodox therapies, nanoparticles have the additional advantages of active/passive targeting, bioavailability, and biocompatibility. Both nanoparticle technology and cold plasma technology offer exceptional opportunities for biomedicine.

Over the last few years, a number of important benefits have been shown to emerge, such as reduced toxicity through combinatorial antimicrobial or anti-cancer effects with the combination of nanoparticle and plasma technology. In view of the current focus on the safe use of nanoparticles, this synergy has proven to be particularly beneficial in reducing the minimum inhibitory concentration of nanoparticles on cancer cells or pathogens [51].

A synergistic combination of plasmas and nanoparticles could contribute to improving the selective penetration by CAP-generated ROS species. It is known that nanoparticles may preferentially deposit near cancer cells rather than healthy cells [19]. Therefore, the combined use of plasma and nanoparticles may enhance the directionality of plasma and nanoparticles to the lesions in the tissue, leading to the intracellular diffusion of plasma and nanoparticles towards diseased sites within tissues [51].

Using gold nanoparticles and cold atmospheric plasma has shown some very promising results compared to their single use. A recent study by Manish *et al* demonstrated that these results present evidence of a plausible potential role of the CAP for improving targeted SN delivery, ultimately to inhibit the progress of melanoma [52].

8.4.3 Synergies between plasma and nanoparticles in the treatment of lung cancer

Our previous studies have shown that CAP and iron oxide based MNPs have synergistic and potent cytotoxicity against lung cancer cells, and significantly inhibited cell proliferation by lowering cell viability and inducing cell apoptosis. Importantly,

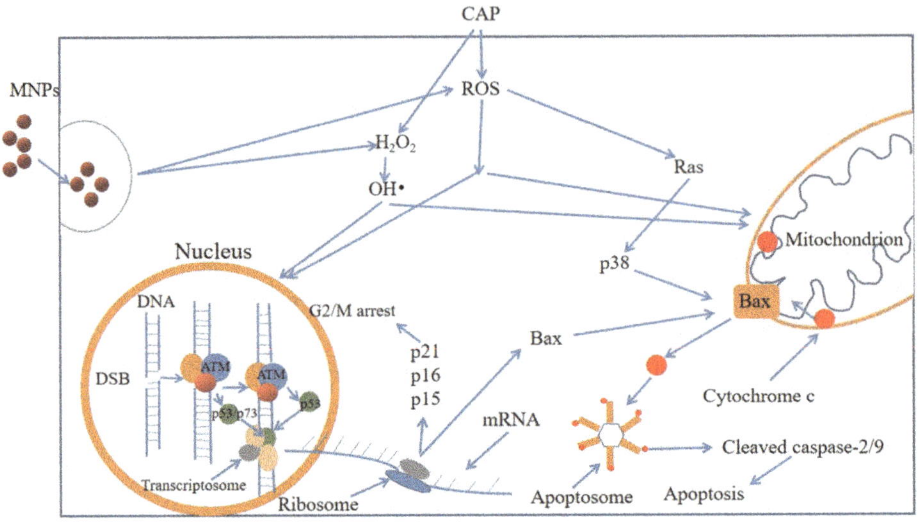

Figure 8.2. Molecular mechanisms of MNPs enhancing the tumor-selective killing effect of CAP.

the binding of CAP with iron oxide based MNPs induced EGFR downregulation while CAP inhibited lung cancer cells by inhibiting pERK and pAKT. Transforming these findings into the *in vivo* environment demonstrates that CAP combined with iron oxide based MNPs is effective at preventing xenograft tumors. Overall, H_2O_2 was produced in CAP-treated A549 cancer cells, while Fe^{2+}/Fe^{3+} from iron oxide based MNPs wa converted H_2O_2 to •OH by Fenton's reaction. Iron oxide based MNP can enhance the tumor killing effect of CAP through this mechanism (figure 8.2). The same study also concluded that even at low plasma doses, CAP can stimulate nanoparticles in cells, leading to cell death [15].

CAP-originated reactive species will cause a noticeable increase of intracellular H_2O_2. Fe^{2+} could catalyze H_2O_2 into •OH, which causes injury to cancer cells, such as inducing mitochondria-mediated apoptosis and double strand DNA breaks.

Selectivity is the most important consideration for the treatment of diseases such as cancer. The working mechanisms of nanoparticles and CAP reveal their potential selectivity for cancer cells. The main downstream effect inside cells after exposure would be the production of ROS/RNS [51]. Intracellular oxidative stress may be attributed to cellular processes, such as mitochondrial respiration and immune cell activation, or cell nanoparticle interactions [40]. Furthermore, in general, the amount of reactive oxygen species produced in cancer cells is much higher than in normal cells [53, 54]. Another possible reason is that the metabolic rate in cancer cells is higher than that in normal cells [54]. This can increase the potential selectivity of ROS/RNS for cancer cells.

In conclusion, we may see an effective synergy between the effects of nanoparticles and cold atmospheric plasma, providing a greater impetus for their use in the treatment of cancer.

8.5 The synergistic therapeutic effect of cold atmospheric plasma and drug-loaded magnetic nanoparticles in lung cancer

8.5.1 Methods for preparing magnetic nanoparticles loaded with drugs

Cytotoxic drugs, while potent, have the enormous drawback of limited selective entry into the lung, thus causing collateral damage to other tissues. To overcome these shortcomings, we report here the development of magnetic nanoparticles loaded with drugs, which target the lung over other tissues five-fold [55]. These nanocarriers have the potential of improving hydrophobic drug delivery, reducing drug degradation, targeting target sites in the body, and presenting sustained and triggered release, which improve therapeutic efficacy and minimize undesired side effects [50]. Therefore, the delivery of anti-cancer agents using nanoparticle carriers has been extensively investigated.

A wide variety of techniques including etching, milling or machining, emulsion solvent evaporation processes and self-assembly have been reported for the synthesis of polymeric magnetic nanoparticles. A very recent study by José *et al* showed that 5-fluorouracil-loaded iron/ethylcellulose (core/shell) nanoparticles could be synthesized by an emulsion solvent evaporation process. They found that the incorporation of 5-fluorouracil into the magnetic composites resulted in a higher drug loading and yielded a slower drug release profile, compared to single 5-fluorouracil surface adsorption [56]. Another study also indicated that fluorescent/magnetic nanoparticles could be fabricated in a one-pot method via the process of mini-emulsification and self-assembly. Furthermore, nanoparticles have excellent dispersibility, storage stability and cell compatibility, which may be beneficial for their potential applications in the biomedical field [57].

Among various fabrication methods, electrospraying is one of the most versatile and cost-effective techniques for nanoparticle fabrication. In the electrospraying process, the polymer solution distributed from the nozzle can easily form core–shell droplets with a diameter of several nanometers under an increasing electric field. Moreover, electrospraying has several unique advantages including enhanced encapsulation efficiency, generating drug-loaded particles with a controlled composition, ease of control of the operating parameters, the ability to produce small and uniform particle size, and scalability [58, 59]. In particular, coaxial electrospraying can be applied to prepare core–shell structured particles [60].

8.5.2 Synergistic effect between cold atmospheric plasma and magnetic nanoparticles loaded with drugs in the treatment of lung cancer

The main disadvantage of cytotoxic drugs is that because they cannot distinguish between cancer cells and normal healthy cells, they kill all cells in contact with them [61]. Due to a lack of selectivity, several tissues along with the tumors suffer collateral damage, leading to adverse side effects. One way to make these drugs more effective and reduce their side effects is to target them primarily to specific organs. To this end, we can further use nanoparticles containing iron to retain the drug in the lungs to maximize its effectiveness using external magnets. Magnetic nanoparticles loaded with drugs for targeted therapy have been considered promising anti-tumor methods in the field of plasma medicine [62].

A recent study by Yu *et al* showed that a PTX-loaded core–shell magnetic electrospraying nanoparticle and CAP combination could be used as a new dual cancer treatment for synergistic inhibition of non-small cell lung cell growth compared to separate treatment. CAP can also induce more effective concentrations of PTX-loaded nanoparticles in cells, thereby increasing ROS production and enhancing the killing effect on cells [15]. Additionally, current successes in nanoparticle cancer research revealed that magnetic nanoparticles loaded with drugs targeted lung cancer cells and promoted the selectivity of CAP. Studies have reported that the combination of CAP and nanoparticles can also be used in the treatment of other cancers. Pretreatment with gold nanoparticles without careful processing and transformation can enhance the anti-cancer effect of CAP, thus it is possible that synergistic effects exist between CAP and gold nanoparticles [48]. The dual treatment of gold nanoparticles coated with polyethylene glycol (PEG) and CAP increases the number of dead cells in glioblastoma and lung adenocarcinoma and reverses EMT [30]. Therefore, the combination of drug delivery and CAP may lead to a paradigm shift in cancer therapy.

8.6 Conclusions

The study of magnetic nanoparticles and atmospheric cold plasma on tumor response has increased our understanding regarding their critical roles in improving cancer progression. Cancer researchers are increasingly focusing on this area. In essence, the synergy of low temperature plasma and magnetic nanoparticles is designed to take advantage of the distinct and different advantages of each of the two technologies in terms of reactivity, selectivity, safety, and disease targeting. Its advantage is not only the simple combination of the two technologies, but in fact, only when the magnetic nanoparticles are synthesized and then post-treated/functionalized in the plasma environment, can they be fully utilized to achieve the best therapeutic effect.

There remain many challenges, such as developing an effective delivery system, optimizing the safe concentration of both magnetic nanoparticles and CAP, and enhancing the effective coupling of magnetic nanoparticles and CAP to ultimately improve the therapeutic effects. However, the plasma–nanoparticle interaction can not only change the performance matrix of its biomedical applications, but also open up many unexpected doors for many currently unknown opportunities. Both nanoparticle technology and cold plasma technology offer an exceptional grand opportunity with potentially enormous impacts on modern medicine.

References

[1] Siegel R L, Miller K D and Jemal A 2018 Cancer statistics *CA Cancer J. Clin.* **60** 277–300

[2] Jemal A, Bray F, Center M M, Ferlay J, Ward E and Forman D 2011 Global cancer statistics *CA Cancer J. Clin.* **61** 69–90

[3] Qin X, Xu H, Gong W and Deng W 2014 The tumor cytosol miRNAs, fluid miRNAs, and exosome miRNAs in lung cancer *Front. Oncol.* **4** 357

[4] Landesman-Milo D, Ramishetti S and Peer D 2015 Nanomedicine as an emerging platform for metastatic lung cancer therapy *Cancer Metastasis Rev.* **34** 291–301

[5] Kleczko E K, Kwak J W, Schenk E L and Nemenoff R A 2019 Targeting the complement pathway as a therapeutic strategy in lung cancer *Front. Immunol.* **10** 954

[6] Piperdi B, Merla A and Perez-Soler R 2014 Targeting angiogenesis in squamous non-small cell lung cancer *Drugs* **74** 403–13

[7] Lovly C M 2015 Combating acquired resistance to tyrosine kinase inhibitors in lung cancer *American Society of Clinical Oncology Educational Book. American Society of Clinical Oncology. Annual Meeting* pp e165–73

[8] Gadgeel S M 2016 Personalized therapy of non-small cell lung cancer (NSCLC) *Adv. Exp. Med. Biol.* **890** 203–22

[9] Chen Y, Liu X, Li Y, Quan C, Zheng L and Huang K 2018 Lung cancer therapy targeting histone methylation: opportunities and challenges *Comput. Struct. Biotechnol. J.* **16** 211–23

[10] Gay-Mimbrera J, Garcia M C, Isla-Tejera B, Rodero-Serrano A, Garcia-Nieto A V and Ruano J 2016 Clinical and biological principles of cold atmospheric plasma application in skin cancer *Adv. Ther.* **33** 894–909

[11] Babington P, Rajjoub K, Canady J, Siu A, Keidar M and Sherman J H 2015 Use of cold atmospheric plasma in the treatment of cancer *Biointerphases* **10** 029403

[12] Gumbel D, Bekeschus S, Gelbrich N, Napp M, Ekkernkamp A, Kramer A and Stope M B 2017 Cold atmospheric plasma in the treatment of osteosarcoma *Int. J. Mol. Sci.* **18** E2004

[13] Graves D B 2012 The emerging role of reactive oxygen and nitrogen species in redox biology and some implications for plasma applications to medicine and biology *J. Phys. D: Appl. Phys.* **45** 263001

[14] Dubuc A, Monsarrat P, Virard F, Merbahi N, Sarrette J P, Laurencin-Dalicieux S and Cousty S 2018 Use of cold-atmospheric plasma in oncology: a concise systematic review *Ther. Adv. Med. Oncol.* **10** 1758835918786475

[15] Yu H, Wang Y, Wang S, Li X, Li W, Ding D, Gong X, Keidar M and Zhang W 2018 Paclitaxel-loaded core–shell magnetic nanoparticles and cold atmospheric plasma inhibit non-small cell lung cancer growth *ACS Appl. Mater. Interfaces* **10** 43462–71

[16] Wagner H E, Brandenburg R, Kozlov K V, Sonnenfeld A, Michel P and Behnke J F 2003 The barrier discharge: basic properties and applications to surface treatment *Vacuum* **71** 417–36

[17] Panngom K, Baik K Y, Nam M K, Han J H, Rhim H and Choi E H 2013 Preferential killing of human lung cancer cell lines with mitochondrial dysfunction by nonthermal dielectric barrier discharge plasma *Cell Death Dis.* **4** e642

[18] Kaushik N K, Uhm H and Ha Choi E 2012 Micronucleus formation induced by dielectric barrier discharge plasma exposure in brain cancer cells *Appl. Phys. Lett.* **100** 084102

[19] Cheng X, Murphy W, Recek N, Yan D, Cvelbar U, Vesel A, Mozetič M, Canady J, Keidar M and Sherman J H 2014 Synergistic effect of gold nanoparticles and cold plasma on glioblastoma cancer therapy *J. Phys. D: Appl. Phys.* **47** 335402

[20] Keidar M, Walk R, Shashurin A, Srinivasan P, Sandler A, Dasgupta S, Ravi R, Guerrero-Preston R and Trink B 2011 Cold plasma selectivity and the possibility of a paradigm shift in cancer therapy *Br. J. Cancer* **105** 1295–301

[21] Keidar M, Shashurin A, Volotskova O, Ann Stepp M, Srinivasan P, Sandler A and Trink B 2013 Cold atmospheric plasma in cancer therapy *Phys. Plasmas* **20** 057101

[22] Yan D, Sherman J H, Cheng X, Ratovitski E, Canady J and Keidar M 2014 Controlling plasma stimulated media in cancer treatment application *Appl. Phys. Lett.* **105** 224101

[23] Graves D B 2014 Reactive species from cold atmospheric plasma: implications for cancer therapy *Plasma Process. Polym.* **11** 1120–7

[24] Arndt S *et al* 2013 Cold atmospheric plasma (CAP) changes gene expression of key molecules of the wound healing machinery and improves wound healing *in vitro* and *in vivo PLoS One* **8** e79325

[25] Keidar M, Yan D, Beilis I I, Trink B and Sherman J H 2018 Plasmas for treating cancer: opportunities for adaptive and self-adaptive approaches *Trends Biotechnol.* **36** 586–93

[26] Li W, Yu H, Ding D, Chen Z, Wang Y, Wang S, Li X, Keidar M and Zhang W 2019 Cold atmospheric plasma and iron oxide-based magnetic nanoparticles for synergetic lung cancer therapy *Free Radic. Biol. Med.* **130** 71–81

[27] Bauer G and Graves D B 2016 Mechanisms of selective antitumor action of cold atmospheric plasma-derived reactive oxygen and nitrogen species *Plasma Process. Polym.* **13** 1157–78

[28] Hanahan D and Weinberg R A 2011 Hallmarks of cancer: the next generation *Cell* **144** 646–74

[29] Suarez-Carmona M, Lesage J, Cataldo D and Gilles C 2017 EMT and inflammation: inseparable actors of cancer progression *Mol. Oncol.* **11** 805–23

[30] Kaushik N K, Kaushik N, Yoo K C, Uddin N, Kim J S, Lee S J and Choi E H 2016 Low doses of PEG-coated gold nanoparticles sensitize solid tumors to cold plasma by blocking the PI3K/AKT-driven signaling axis to suppress cellular transformation by inhibiting growth and EMT *Biomaterials* **87** 118–30

[31] Kamiya T, Goto A, Kurokawa E, Hara H and Adachi T 2016 Cross talk mechanism among EMT, ROS, and histone acetylation in phorbol ester-treated human breast cancer MCF-7 cells *Oxid. Med. Cell. Longev.* **2016** 1284372

[32] Kang T, Li F, Baik S, Shao W, Ling D and Hyeon T 2017 Surface design of magnetic nanoparticles for stimuli-responsive cancer imaging and therapy *Biomaterials* **136** 98–114

[33] Fang X, Cheng X, Zhang Y, Zhang L G and Keidar M 2018 Single-step synthesis of carbon encapsulated magnetic nanoparticles in arc plasma and potential biomedical applications *J. Colloid Interface Sci.* **509** 414–21

[34] Khan M I, Mohammad A, Patil G, Naqvi S A, Chauhan L K and Ahmad I 2012 Induction of ROS, mitochondrial damage and autophagy in lung epithelial cancer cells by iron oxide nanoparticles *Biomaterials* **33** 1477–88

[35] Wu W, He Q and Jiang C 2008 Magnetic iron oxide nanoparticles: synthesis and surface functionalization strategies *Nanoscale Res. Lett.* **3** 397–415

[36] Cheng F Y, Su C H, Yang Y S, Yeh C S, Tsai C Y, Wu C L, Wu M T and Shieh D B 2005 Characterization of aqueous dispersions of Fe_3O_4 nanoparticles and their biomedical applications *Biomaterials* **26** 729–38

[37] Wu Y N, Chen D H, Shi X Y, Lian C C, Wang T Y, Yeh C S, Ratinac K R, Thordarson P, Braet F and Shieh D B 2011 Cancer-cell-specific cytotoxicity of non-oxidized iron elements in iron core-gold shell NPs *Nanomed. Nanotechnol. Biol. Med.* **7** 420–7

[38] Mohammadinejad R, Moosavi M A, Tavakol S, Vardar D O, Hosseini A, Rahmati M, Dini L, Hussain S, Mandegary A and Klionsky D J 2019 Necrotic, apoptotic and autophagic cell fates triggered by nanoparticles *Autophagy* **15** 4–33

[39] Ou L, Song B, Liang H, Liu J, Feng X, Deng B, Sun T and Shao L 2016 Toxicity of graphene-family nanoparticles: a general review of the origins and mechanisms *Part. Fibre Toxicol.* **13** 57

[40] Manke A, Wang L and Rojanasakul Y 2013 Mechanisms of nanoparticle-induced oxidative stress and toxicity *BioMed. Res. Int.* **2013** 942916

[41] Bauer A T, Strozyk E A, Gorzelanny C, Westerhausen C, Desch A, Schneider M F and Schneider S W 2011 Cytotoxicity of silica nanoparticles through exocytosis of von Willebrand factor and necrotic cell death in primary human endothelial cells *Biomaterials* **32** 8385–93

[42] Lee N and Hyeon T 2012 Designed synthesis of uniformly sized iron oxide nanoparticles for efficient magnetic resonance imaging contrast agents *Chem. Soc. Rev.* **41** 2575–89

[43] Pan Y, Du X, Zhao F and Xu B 2012 Magnetic nanoparticles for the manipulation of proteins and cells *Chem. Soc. Rev.* **41** 2912–42

[44] Zhou Z, Wang L, Chi X, Bao J, Yang L, Zhao W, Chen Z, Wang X, Chen X and Gao J 2013 Engineered iron-oxide-based nanoparticles as enhanced T_1 contrast agents for efficient tumor imaging *ACS Nano* **7** 3287–96

Li J, He Y, Sun W, Luo Y, Cai H, Pan Y, Shen M, Xia J and Shi X 2014 Hyaluronic acid-modified hydrothermally synthesized iron oxide nanoparticles for targeted tumor MR imaging *Biomaterials* **35** 3666–77

[45] Gao P, Mei C, He L, Xiao Z, Chan L, Zhang D, Shi C, Chen T and Luo L 2018 Designing multifunctional cancer-targeted nanosystem for magnetic resonance molecular imaging-guided theranostics of lung cancer *Drug Deliv.* **25** 1811–25

[46] Huang Y, Mao K, Zhang B and Zhao Y 2017 Superparamagnetic iron oxide nanoparticles conjugated with folic acid for dual target-specific drug delivery and MRI in cancer theranostics *Mater. Sci. Eng.* C **70** 763–71

[47] Gumbel D, Gelbrich N, Napp M, Daeschlein G, Kramer A, Sckell A, Burchardt M, Ekkernkamp A and Stope M B 2017 Peroxiredoxin expression of human osteosarcoma cells is influenced by cold atmospheric plasma treatment *Anticancer Res.* **37** 1031–8

[48] Aryal S and Bisht G 2017 New paradigm for a targeted cancer therapeutic approach: a short review on potential synergy of gold nanoparticles and cold atmospheric plasma *Biomedicines* **5** E38

[49] Ratovitski E A, Cheng X, Yan D, Sherman J H, Canady J, Trink B and Keidar M 2014 Anti-cancer therapies of 21st century: novel approach to treat human cancers using cold atmospheric plasma *Plasma Process. Polym.* **11** 1128–37

[50] Zhu W, Lee S J, Castro N J, Yan D, Keidar M and Zhang L G 2016 Synergistic effect of cold atmospheric plasma and drug loaded core–shell nanoparticles on inhibiting breast cancer cell growth *Sci. Rep.* **6** 21974

[51] Kong M G, Keidar M and Ostrikov K 2011 Plasmas meet nanoparticles—where synergies can advance the frontier of medicine *J. Phys. D: Appl. Phys.* **44** 174018

[52] Adhikari M, Kaushik N, Ghimire B, Adhikari B, Baboota S, Al-Khedhairy A A, Wahab R, Lee S J, Kaushik N K and Choi E H 2019 Cold atmospheric plasma and silymarin nanoemulsion synergistically inhibits human melanoma tumorigenesis via targeting HGF/c-MET downstream pathway *Cell Commun. Signal.* **17** 52

[53] Minai L, Yeheskely-Hayon D and Yelin D 2013 High levels of reactive oxygen species in gold nanoparticle-targeted cancer cells following femtosecond pulse irradiation *Sci. Rep.* **3** 2146

[54] Bisht G and Rayamajhi S 2016 ZnO nanoparticles: a promising anticancer agent *Nanobiomedicine* **3** 9

[55] Kulkarni P, Rajadurai M, Sevilimedu A, Basaveni S, Yellanki S, Medishetti R and Saxena U 2018 Magnetic nanoparticle formulation for targeted delivery of chemotherapeutic irinotecan to lungs *Drug Deliv. Transl. Res.* **8** 1450–9

[56] Arias J L, Lopez-Viota M, Delgado A V and Ruiz M A 2010 Iron/ethylcellulose (core/shell) nanoplatform loaded with 5-fluorouracil for cancer targeting *Colloids Surf.* B **77** 111–6

[57] Li B, Shao W, Wang Y, Xiao D, Xiong Y, Ye H, Zhou Q and Jin Q 2019 Synthesis and morphological control of biocompatible fluorescent/magnetic janus nanoparticles based on the self-assembly of fluorescent polyurethane and Fe_3O_4 nanoparticles *Polymers* **11** 272

[58] Sridhar R, Lakshminarayanan R, Madhaiyan K, Amutha Barathi V, Lim K H and Ramakrishna S 2015 Electrosprayed nanoparticles and electrospun nanofibers based on natural materials: applications in tissue regeneration, drug delivery and pharmaceuticals *Chem. Soc. Rev.* **44** 790–814

[59] Cao L, Luo J, Tu K, Wang L Q and Jiang H 2014 Generation of nano-sized core–shell particles using a coaxial tri-capillary electrospray-template removal method *Colloids Surf. B, Biointerfaces* **115** 212–8

[60] Rasekh M, Ahmad Z, Cross R, Hernandez-Gil J, Wilton-Ely J and Miller P W 2017 Facile preparation of drug-loaded tristearin encapsulated superparamagnetic iron oxide nanoparticles using coaxial electrospray processing *Mol. Pharm.* **14** 2010–23

[61] Winkler G C, Barle E L, Galati G and Kluwe W M 2014 Functional differentiation of cytotoxic cancer drugs and targeted cancer therapeutics *Regul. Toxicol. Pharmacol.* **70** 46–53

[62] Jalili A, Irani S and Mirfakhraie R 2016 Combination of cold atmospheric plasma and iron nanoparticles in breast cancer: gene expression and apoptosis study *OncoTargets Ther.* **9** 5911–7

IOP Publishing

Lung Cancer and Imaging

Ayman El-Baz and Jasjit S Suri

Chapter 9

Exploiting exhaled aerosol fingerprints to detect lung cancers and obstructive respiratory diseases

Jinxiang Xi and Xiuhua April Si

9.1 Introduction

Early detection of lung cancer is critical to patient survivability. More than 70% of patients with non-small cell lung cancer (NSCLC) can be cured if it is detected at stage I, while less than 25% are cured at stage III [1, 2]. Current techniques to detect lung cancer and respiratory diseases include the spirometer for pulmonary function tests, x-rays for screening, CT/PET/SPET to identify airway remodeling, and biopsy to evaluate the disease type and extent [3]. These diagnostic tools are reliable in general, but are also expensive and require professional operation. Some have radiological risks (CT/PET/SPET) and can be invasive (biopsy).

In recent years, new diagnostic devices for lung diseases have surfaced that utilize exhaled breath, which contains clues on lung health. A growing tumor cell is also accompanied by metabolic changes, which produce certain chemicals and generates a signature breath 'fingerprint'. This breath fingerprint can be exploited to decide if a specific disease is present and at which stage [4]. As the breath test provides a non-invasive alternative to conventional diagnostic tools, extensive studies have been carried out to analyze the breath contents and identifying signature breath biomarkers. Elevated levels of nitric oxide have been reported in the breath of patients with asthma [5], cytokines for cystic fibrosis [6], antioxidants for chronic obstructive pulmonary disease (COPD) [7], and decane, H_2O_2, and isoprene for NSCLC [8, 9]. While some biomarkers have already been applied in clinical practice, such as nitric oxide for asthmatic patients, other biomarkers are still being developed (e.g. profiles of volatile organic compounds (VOC)) [10]. Reviews of using VOC breath tests for lung cancer diagnosis and the development of associated medical devices are presented in [11–14].

One critical limitation of the gas-signature based approaches is that they can only determine the presence and concentration of certain exhaled chemicals. No

doi:10.1088/978-0-7503-2540-0ch9

information on the carcinogen site can be retrieved from such breath tests, which is also essential to cancer treatment planning. At the current stage, such information can only be attained using imaging tools such as MRI, CT, or PET, which are accurate but also suffer from high cost and potential health risks. Moreover, targeted drug delivery can only live up to its name if the site of the disease can be found beforehand. It is, therefore, highly desirable to have alternative tools that can pinpoint the malignant sites in a non-invasive and less costly manner.

Computational simulations of respiratory dynamics have persistently indicated that the patterns of the exhaled aerosol distributions, even though seemingly chaotic, are indeed unique with respect to the airway geometry [15–17]. These patterns will differ whenever there is a change to the airway geometry. It is hypothesized that each lung gives a signature exhaled aerosol fingerprint (AFP), as opposed to the aforementioned gas fingerprint. The AFP pattern, which resembles an actual human fingerprint, is a collective image of the expiratory aerosols traveling through the entire respiratory tract. As such, a deviation from the normal profile indicates an airway remodeling within the respiratory tract, and should be able to be retrieved using the inverse approaches that were proposed in Xi *et al* [15–21].

The proposed concept of AFP based breath testing has two characteristics that are desirable in lung disease diagnosis and treatment: (i) detecting and locating the disease site and (ii) targeted drug delivery to the disease site. If the concept were proven feasible, a combined diagnosis–drug-delivery device could be further developed. The device will be non-invasive, give real-time diagnosis feedback, be capable of precise drug delivery, and at the same time it will be easy-to-use and low-cost. The vision is that the patient takes a breath test for diagnosis purposes, and a patient-specific drug delivery protocol can be subsequently developed that targets therapeutic aerosols at the diseased site only, thereby optimizing the medical outcome and minimizing side effects. The proposed AFP based breath testing works best for lung diseases where the airway structural remodeling is not small, and therefore could be suited for asthma, COPD, and NSCLC. The proposed breath testing will be particularly suitable for respiratory disease screening for those under elevated and prolonged exposures, such as textiles and coal mine workers. Due to its easy-to-use and low-cost features, the workers can be tested more frequently. Regular testing will develop a record of the changes in the patient's lung health condition. Disease localization can facilitate a personalized treatment protocol, such as targeted pulmonary drug delivery.

Previous studies also attempted to use exhaled aerosols as diagnostic tools, which is termed as aerosol bolus dispersion (ABD) [22–26]. The similarities and differences between the method presented in this study and the ABD method are discussed below. Both methods are based on the concept that a patient with a remodeled lung will exhale differently, which will manifest itself in expiratory fine-regime aerosols. However, at least three factors establish the novelty of the proposed method: (i) test procedures, (ii) variables to measure, and (iii) the information that we can obtain from the test. Concerning the test procedures, ABD needs only one step, i.e. inhalation–exhalation. In contrast, the AFP based test needs up to three steps. In the first step, a bolus aerosol is inhaled to a predefined depth and then exhaled for screening purposes. In the second step, aerosol tracers are released selectively to the suspected regions of the lung in order to localize the disease site. In the third step, a personalized drug delivery protocol can be developed that targets pharmaceuticals at the malignant site only. Regarding the variables to measure, ABD records the aerosol concentration as a function of the flow volume to evaluate several bolus variables that are useful in detecting airway remodeling [22, 25]; on the other hand, the AFP based approach directly uses the images (particle distribution pattern) of the exhaled aerosols collected on a mouth filter. Finally, concerning what new information we can obtain from the test, ABD tests will not generate new information on lung health compared to current functional tests. In contrast, new light can be shed on the disease site from the proposed AFP based tests, which is crucial in achieving targeted drug delivery to the diseased site.

In this chapter, we will describe the recent developments in feature extraction and classification of the exhaled aerosol images to establish the relationship between the images and the underlying airway remodeling. Different feature extraction algorithms (aerosol density, fractal dimension, principal mode analysis, and dynamic mode decomposition) and machine learning approaches (SVM, random forest, and convolutional neural network) will be discussed.

9.2 Methods and materials

9.2.1 Healthy and diseased airway models

In this study, images of exhaled aerosols, or AFP, were numerically generated using physiology-based modeling and simulations in anatomically accurate airway models, as shown in figure 9.1. To this aim, two respiratory airway models have been developed. The first model was a simplified geometry that included the respiratory tract from the oral cavity to the third generation (G3) of lung bifurcations (figures 9.2(a) and (b)), while the second model was a more complex, realistic geometry that extended to the ninth generation (G9) of lung bifurcations (figure 9.2(c)). The first model was developed based on MRI scans of a 53-year-old male [15]. There were 23 outlets in the geometry. The detailed procedures of model development and airway dimensions can be found in Xi and Longest [15]. The second model shared the mouth–throat geometry with the first model, which was connected to a more complex lung model [29]. The volume of the lung model was scaled to be 3.5 l, which is consistent with the functional residual capacity (FRC) [30, 31]. There were 115 outlets in this lung model. The two airway models were further modified using HyperMorph (Troy, MI) to generate airway geometries that represented different types of diseases with varying severities (figures 9.1(b) and (c)). High-quality computational mesh was generated for each airway model (figure 9.1(d)). Three test cases were designed, as described below.

In the first test case (figure 9.2(a)), we aimed to test if there are significant differences among the exhaled aerosol images from healthy (model A) and diseased lungs (models B–D). Specifically, model B has a 10 mm sized tumor at the carina ridge of the trachea, while model C has a 4 mm sized tumor located at G3 (i.e. segmental bronchus) in the left lower lobe. In both models, the ratios of the tumor

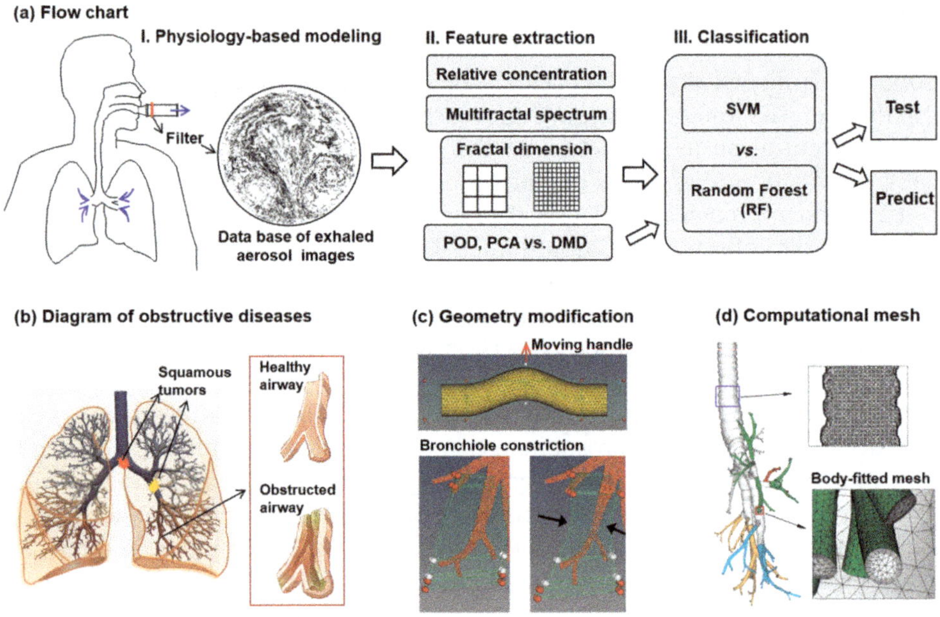

Figure 9.1. Study methodology. (a) A flow chart of this study, which consists of three steps: physiology-based modeling and simulation, feature extraction, and classification. (b) Diagram of respiratory obstructive diseases. (c) Disease model via geometry modification using Hypermesh. (d) Computational mesh with near-wall body-fitted cells. (Adapted from [27], CC BY-NC 4.0, and [28] with permission from Elsevier.)

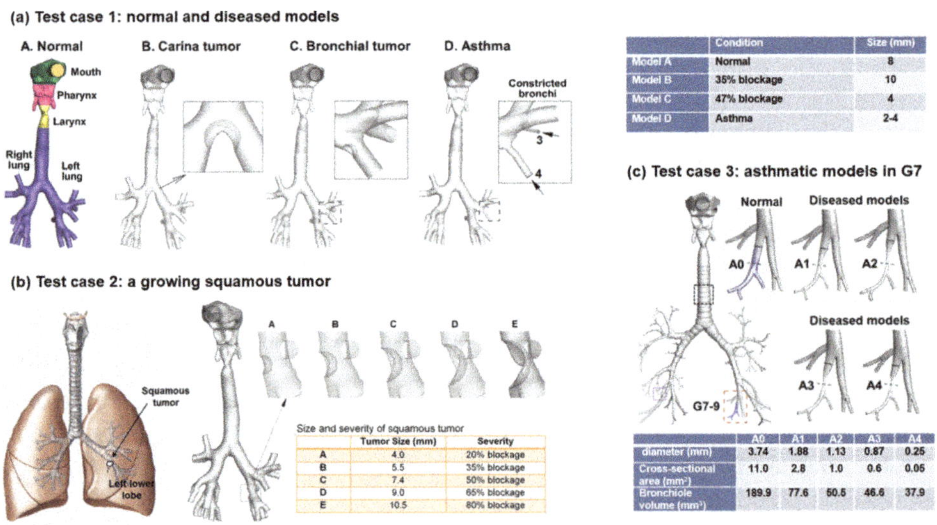

Figure 9.2. Airway models used in three test cases. (a) Test case 1: normal versus diseased models in large airways. (b) Test case 2: a growing squamous tumor at the segmental bronchus (G3). Reproduced from [27]. CC BY-NC 4.0. (c) Asthmatic model in small airways (G7). Reproduced from [45]. CC BY-NC 4.0. The morphological dimensions of the airway in three test cases are also shown.

sizes to the host airway diameters followed those in Segal *et al* [32], who investigated the influence of the location and size of tumors on respiratory airflows. In model D, there are two constricted bronchi in the left upper lobe (number 3 and 4 in figure 9.2(a)) and it is intended to represent local asthmatic airways.

In the second test case, we aimed to characterize the differences of the exhaled aerosol images due to a growing tumor at the segmental bronchus (G3) (figure 9.2(b)). A squamous tumor results from uncontrolled growth of round cells [33]. They can grow in size and constitute cavities in the lung parenchyma. These kinds of tumors are often observed in the larger central airways, either in the main bronchi or major lobes [33]. In this case (figure 9.2(b)), the tumor was in the segmental bronchus of the lower left lobe and had five different diameters to model the varying stages of the tumor [27].

In the third test case, we aimed to test whether the proposed diagnostic method can detect the geometrical changes in small airways with diameters less than 2 mm (figure 9.2(c)). The rationale behind this test is that a diagnostic tool should be sensitive (and robust) enough to work reliably in clinical settings, which can have more compounding factors. To this aim, four levels of airway constrictions (A1, A2, A3, A4) were generated by progressively narrowing the diameters of the bronchioles at G7 in the lower left lobe using Hypermesh [28, 34]. The minimal diameter and cross-sectional area of the constricted bronchioles are listed in the table in figure 9.2(c), along with the bronchiolar volumes that are affected by the constriction.

9.2.2 Acquisition of exhaled aerosol images

Physiology-based simulations were undertaken to mimic the breath tests and generate the exhaled aerosol images. A bolus of aerosol tracers was inhaled to a certain depth and was subsequently exhaled to a filter positioned at the mouth opening. The aerosol bolus was generated using a stochastic scheme and consisted of 30 000 particles [19]. The respiratory airflow was simulated using the low Reynolds number (LRN) k–ω model [35], which has been demonstrated to capture flow transitions accurately [36].

A discrete-phase Lagrangian tracking model with near-wall treatment was implemented to simulate the behavior and fate of particles [37]. The governing equation for the particle motion is expressed as [15],

$$\frac{dv_i}{dt} = \frac{f}{\tau_p C_c}(u_i - v_i) + g_i(1 - \alpha) + f_{i,\,\mathrm{Brownian}} + f_{i,\,\mathrm{lift}}, \tag{9.1}$$

where u_i and v_i are velocities of the flow and particle, respectively. τ_p $(= \rho_p\, d_p^{\,2}/18\mu)$ is the particle transient time, with d_p being the particle diameter and μ the flow viscosity. f is the drag factor [38] and C_c is the Cunningham factor as formulated in Allen and Raabe [39]. User-defined functions (UDFs) were applied to take into account the effects of finite particle inertial [40] and near-wall damping [41]. This model had been well validated in our previous studies, which provided a close match with *in vitro* experimental data for both nanoparticles [40] and micron-sized particles

[17]. ANSYS ICEM CFD (Ansys, Inc.) was utilized to prepare the computational mesh (figure 9.1(d)). A mesh sensitivity analysis was performed with incrementally increasing mesh densities [16] until the variation in the variable of interest was less than 1%.

9.2.3 Feature extraction of exhaled aerosol images

9.2.3.1 Relative concentration

Although the particle distributions can be visually differentiated between different models, particle overlapping may prevent an accurate quantification of particle concentrations. To remedy this drawback, the relative concentration will be calculated as the ratio of local aerosol accumulations over the averaged concentration [42]. For a given airway model, the exhaled aerosol profile and local relative concentrations appear similar. However, the concentration map can readily pinpoint the sites of peak aerosol localization, which should also be the most susceptible sites for tumorigenesis.

9.2.3.2 Fractal dimension and multifractal spectrum analysis

The exhaled aerosol images exhibit a complex profile and can be characterized using the box-counting fractal dimension (D_B), which quantifies the complexity of the image at varying resolutions. Mathematically, D_B is computed as the gradient between the number of grids containing pixels (box-count) N_ε and the resolution scale ε in the log–log plot:

$$D_B = \ln N_\varepsilon / \ln \varepsilon. \tag{9.2}$$

The multifractal spectrum analysis is another approach to measure the complexity of a system. This method rests on the fact that a natural system usually has multiple scaling probabilities. To compute the multifractal spectrum, a normalized parameter $\mu_i(q, \varepsilon)$ can be calculated from a group of scaling exponents, q [43]:

$$\mu_i(q, \varepsilon) = [P_i(\varepsilon)]^q / \sum [P_i(\varepsilon)]^q. \tag{9.3}$$

Here $P_i(\varepsilon)$ is the possibility of pixels found in the ith box with a resolution scale of ε. The singularity strength $\alpha(q)$ and the multifractal function $f(\alpha)$ in relation to $\mu_i(q, \varepsilon)$ can be calculated as

$$\alpha(q) = \lim_{\varepsilon \to 0} \frac{\sum \mu_i(q, \varepsilon) \ln P_i(\varepsilon)}{\ln \varepsilon} \tag{9.4}$$

$$f(\alpha_q) = \lim_{\varepsilon \to 0} \frac{\sum \mu_i(q, \varepsilon) \ln \mu_i(q, \varepsilon)}{\ln \varepsilon}. \tag{9.5}$$

The plot between $\alpha(q)$ and $f(q)$ shows the multifractal spectrum of the image. The multifractal variables $\alpha(q)$ and $f(q)$ will be calculated using the open-source codes *ImageJ* and *FracLac* [44].

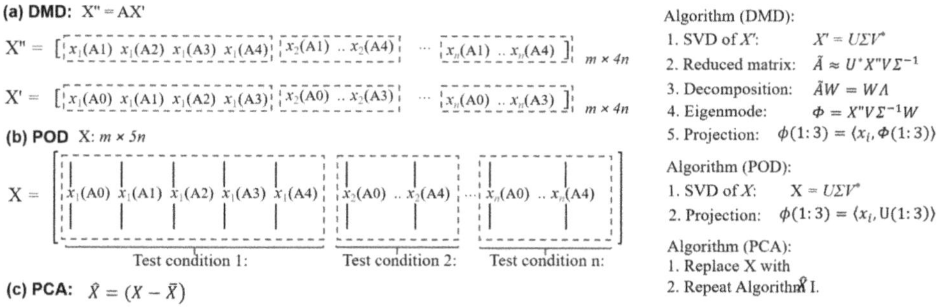

Figure 9.3. Schematic of feature extraction using SVD-based algorithms: (a) DMD, (b) POD, and (c) PCA. Here x_1 (A0) represents the aerosol image as a single-column vector. The parameter m is the size of the image (e.g. a 600 by 600 image gives m = 360 000), and n is the amount of test with each model. (Adapted from [45] CC BY 4.0.)

9.2.3.3 Dynamic mode decomposition (DMD)

Disease growth is inherently a dynamic process. It is therefore desirable to extricate the time-varying features from the exhaled aerosol images and use these features to determine the stage of the disease. Dynamic mode decomposition (DMD) directly takes into account the temporal dynamics of a system through the equation $X'' = A*X'$. In this equation, X'' = [A1, A2, A3, A4] and X' = [A0, A1, A2, A3], where A0–4 are the five stages of the disease (figure 9.3(a)). For comparison purposes, proper orthogonal decomposition (POD) and principal component analysis (PCA) were also considered. The major difference between these two algorithms is that POD studies the original image matrix X = [A0, A1, A2, A3, A4] (figure 9.3(b)), while PCA studies the corrected matrix $\hat{X} = (X - \overline{X})$, where each image was subtracted by the mean (figure 9.3(c)). Compared to POD, the DMD algorithm has three additional steps, which extracts the temporal features from X' to X'', as displayed in figure 9.3(c). After the eigenmodes (i.e. features) are obtained, each image will be expressed as a linear combination of a number of eigenmodes. The eigenmode coefficients constitute a vector that represents the image, which will be further used for classification training and testing. To assess the impact from the retained eigenmodes on classification accuracy, six tests will be compared that retain 3, 5, 10, 25, 75, and 100 eigenmodes, respectively.

9.2.4 Image classification of exhaled aerosol images

Two classification methods, support vector machine (SVM) [46, 47] and random forest (RF) [48], will be used in this study to classify healthy and abnormal airway models [49]. A ten-fold cross-validation method will be adopted, where the data are randomly split into ten equal-sized groups. In each step, nine groups will be used for training and one for testing. This step will be repeated ten times. In other words, each group will be used for the training nine times and for testing once. The classification accuracy is expressed as follows:

$$\text{Accuracy} = 1 - \frac{\text{total number of misclassified samples}}{\text{total number of samples}}. \tag{9.6}$$

To obtain a classification accuracy of statistical significance, the ten-fold cross-validation test will be iterated one hundred times. The *R* package 'e1071' is used to train and test the SVM and RF models. Statistics package Minitab 18 (State College, PA) will be used to calculate the classification variability by means of one-way analysis of variance (ANOVA).

9.3 Results

Three test cases are presented herein. The first test case demonstrated that significant differences existed in exhaled aerosols between healthy and diseased patients, as well as between different types of disease. The second test case demonstrated that such differences could also be measurable at different stages of one disease (e.g. a growing squamous tumor in G3). The third test case showed that even airway remodeling in deep lungs (G7–9) could be detected using the proposed fractal-machine-learning method. In section 9.3.4, the third test case was further explored using DMD-extracted features, which further improved the classification accuracy.

9.3.1 AFP differences in healthy and diseased airways

9.3.1.1 Image acquisition from physiology-based modeling

The AFP pattern, which resembles an actual human fingerprint, collectively results from the aerosol motions through the lungs. In order to predict lung structure remodeling via exhaled aerosol breath tests, the AFPs should be adequately sensitive to variations in lung geometries. Figures 9.4(a) and (b) show the expiratory airflow and aerosol patterns at the mouth, respectively, in the four models that represent one healthy and three diseased airways (carinal tumor, squamous tumor at the left segmental bronchus, and constricted bronchioles) [50]. The sizes of tracer particles were 1 μm and 5 μm under a steady breathing condition of 30 L min^{-1}. There are substantial differences in particle distributions between healthy and diseased patients, as well as among diseases with different sites and levels of severity. As the particle size increased from 1 μm to 5 μm, such differences become even more pronounced.

Figure 9.4(c) shows the exhaled aerosol distributions (red) when aerosols were released only from the two constricted bronchi (red particles) of model D and were superimposed onto the asthma case [50]. The red particles had a clear pattern and could be viewed as a biomarker for that diseased condition. In this sense, these tagged trace particles can be employed to detect the position of the airway abnormality and estimate the seriousness of the air passage obstruction. The plot of the normal case (model A) is also shown in figure 9.4(c) for comparison purposes, with the tracer aerosols released from corresponding healthy bronchioles being visualized in red.

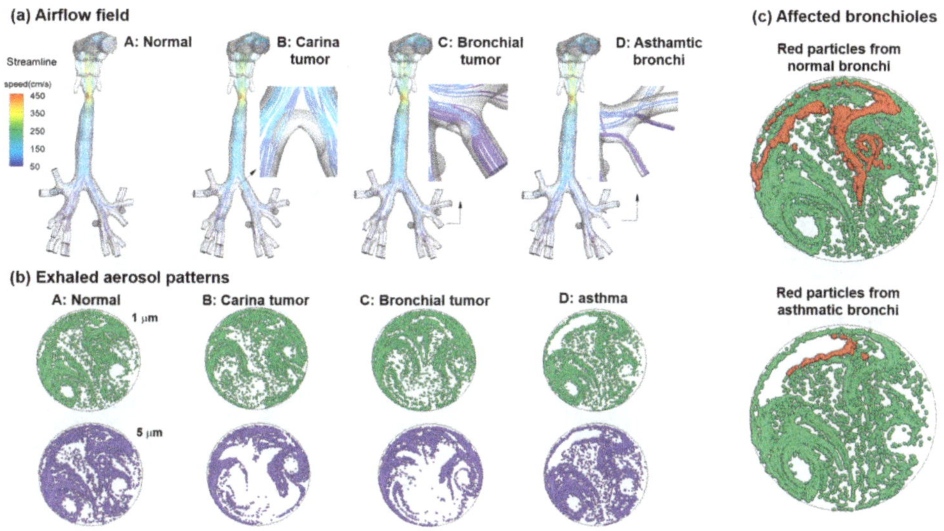

Figure 9.4. Test case 1: (a) airflow, (b) exhaled aerosol patterns, and (c) comparison of particles that were originally released from the normal and constricted bronchi. One normal (model A) and three diseased (models B–D) were considered. The three diseased models are carina tumor, bronchiolar tumor at G3 of the left lower lobe, and constricted bronchi in the left upper lobe (or asthma), respectively.

9.3.1.2 Relative concentration

Although the particle distributions in figure 9.4(b) are visually distinct between models, particle overlapping may prevent an accurate quantification of particle concentration. Figure 9.5 displays the ratio of local aerosol accumulations over the averaged concentration, with the blue color representing zero and the red color representing high aerosol concentrations [42]. The concentration map can readily pinpoint the sites of peak aerosol localization (red color), which should also be the most susceptible sites for tumorigenesis.

9.3.1.3 Fractal and multifractal feature extraction

The fractal dimension quantifies the complexity of an image by measuring the pixels occupied by the particles, whereas the multifractal spectrum quantifies both the heterogeneity (space versus particles) and complexity [18], as shown in figure 9.6 [42]. Human lungs resemble an upside-down tree and can be considered as a fractal structure [25, 26] with a fractal dimension of approximately 1.57 [29, 30]. During respiration, inhaled aerosols constantly fill and empty the lung trees. It is expected that the exhaled particles, which travel back from the deep lung to the mouth by passing through the bifurcation networks, should also show fractal features and therefore, are suitable for fractal analysis. Figure 9.6(a) shows the box-counting method to calculate fractal dimension (FD) of model A (right panel), as well as the comparison of FDs among the four models for the whole image (middle panel) and a prespecified region of interest (ROI, left panel). It is observed that the whole-image FDs do not show significant differences from the normal case except for model D. Instead, significant differences are found in the regional FDs among the four

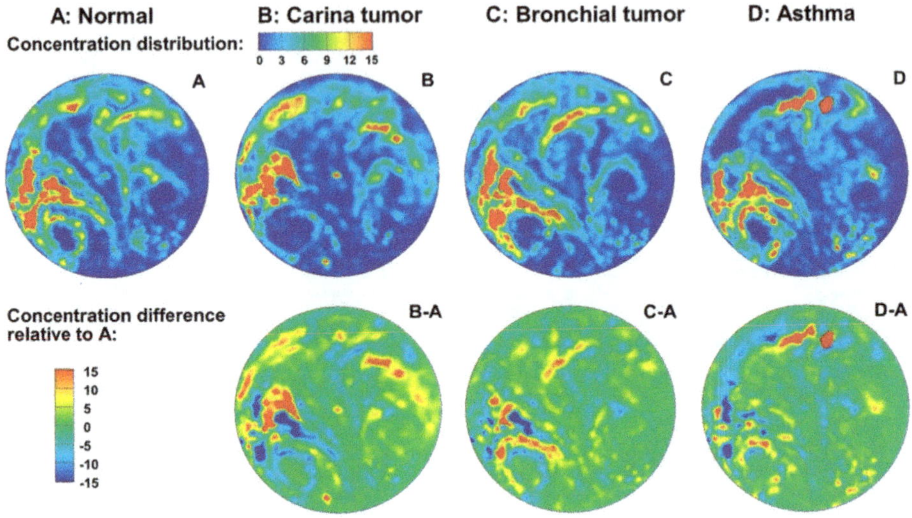

Figure 9.5. Relative concentrations of exhaled aerosols from the normal and three diseased airway models. The concentration difference in the second row was calculated by subtracting the relative concentration of each model by that of model A.

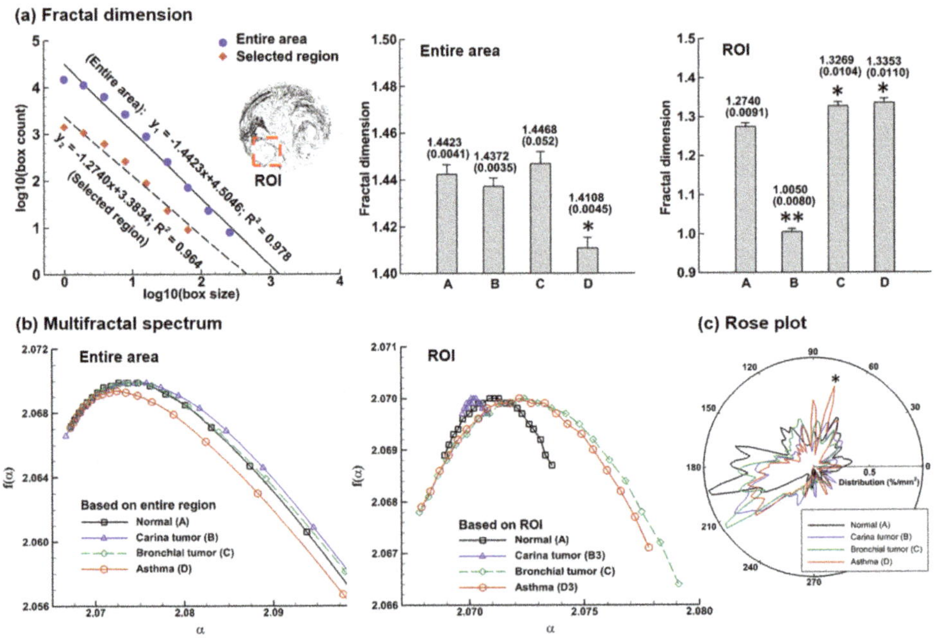

Figure 9.6. Fractal and multifractal analyses of exhaled aerosols from the normal and three diseased airway models. (a) Box-counting method to calculate fractal dimension, FD (left), and FDs of the whole image (middle) and ROI (right). (b) Multifractal spectra for the whole image (left) and ROI (right). The spatial distribution of aerosols was also visualized as a rose plot in (c).

models. Similar results are also observed in the multifractal spectrum (figure 9.6(b)), where significant differences among models are absent for the whole image but prevail for the ROI. This indicates that FD in sub-regions, not the whole image, should be used for later pattern recognition and disease classification [31]. The aerosol distribution is also visualized in figure 9.6(c) as a rose plot, which also exhibits large differences among the four models. It is therefore inferred that variations in lung structures appear to generate sufficient large differences in the exhaled aerosols, which can be explored to correlate to the underlying lung diseases.

9.3.2 Growing bronchial tumor

9.3.2.1 Perturbed airflow field

Figure 9.7(a) shows the airflows during exhalation among the five stages of a squamous tumor located at a segmental bronchus (G3) of the left lower lobe. The airway obstruction due to the bronchial tumor noticeably modifies the airflow field near the tumor as illustrated by the distorted streamlines. The flow perturbation will be transported by the exhalation flows to downstream of the respiratory tract. As the tumor grows from case A to E, more airway obstruction and higher flow resistance are expected, which give a lower volumetric flow rate under the same respiration effort. Due to airway obstruction, the trajectories of aerosols are also disturbed, which can perceivably change the distribution of exhaled aerosols. Figure 9.7(b) compares the velocity contours at slice 1–1′ in two different orientations (a–a′ and b–b′) across the five stages of the growing tumor. As expected, the flow speed progressively drops with increasing tumor size. As the air moves toward the mouth,

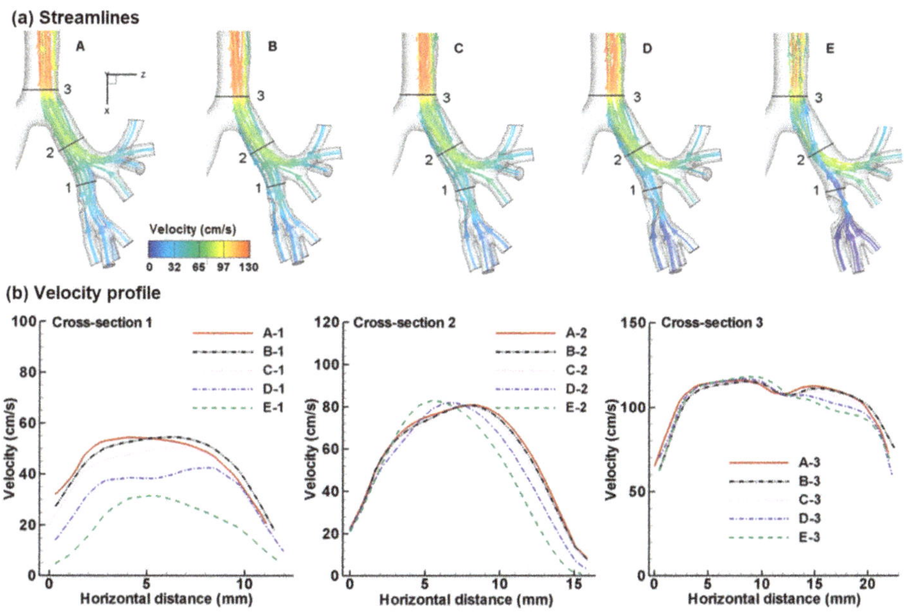

Figure 9.7. Test case 2: comparison of airflow fields among the five stages of a growing squamous tumor in terms of (a) streamlines and (b) velocity profiles. (Adapted from [27] CC BY-NC 4.0.)

the difference in airflows gradually decreases due to the mingling of flows joining from neighboring branches. It is recalled that the aerosol profile is determined by both local flows and their upstream histories. Even though the downstream flow field may look indistinguishable, the aerosol patterns can be highly distinct because of their time-integrative properties.

9.3.2.2 Patterns of exhaled aerosol fingerprints

Distributions of the tracer particles collected at the mouth opening are visualized in figure 9.8(a). Both differences and similarities are observed in particle distributions among the five stages of the bronchial tumor. Among many differences in figure 9.8(a), two are noteworthy. First, a recirculation zone is observed in the left lower part that persists for all stages of the tumor, while a smaller recirculation zone in the right part shrinks in size gradually from case A to E (figure 9.8(a)). These two recirculation zones are not symmetric relative to the centerline of the circular filter, which may be attributed to the left–right asymmetry of the lungs. Second, large differences exist in the particle distributions between the two regions outlined by a dashed red circle and a box (figure 9.8(a)). In both regions, the particle concentration decreases with increasing tumor size. Moreover, increasingly scattered particle distributions are observed in the dashed red box with increasing tumor size from A to E.

Figure 9.8(b) shows the relative concentrations (or local density) of exhaled particles on the mouth filter, with zero concentration in blue and maximum concentration in red. Compared to particle profiles (figure 9.8(a)), the concentration image (figure 9.8(b)) identifies the peak particle accumulations (red), which cannot be identified in the exhaled aerosol images *per se* due to particle overlapping. In this test case, both the left recirculation zone and the lower-right corner (red dashed circle) exhibit elevated levels of aerosol accumulations. The accumulation levels in left recirculation remain relatively unchanged for all stages herein, while that in the lower-right corner decreases continuously as the tumor grows from A to E. A similar

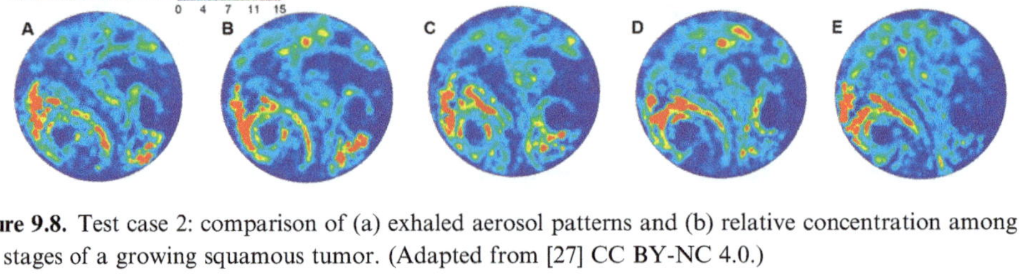

Figure 9.8. Test case 2: comparison of (a) exhaled aerosol patterns and (b) relative concentration among the five stages of a growing squamous tumor. (Adapted from [27] CC BY-NC 4.0.)

decline is also observed in figure 9.8(a) in the right-middle region (red rectangle). These time-varying correlations can be utilized as biomarkers to probe the progression of the tumor, which will be further discussed in later sections.

9.3.2.3 Fractal dimension

Fractal dimensions (FDs) were computed for exhaled aerosol images both in the whole image and specified ROIs (figure 9.9). In each case, the standard deviations in FD were computed from aerosol images that were predicted based on stochastically generated inlet particle profiles ($n = 5$). A consistent FD variation with growing tumor sizes was not observed for the whole images, as indicated by the erratic change of the FD values in figure 9.9(a). Rather, a constant decrease in FD was noted for the two selected regions of interest (ROI_1 and ROI_2) with tumor growth. This finding confirms the previous observation that malignant lungs gave lower FDs than those in normal lungs [51]. Different from the small FD variations for the whole images, large variations in the FD were predicted in both ROIs across the five disease stages. Moreover, the derivation of FD from the control case (case A) increases steadily in the diseased models from B to E. Accordingly, the ROI-based FD seems to be a feasible biomarker to monitor tumor growth and gauge tumor severity. Considering that FDs in sub-regions may carry more concentrated information from the disease, each aerosol image was further split into a 6 × 6 grid. Figure 9.9(b) shows the FD values in each grid. As expected, large differences in color patterns are observed across the five tumor stages, with a unique pattern in each stage.

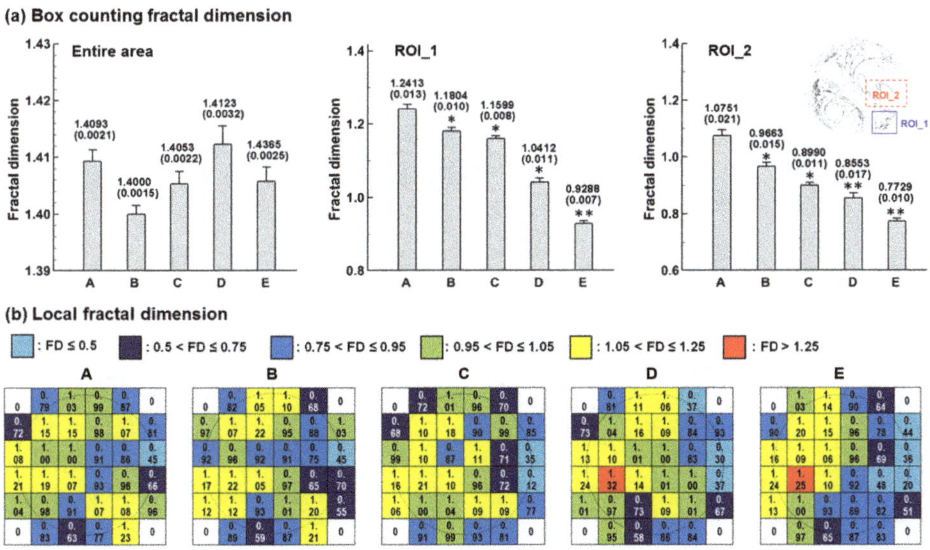

Figure 9.9. Fractal analysis in the test case 2: (a) comparison of fractal dimensions among the five tumor stages for the entire image (left), ROI_1 (middle), and ROI_2 (right); (b) FD distribution by dividing the image into a 6 × 6 lattice for the five tumor stages. (Adapted from [27] CC BY-NC 4.0.)

9.3.2.4 *Multifractal spectrum analysis*

The multifractal spectra of the exhaled AFP images are shown in figure 9.10 for the five stages of the growing tumor. Interesting transition patterns can be observed across the stages (figure 9.10(a)), as illustrated in the 3D surface plots of particle localization at the mouth. First, the height of the peaks in the left corner (solid black arrow) decreases continuously from case A to E. Second, the aerosol concentration in the left-middle zone (red rectangle) decreases as the tumor grows from case A to E. These two outlined regions will be used as the ROIs in this test case for multifractal spectrum analysis, as shown in figures 9.10(b) and (c), respectively.

Again, apparently different profiles among the five disease stages are observed in the multifractal spectra in both ROIs (figures 9.10(b) and (c)), lending support that the differences in exhaled aerosols can be significant and are quantitatively comparable between health and disease. Differences between the two ROIs were also predicted in their multifractal spectra. As illustrated in figure 9.10(b), the $f(\alpha)$-spectra in the first ROI converge to a single point ($q = 0$), which is not observed in the second ROI (figure 9.10(c)). As a result, the first ROI is mono-fractal, while the second ROI_2 is considered to be multifractal. Comparing the right panels in figures 9.10(b) and (c), the discrepancy ($\alpha_{max} - \alpha_{min}$) is associated with the heterogeneity of the aerosol images. This discrepancy decreases persistently for both ROIs considered as the tumor grows in size from case A to E, indicating a decrease of heterogeneity with disease deterioration. This result corroborates findings in previous studies [52, 53] that a narrower range of α often gives a lower value of lacunarity, which is an alternative indicator of image heterogeneity. Similar

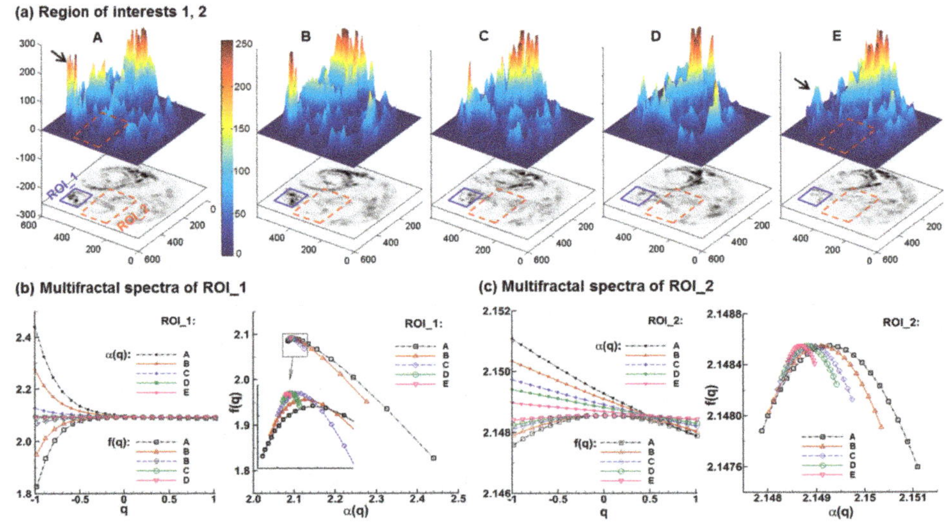

Figure 9.10. Multifractal spectrum analysis in test case 2. (a) 3D plot of aerosol concentrations. (b) Comparison of the multifractal spectra in ROI_1 across the five tumor stages. (c) Comparison of the multifractal spectra in ROI_2 across the five tumor stages. (Reproduced from [27] CC BY-NC 4.0.)

examples include vascular networks with high density [53] and soils with low porosity [52].

9.3.3 Asthmatic bronchioles in small airways

9.3.3.1 Airflow field and exhaled aerosol images

Figure 9.11 compares the exhalation flows and aerosol distributions among the five stages of an asthmatic bronchiole at G7. The bronchiolar constriction significantly alters the velocity field in the bronchiole (figure 9.11(a)). These flow perturbations are convected by exhalation flows downstream to approximately four bifurcations beyond the constriction site. Disturbances to solid particles will persist for an even longer distance because of their inertia. The constricted bronchioles also increase the flow resistance and decrease the volumetric flow rate through it, which further modifies the exhaled aerosol behaviors. It is emphasized that even though the downstream airflow fields may be similar, the aerosol profiles can be highly different because of upstream particle perturbations. This is evident in the strikingly distinct patterns of exhaled aerosols that originated from the disease-affected bronchioles at five stages (figure 9.11(b)).

9.3.3.2 Fractal-feature extraction

To vectorize the exhaled AFPs, the aerosol image shown in figure 9.12(a) was split into an $n \times n$ matrix, and the FD in each grid was computed. Figure 9.12(b) shows the FDs in a 3×3 matrix while figure 9.12(c) shows the FDs in a 6×6 matrix. The color code was calculated as the ratio $\alpha(i) = \text{FD}(i)/\text{FD}(\text{A0})$, i = A0, A1, A2, A3, A4,

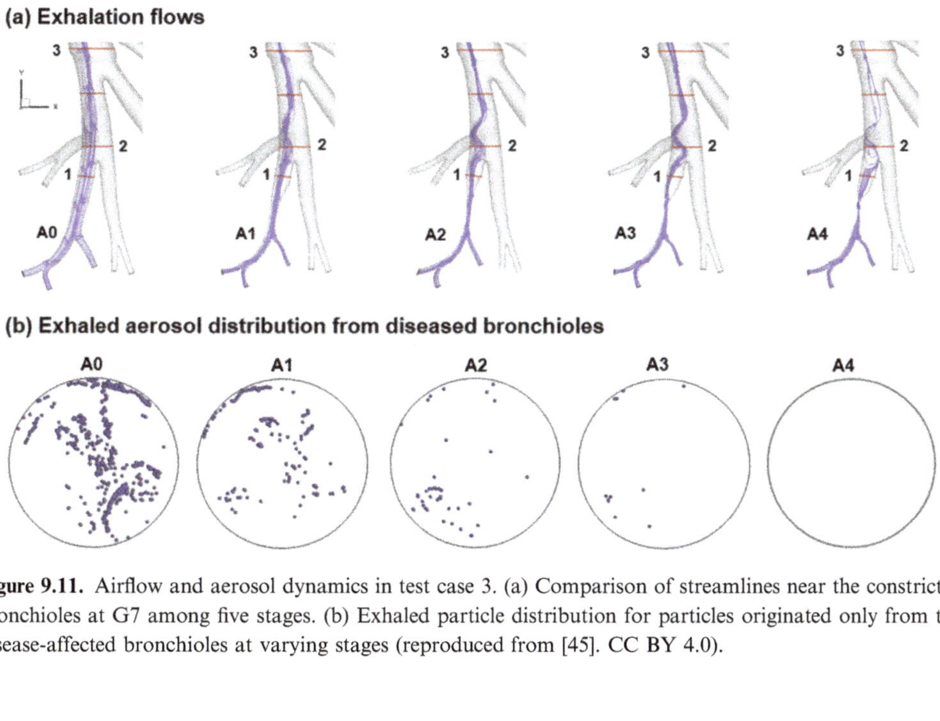

Figure 9.11. Airflow and aerosol dynamics in test case 3. (a) Comparison of streamlines near the constricted bronchioles at G7 among five stages. (b) Exhaled particle distribution for particles originated only from the disease-affected bronchioles at varying stages (reproduced from [45]. CC BY 4.0).

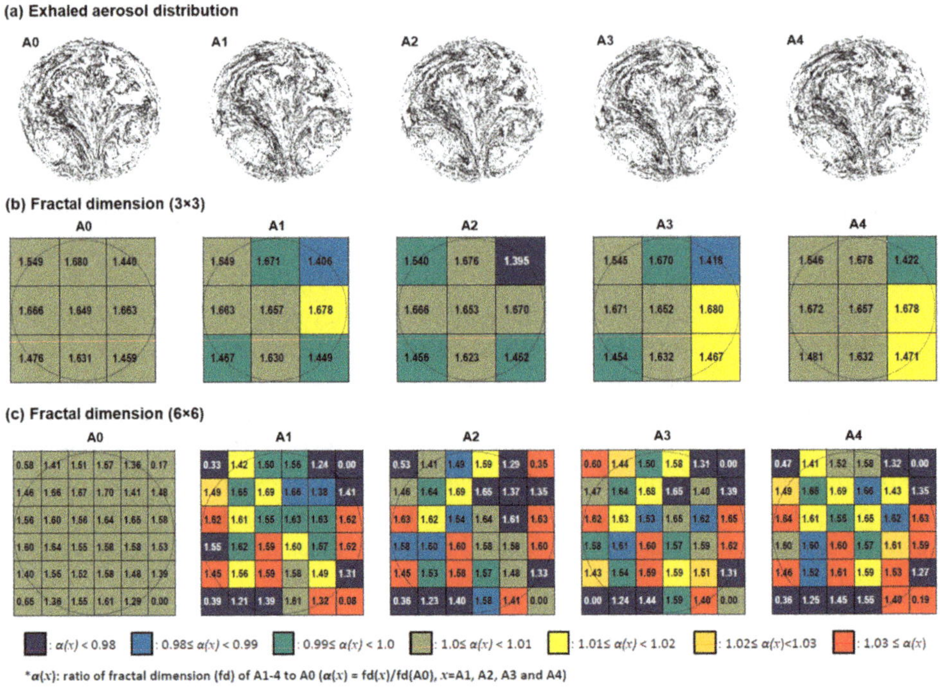

Figure 9.12. Exhaled aerosol patterns and FD-based feature extraction in test case 3. (a) Exhaled AFPs for the five stages of the bronchiolar tumor. (b) FD distribution at 3 × 3 resolution. (c) FD distribution at 6 × 6 resolution. (Reproduced from [28] with permission from Elsevier.)

with dark blue being the lowest ratio and red the highest. The pattern of color arrays was observed to be distinct for each model and at each matrix resolution ($n \times n$). Each image was expressed as a vector consisting of n^2 features by stacking the $n \times n$ FD values in one row. The distinct color patterns between different matrix resolutions for the same image can impart more information in revealing the subtle variations that are hidden in the images.

9.3.3.3 Database quality check

Principal component analysis (PCA) was carried out to check the quality of the 9 × 9 dataset, as shown in figure 9.13. It is observed that the first principal component (PC1) accounts for 20.6% of the total variance and has an eigenvalue of 15.5 (figure 9.13(a)). The PC2 accounts for 14.0% of the data variance and has an eigenvalue of 10.5. Together, the first two PCs capture 34.6% of the data variance. The first five PCs capture 56.8%, whereas the other 85 PCs capture the remaining variance of 43.2% (100 PCs retained in this case). As a result, unimportant components can be safely neglected without noticeably compromising classification accuracies. To identify outliers in the image database, the Mahalanobis distances are plotted in figure 9.13(b) for all images in the database [54]. No obvious outlier is found in this database because all data points fall below 10.65, the reference line for outlier existence [54].

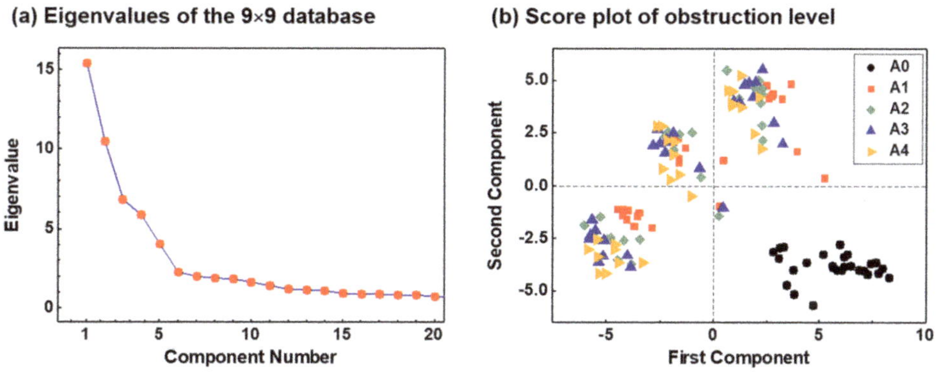

Figure 9.13. PCA-based quality check of images in test case 3 that was mapped in a 9 × 9 matrix. (a) Eigenvalues of the first 20 principal components. (b) Score plot of the airway obstruction level as a function of the first two principal components.

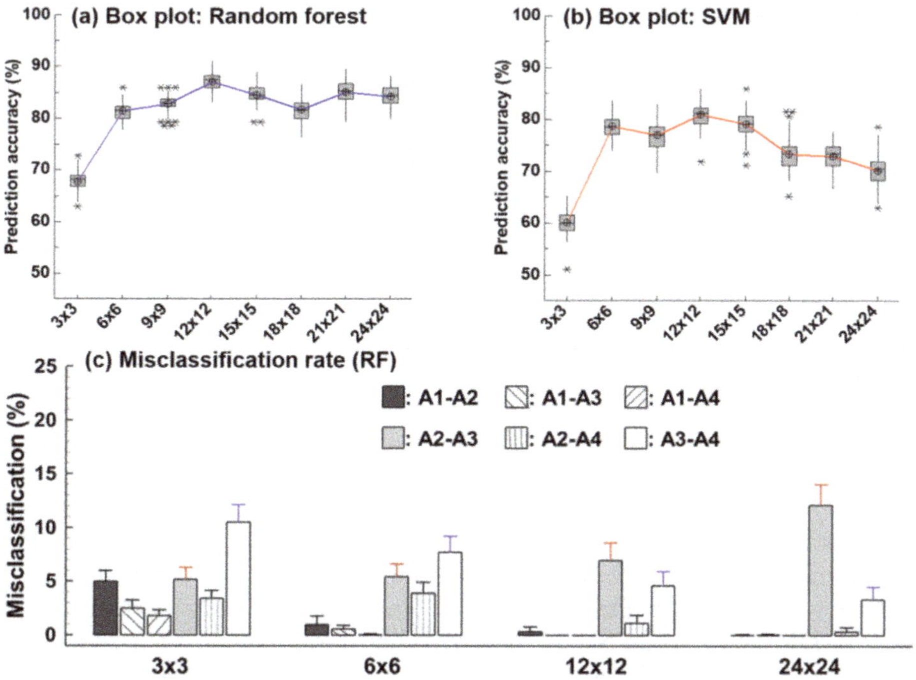

Figure 9.14. Image classification in test case 3. (a) The predicted five-class classification accuracies based on RF at different sampling resolutions, (b) those based on SVM, and (c) the misclassification rate based on RF. (Adapted from [28] with permission from Elsevier.)

9.3.3.4 Classification using RF and SVM algorithms

Two classification methods, SVM and random forest (RF), were applied to train and test the image data at varying matrix resolutions. Figures 9.14(a) and (b) show the statistical results of the five-class classification (A0–4) using RF and SVM, respectively. As expected, the lowest classification accuracy was predicted at 3 × 3 resolution because of its low sampling resolution. The classification accuracy improves with increasing sampling resolutions until reaching the optimal accuracy at 12 × 12, and drops thereafter as the sampling resolution becomes even finer (figures 9.14(a) and (b)). This accuracy deterioration may suffer from the probability that a too-small sampling grid may miss the disturbance signals from the small airways. The highest accuracy with SVM is found at 12 × 12 as well. Overall, RF persistently outperformed SVM in this test case (figure 9.14(a) versus 9.14(b)).

9.3.3.5 Misclassification analysis

Figure 9.14(c) shows the misclassification rates using RF in this test case. The highest rates of misclassification are observed for the pairs A2–A3 and A3–A4, indicating its strong association with structural similarities. Conversely, misclassifications are much reduced for A2–A4, whose geometrical difference is more pronounced than that of A2–A3 or A3–A4. Regarding different resolutions, extensive misclassifications are found at either highly coarse (3 × 3) or highly fine (24 × 24) resolutions. Misclassification spikes are absent at 6 × 6 and 12 × 12, although there are still misclassifications for A2–A3 and A3–A4 at these two resolutions (figure 9.14(c)). It is conjectured that the best classification accuracy at 12 × 12 can result from the disease site at G7 that has 128 (2^7) sister bronchioles and, if being evenly mapped, needs an 11.3 × 11.3 matrix. However, the verification of this hypothesis needs future investigation.

9.3.4 Dynamic mode decomposition (DMD) to catch disease growth

9.3.4.1 DMD versus conventional algorithms

In this section, we will explain the usage of dynamic mode decomposition (DMD) to extract features of the images and demonstrate the superiority of our method over conventional algorithms, such as fractal dimension, proper orthogonal decomposition (POD), and principal component analysis (PCA). As a quick explanation, both POD and PCA are based on the singular value decomposition (SVD) that can handle non-square matrices. POD decomposes the system into mutually orthogonal eigenmodes that are spatially independent of each other. PCA is similar to POD, while it eliminates the average in order to emphasize the image contrast. PCA has been widely used in machine learning for dimensionality reduction and feature extraction. DMD is also an SVD-based decomposition method such as POD and PCA. However, the DMD modes directly capture the temporal evolution of the system and are inherently suitable for studying time-varying systems, which develop around an attractor (e.g. one type of lung disease) with transient oscillators (e.g. diseases at different stages). Details of the mathematical algorithms for DMD, POD, and PCA can be found in Xi and Zhao [45].

9.3.4.2 DMD feature extraction of exhaled AFP images

Figure 9.15(a) displays DMD-predicted dynamic eigenvalues in the complex plane, with each dot representing one eigenmode. Most modes are observed to be within the unit circle, while a small number of eigenmodes are lying on or in close proximity

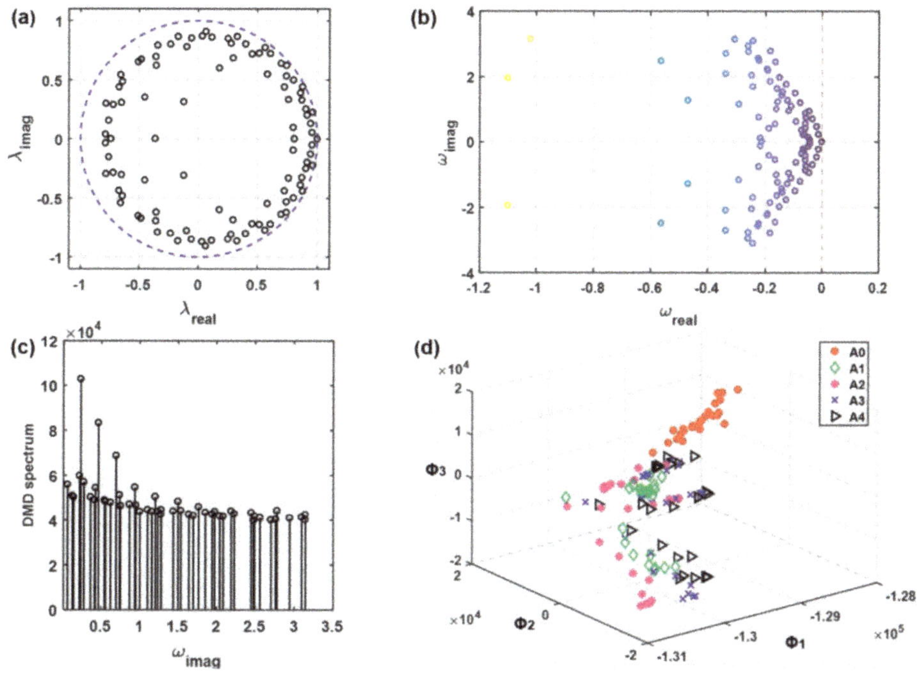

Figure 9.15. DMD analysis of exhaled aerosol images in test case 3: (a) DMD eigenvalues λ, (b) the transformed eigenvalues $\omega = \log(\lambda)/(2\pi)$, (c) DMD energy spectrum, and (d) eigenspace spanned by the first three DMD modes. (Adapted from [45] CC BY 4.0.)

to the right side of the circle. The radius of each mode (i.e. distance from the center) denotes its dynamic characteristics, growing if the radius is larger than one while decaying if the radius is less than one. In figure 9.15(a), nearly all eigenvalues fall within the circle, which signifies a strong damping and a stable system in this test case.

The transformed eigenvalues are shown in figure 9.15(b), which is expressed as $\omega = \log(\lambda)/(2\pi)$. The real part of ω_i in each point represents the response of the eigenmode to inputs (e.g. disease types and stages). Similar to figure 9.15(a), while decay occurs for most modes, several modes lay on or in the proximity of the red line, suggesting neutral stability and slow decay for these modes. Figure 9.15(c) shows the DMD spectrum. Three spikes are observed at frequencies *f*0, *f*1, and *f*2. It is no surprise that *f*0 is related to the respiration flow rate (repeated every three cases), *f*1 to the disease stage (repeated every five cases), and *f*2 to the diameter of tracer particles (repeated every nine cases). It is noted that that three inhalation rates and nine particle sizes were considered in this test case.

The test images were subsequently projected into the eigenspace spanned by the leading eigenmodes. Figure 9.15(d) shows the images in the eigenspace spanned by the first three modes. Reasonable clustering and separation of data points were observed according to the disease stage. It is emphasized that eigenvalues from DMD are complex numbers, with the real part signifying the growth/decay and the imaginary part signifying the oscillation. This capacity to characterize both the

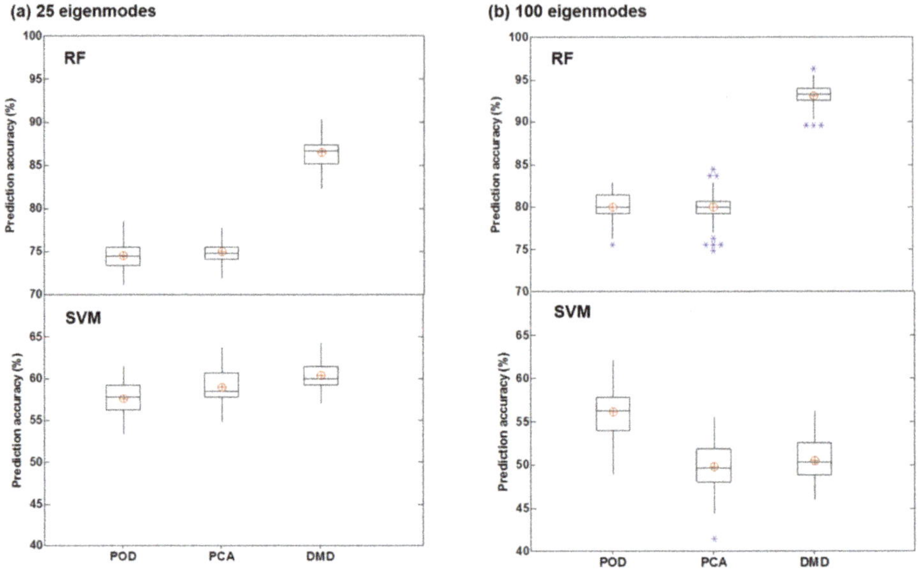

Figure 9.16. Classification accuracy of the five stages of an asthmatic bronchiole (A0–4) by retaining a varying amount of eigenmodes: (a) 25 and (b) 100. Various combinations between feature extraction (POD, PCA, DMD) and classification (SVM and RF) algorithms were compared. (Reproduced from [45] CC BY 4.0.)

growth/decay and oscillation behaviors is highly advantageous when studying temporal signals and progressive systems.

9.3.4.3 SVM and RF classification based on DMD features

The classification accuracies for five stages of an asthmatic bronchiole (A0–4) at G7 are shown in figure 9.16. This figure was plotted from the ten-fold cross-validation tests that were iterated one hundred times. To evaluate the effects of extracted features, one retained twenty-five eigenmodes and the other retained one hundred (figure 9.16(a) versus (b)). To study the effect of classification algorithms, SVM and RF were considered. Overall, RF outperformed SVM for all tests. When using the RF classification algorithm, the classification accuracy using DMD-extracted features is significantly higher than that using POD- or PCA-extracted features (figures 9.16(a) and (b), upper panel). When using the SVM, however, an insignificant discrepancy was observed in the classification accuracy among the three features (figures 9.16(a) and (b), lower panel). It is also observed that retaining more features could increase classification uncertainty, as indicated by the outliers presented in the 100 mode case (figure 9.16(b)) versus no outlier with 25 modes (figure 9.16(a)). This uncertainty might be caused by noisy data and associated features that contaminated the disease stage related features.

9.4 Discussion

In many circumstances, it is nontrivial to find a subset of features that can effectively characterize the system of interest. In this chapter, we introduced a non-invasive method for lung disease diagnosis based on exhaled aerosols and presented the latest developments in extracting features from the exhaled aerosols. The performance of extracted features in correlating to underlying respiratory obstructive diseases was compared in terms of classification accuracy in both the tracheobronchial region (G3) and small airways (G7). It was found that the DMD-extracted features, in combination with the RF classification algorithm, gave the highest prediction accuracy.

Why DMD can extract more informative features and give improved classification accuracy than POD or PCA is discussed below. DMD considers the time-varying features related to different stages of a squamous tumor and an asthmatic bronchiole and therefore captures the phase transition from one stage to another. Instead, POD and PCA extract mutually orthogonal eigenmodes from the image matrix; loss of information associated with the disease growth often occurs during the averaging process to construct the correlation matrix. Furthermore, the POD- and PCA-extracted eigenmodes are not temporally independent of each other [55], which would also adversely affect their classification accuracies.

The newly proposed DMD–RF method outperformed the fractal–RF method by a large margin (7.8%). Fractal dimensions have been explored in previous studies [28, 56] to vectorize exhaled aerosol images at different sampling resolutions. The best fractal–RF classification accuracy for five-class classification of an asthmatic bronchiole was 87.0% [28]. Despite the ability of fractals in quantifying complex patterns, information losses are inevitable due to the box-counting principle underlying the fractal dimensions. It is not clear yet how the information loss impacts the disease classification. In contrast, DMD-based features (eigenmodes) are directly extracted from raw images (i.e. pixel values) using singular value decomposition (SVD) to find the leading coherent structures, thus minimizing information loss. The second DMD-based enhancement comes from the temporal dynamics that is deeply rooted in disease growth. Time-related features can be disclosed that can be otherwise overlooked using static decomposition approaches such as POD and PCA.

Detecting diseases in small airways is more challenging than in the central and large airways owing to their much weaker perturbation signals. There are two factors that can contribute to these weak signals: small perturbations due to small airway sizes in deep lungs and a longer period of signal decay during exhalation. It is critical to know whether these signals can be captured by the mouth filter and can be subsequently traced back to the origin of these signals. In this chapter, we demonstrated that the DMD–RF method was sensitive enough to detect even subtle variations in AFP images. In the test case of the asthmatic bronchiole with a diameter less than 1.87 mm, the five-class classification accuracy was 94.8% when using 100 features. In addition, this asthmatic bronchiole model has only one deformed bronchiole and is expected to generate much weaker disturbance signals relative to real-life asthma, where often a large area is affected and thus is more suitable for diagnosis. It is acknowledged that the high accuracy in this test case is because of many idealized assumptions; the classification accuracy is expected to be lower in clinical settings due to numerous compounding factors.

Convolutional neural networks (CNNs) have gained ever-increasing popularity in recent years with mounting evidence of improved performance over conventional machine learning methods [57, 58]. One major advantage of CNNs is that they can automatically learn the features from the training images and thus can directly use the input images. In addition, the rich features that CNNs can learn at multiple levels has given rise to many successful applications in medical image analysis [59, 60]. However, there are specific challenges in using CNN models. Due to its self-learning nature, a CNN model needs a large dataset to capture the image features effectively; however, high-quality medical images are usually not readily available. In this test case, a dataset of 405 exhaled aerosol images was, which might have been enough for classifications with SVM and RF, but was still far from adequate for meaningful CNN training and testing. Future assessment of CNN performance in automatic feature extraction and classification of exhaled aerosol images is warranted as more AFP images become available.

In this chapter, local bronchiolar constrictions in G3 (a growing tumor) and G7 (asthmatic bronchioles) in the left lung were selected to demonstrate the applicability of exhaled AFP based breath tests in lung diagnosis. It is noted that disease-induced airway remodeling can happen anywhere in the respiratory tract and at multiple places. Will the overlaying of particle perturbations from different disease sites makes it too complex to differentiate by the proposed fractal–RF or DMD–RF methods? Our best guess is that it will not. All AFP images, regardless of how complicated they appear, can simply be characterized as feature vectors for classification purposes. As different types of diseases will give rise to unique patterns of exhaled aerosols, a database of common respiratory obstructive diseases can be developed to train and validate a generic diagnostic system. The database can be extended by including AFP images of new or uncommon diseases. As new AFP images are becoming available, the existent diagnostic system can be constantly refined for improved accuracies.

The high accuracy herein was because of a limited number of disease models with idealized test conditions. Results in this study are not applicable to other respiratory diseases, nor can they be directly compared to the diagnostic rate of current diagnostic techniques. Many uncertainties exist that can complicate the training process and reduce classification accuracies. Patient-related uncertainties include the body position, inhalation rate, mouth shape, and tongue position. The lung geometry itself can also differ among patients. The compounding influences from certain factors can be alleviated by careful planning; other factors demand additional investigations. For example, using a mouthpiece is anticipated to minimize the impacts of the oral cavity shape and tongue position. Similarly, standardization of the participant's breathing and sitting position should mitigate compounding influences from the variability in respiration and body position, respectively.

There are several assumptions that restrict the physical realism of this study, such as steady inhalation and exhalation, noncompliant airway walls, uniform outlet pressure, and a small cohort of respiratory disease models. Tidal breathing [17] and compliant walls [61] can exert noticeable impacts on both airflow and aerosol dynamics. Also, the ventilation distribution can differ between the case with a uniform outlet pressure and the case with specific resistance and compliance of downstream airways [62, 63]. It is acknowledged that a uniform pressure was adopted at the outlets in all test cases due to the lack of resistance/compliance data. The impact of this assumption on diagnostic accuracy, however, should be minor, considering the consistency of this assumption for all images herein, as well as the fact that classification was based not on individual patterns, but on similarities/differences among patterns. Considering the high variability in site, size, and type of respiratory diseases, detecting a disease that has not been included in the database is impractical. One advantage of the simulation-based database is that it can be readily extended by simulating more scenarios of obstructive diseases. The development of the training database can be an ongoing process. New sample images will help refine the diagnostic system and improve both its prediction accuracy and statistical power. Considering the respiratory airway models, only two lung geometries were considered, while intersubject variability was neglected. Also, only numerical simulations were undertaken. Complimentary *in vitro* and *in vivo* tests are required to verify the numerical prediction herein.

9.5 Conclusion

In conclusion, exhaled aerosols from the human lungs exhibit unique patterns, and a pattern deviation can be correlated to underlying structural variations in the lungs. Different algorithms of feature extraction were discussed, and their capacity in characterizing airway variations was evaluated in both the upper and lower sections of anatomically accurate lung models. The fractal dimensions of the exhaled aerosol images at multiple resolutions appeared to effectively capture the geometrical variation that accompanies the progression of respiratory diseases. Significantly improved performance was achieved using dynamic algorithms for feature extraction (DMD) than when using static algorithms (fractal, POD, and PCA). Considering machine learning models, RF consistently outperformed SVM for both the static and dynamic features considered in this study.

References

[1] Coate L E *et al* 2011 Treatment of the elderly when cure is the goal the influence of age on treatment selection and efficacy for stage III non-small cell lung cancer *J. Thorac. Oncol.* **6** 537–44

[2] Hubbard M O, Fu P, Margevicius S, Dowlati A and Linden P A 2012 Five-year survival does not equal cure in non-small cell lung cancer: a surveillance, epidemiology, and end results-based analysis of variables affecting 10- to 18-year survival *J. Thorac. Cardiovasc. Surg.* **143** 1307–13

[3] Krause A 2012 Diagnosis of interstitial lung diseases *Z. Rheumatol.* **71** 542–3

[4] Miekisch W, Schubert J K and Noeldge-Schomburg G F E 2004 Diagnostic potential of breath analysis—focus on volatile organic compounds *Clin. Chim. Acta* **347** 25–39

[5] Kostikas K, Koutsokera A, Papiris S, Gourgoulianis K I and Loukides S 2008 Exhaled breath condensate in patients with asthma: implications for application in clinical practice *Clin. Exp. Allergy* **38** 557–65

[6] Colombo C *et al* 2011 Analysis of inflammatory and immune response biomarkers in sputum and exhaled breath condensate by a multi-parametric biochip array in cystic fibrosis *Int. J. Immunopathol. Pharmacol.* **24** 423–32

[7] Loukides S, Bakakos P and Kostikas K 2011 Oxidative stress in patients with COPD *Curr. Drug Targets* **12** 469–77

[8] Chan H P, Tran V, Lewis C and Thomas P S 2009 Elevated levels of oxidative stress markers in exhaled breath condensate *J. Thorac. Oncol.* **4** 172–8

[9] Poli D *et al* 2005 Exhaled volatile organic compounds in patients with non-small cell lung cancer: cross sectional and nested short-term follow-up study *Respir. Res.* **6** 71

[10] Vijverberg S J H, Koenderman L, Koster E S, van der Ent C K, Raaijmakers J A M and Maitland-van der Zee A H 2011 Biomarkers of therapy responsiveness in asthma: pitfalls and promises *Clin. Exp. Allergy* **41** 615–29

[11] Mazzone P J 2008 Analysis of volatile organic compounds in the exhaled breath for the diagnosis of lung cancer *J. Thorac. Oncol.* **3** 774–80

[12] Buszewski B, Kesy M, Ligor T and Amann A 2007 Human exhaled air analytics: biomarkers of diseases *Biomed. Chromatogr.* **21** 553–66

[13] Horvath I, Lazar Z, Gyulai N, Kollai M and Losonczy G 2009 Exhaled biomarkers in lung cancer *Eur. Respir. J.* **34** 261–75

[14] Phillips M *et al* 2003 Detection of lung cancer with volatile markers in the breath *Chest* **123** 2115–23

[15] Xi J and Longest P W 2007 Transport and deposition of micro-aerosols in realistic and simplified models of the oral airway *Ann. Biomed. Eng.* **35** 560–81

[16] Xi J and Longest P W 2009 Characterization of submicrometer aerosol deposition in extrathoracic airways during nasal exhalation *Aerosol Sci. Technol.* **43** 808–27

[17] Xi J, Longest P W and Martonen T B 2008 Effects of the laryngeal jet on nano- and microparticle transport and deposition in an approximate model of the upper tracheobronchial airways *J. Appl. Physiol.* **104** 1761–77

[18] Xi J, Si X, Kim J W and Berlinski A 2011 Simulation of airflow and aerosol deposition in the nasal cavity of a 5-year-old child *J. Aerosol Sci.* **42** 156–73

[19] Si X A, Xi J, Kim J, Zhou Y and Zhong H 2013 Modeling of release position and ventilation effects on olfactory aerosol drug delivery *Respir. Physiol. Neurobiol.* **186** 22–32

[20] Xi J, Si X and Longest P W 2013 Electrostatic charge effects on pharmaceutical aerosol deposition in human nasal-laryngeal airways *Pharmaceutics* **6** 26–35

[21] Xi J, Si X A and Gaide R 2014 Electrophoretic particle guidance significantly enhances olfactory drug delivery: a feasibility study *PLoS One* **9** e86593

[22] Blanchard J D 1996 Aerosol bolus dispersion and aerosol-derived airway morphometry: assessment of lung pathology and response to therapy. 1 *J. Aerosol Med.* **9** 183–205

[23] Goo J and Kim C S 2001 Analysis of aerosol bolus dispersion in a cyclic tube flow by finite element method *Aerosol Sci. Technol.* **34** 321–31

[24] Lee D and Lee J 2002 Dispersion of aerosol bolus during one respiratory cycle in a model lung airway *J. Aerosol Sci.* **33** 1219

[25] Anderson P J and Dolovich M B 1994 Aerosols as diagnostic tools *J. Aerosol Med.* **7** 77–88

[26] Blanchard J D 1996 Aerosol bolus dispersion and aerosol-derived airway morphometry: assessment of lung pathology and response to therapy. 2 *J. Aerosol Med.* **9** 453–76

[27] Xi J *et al* 2015 CFD modeling and image analysis of exhaled aerosols due to a growing bronchial tumor: towards non-invasive diagnosis and treatment of respiratory obstructive diseases *Theranostics* **5** 443–55

[28] Xi J, Zhao W, Yuan J E, Cao B and Zhao L 2017 Multi-resolution classification of exhaled aerosol images to detect obstructive lung diseases in small airways *Comput. Biol. Med.* **87** 57–69

[29] Yeh H C and Schum G M 1980 Models of human lung airways and their application to inhaled particle deposition *Bull. Math. Biol.* **42** 461–80

[30] ICRP 1994 *Human Respiratory Tract Model for Radiological Protection* vol 66 (New York: Elsevier)

[31] Heistracher T and Hofmann W 1995 Physiologically realistic models of bronchial airway bifurcations *J. Aerosol Sci.* **26** 497–509

[32] Segal R A, Guan X, Shearer M and Martonen T B 2000 Mathematical model of airflow in the lungs of children I: effects of tumor sizes and locations *J. Theor. Med.* **2** 199–213

[33] Daisne J F *et al* 2004 Tumor volume in pharyngolaryngeal squamous cell carcinoma: comparison at CT, MR imaging, and FDG PET and validation with surgical specimen *Radiology* **233** 93–100

[34] Xi J, Yuan J E, Si X, Zhou Y and Cheng Y S 2015 Parametric study on mouth-throat geometrical factors on depositions of orally inhaled aerosols *J. Aerosol Sci.* **99** 94–106

[35] Kim J W, Xi J and Si X A 2013 Dynamic growth and deposition of hygroscopic aerosols in the nasal airway of a 5-year-old child *Int. J. Numer. Methods Biomed. Eng.* **29** 17–39

[36] Wilcox D C 2008 Formulation of the *k–w* turbulence model revisited *AIAA J.* **46** 2823–38

[37] Longest P W and Xi J 2007 Computational investigation of particle inertia effects on submicron aerosol deposition in the respiratory tract *J. Aerosol Sci.* **38** 111–30

[38] Morsi S A and Alexander A J 1972 An investigation of particle trajectories in two-phase flow systems *J. Fluid Mech.* **55** 193–208

[39] Allen M D and Raabe O G 1985 Slip correction measurements of spherical solid aerosol particles in an improved Millikan apparatus *Aerosol Sci. Technol.* **4** 269–86

[40] Longest P W and Xi J 2007 Effectiveness of direct Lagrangian tracking models for simulating nanoparticle deposition in the upper airways *Aerosol Sci. Technol.* **41** 380–97

[41] Xi J and Longest P W 2008 Evaluation of a drift flux model for simulating submicrometer aerosol dynamics in human upper tracheobronchial airways *Ann. Biomed. Eng.* **36** 1714–34

[42] Xi J, Si X A, Kim J, Mckee E and Lin E B 2014 Exhaled aerosol pattern discloses lung structural abnormality: a sensitivity study using computational modeling and fractal analysis *PLoS One* **9** e104682

[43] Karperien A, Ahammer H and Jelinek H F 2013 Quantitating the subtleties of microglial morphology with fractal analysis *Front. Cell. Neurosci.* **7** 1–18

[44] Karperien A *Fractal Dimension and Lacunarity* [https://www.imagej.nih.gov/ij/plugins/fraclac/fraclac.html]

[45] Xi J and Zhao W 2019 Correlating exhaled aerosol images to small airway obstructive diseases: a study with dynamic mode decomposition and machine learning *PLoS One* **14** e0211413

[46] Cortes C and Vapnik V 1995 Support-vector networks *Mach. Learn.* **20** 273–97

[47] Ramaswamy S *et al* 2001 Multiclass cancer diagnosis using tumor gene expression signatures *PNAS* **98** 15149–54

[48] Breiman L 2001 Random forests *Mach. Learn.* **45** 5–32

[49] Noble W S 2006 What is a support vector machine? *Nat. Biotechnol.* **24** 1565–7

[50] Xi J, Kim J, Si X A and Zhou Y 2013 Diagnosing obstructive respiratory diseases using exhaled aerosol fingerprints: a feasibility study *J. Aerosol Sci.* **64** 24–36

[51] Boser S R, Park H, Perry S F, Ménache M G and Green F H Y 2005 Fractal geometry of airway remodeling in human asthma *Am. J. Respir. Crit. Care Med.* **172** 817–23

[52] Posadas A N D, Giménez D, Quiroz R and Protz R 2003 Multifractal characterization of soil pore systems *Soil Sci. Soc. Am. J.* **67** 1361–9

[53] Gould D J, Vadakkan T J, PochÉ R A and Dickinson M E 2011 Multifractal and lacunarity analysis of microvascular morphology and remodeling *Microcirculation* **18** 136–51
[54] Xiang S, Nie F and Zhang C 2008 Learning a Mahalanobis distance metric for data clustering and classification *Pattern Recogn.* **41** 3600–12
[55] Hémon P and Santi F 2007 Simulation of a spatially correlated turbulent velocity field using biorthogonal decomposition *J. Wind Eng. Ind. Aerodyn.* **95** 21–9
[56] Xi J, Zhao W, Yuan J E, Kim J, Si X and Xu X 2015 Detecting lung diseases from exhaled aerosols: non-invasive lung diagnosis using fractal analysis and SVM classification *PLoS One* **10** e0139511
[57] Litjens G *et al* 2017 A survey on deep learning in medical image analysis *Med. Image Anal.* **42** 60–88
[58] Suzuki K 2017 Overview of deep learning in medical imaging *Radiol. Phys. Technol.* **10** 257–73
[59] Sharma H, Zerbe N, Klempert I, Hellwich O and Hufnagl P 2017 Deep convolutional neural networks for automatic classification of gastric carcinoma using whole slide images in digital histopathology *Comput. Med. Imaging Graph.* **61** 2–13
[60] Yamashita R, Nishio M, Do R K G and Togashi K 2018 Convolutional neural networks: an overview and application in radiology *Insights Imaging* **9** 911–29
[61] Berg E J, Weisman J L, Oldham M J and Robinson R J 2010 Flow field analysis in a compliant acinus replica model using particle image velocimetry (PIV) *J. Biomech.* **43** 1039–47
[62] Oakes J M, Marsden A L, Grandmont C, Shadden S C, Darquenne C and Vignon-Clementel I E 2014 Airflow and particle deposition simulations in health and emphysema: from *in vivo* to in silico animal experiments *Ann. Biomed. Eng.* **42** 899–914
[63] Oakes J M, Marsden A L, Grandmont C, Darquenne C and Vignon-Clementel I E 2015 Distribution of aerosolized particles in healthy and emphysematous rat lungs: comparison between experimental and numerical studies *J. Biomech.* **48** 1147–57

Chapter 10

A study of ground-glass opacity (GGO) nodules in the automated detection of lung cancer

May Phu Paing, Chuchart Pintavirooj, Kazuhiko Hamamoto and Supan Tungjitkusolmun

10.1 Introduction

Cancer is one of the most serious diseases because the number of cancer deaths is increasing day by day. Recently, the World Health Organisation (WHO) reported that the global cancer burden increased to 1.8 million new cases and 9.6 million deaths in 2018 [1]. Among various types of cancer, lung cancer shows the highest mortality rate. Approximately one in five cases of cancer death is related to lung cancer and 1.8 million deaths usually occur every year [2].

Lung cancer begins when the cells in the lung tissues proliferate uncontrollably. Smoking is the primary risk factor of lung cancer, and it leads to over two-thirds of lung cancer deaths globally. Smoking controls, early detection, and effective treatments have significantly reduced the mortality rate of lung cancer over the last two decades. During the years 1990–2016, the mortality rate declined by 48% in males and from 2002 to 2016, it decreased by 23% in females [2]. Lung cancer, however, occurs not only in smokers but also in non-smokers due to other risk factors such as passive smoking, radon gas, asbestos and other industrial chemicals, air pollution, related lung diseases, and genetic predisposition. Once a lung cancer starts, a patient may suffer some common symptoms such as trouble with breathing, wheezing, persistent cough, chest pain, and hemoptysis (coughing up blood). However, these symptoms may vary depending upon when and how much the cancer spreads. Sometimes, it even shows no suspicious signs, in particular at the early stages of the disease.

In clinical practice, physicians usually use a variety of image screening techniques to diagnose lung cancer. Among them, the most traditional one is the chest x-ray. It is a photon–atom interaction which projects radiation into the patient's body to take pictures of the internal organs. Although x-ray is a simple and inexpensive modality,

doi:10.1088/978-0-7503-2540-0ch10

it has the side effect of radiation damage, ionizing tissue along the beam path. An improved pattern of x-ray is computed tomography (CT), which combines the x-ray procedure with computer technology. Unlike traditional x-rays, CT can produce a sequence of multiple 2D cross-sectional images taken from 360 degrees around the body. These images are called slices, and they can be reconstructed as a 3D volumetric image for more detailed information about the shape and size of the cancerous region. Compared to x-rays, the CT modality can give better quality, contrast, and spatial resolution images while using a lower amount of radiation.

Moreover, the effectiveness of CT has been proved by several studies and is highly recommended for early diagnosis of lung cancer. For instance, the National Lung Screening Trial (NLST) reported a 20% decrease of lung cancer mortality in patients who received low-dose CT screening [3]. Similar to CT screening, magnetic resonance imaging (MRI) can also provide volumetric images. However, it differs from CT in using a strong magnetic field instead of an x-ray beam [4], thus it has no harmful side effect of radiation. In addition, the image quality produced by MRI is also superior to CT. However, MRI screening takes significantly longer and costs more compared to CT. Moreover, it is only available in some well-equipped hospitals.

For this reason, CT imaging is preferred over MRI and became a standard modality for lung cancer diagnosis. Whatever the differences, the shared objective of all the screening modalities mentioned above is to detect lung cancer at an earlier stage. If lung cancer is identified at the immature stage and before it spreads, it has a higher potential to be cured through providing effective treatment. In the real-world, up to 25% of lung cancer cases are unexpected findings of abnormal lesions while performing routine chest exams. These lesions appear as round or oval opacities on the chest scans, and they are termed as pulmonary nodules in radiology. As they are the earliest signal for suspecting lung cancer, detection of them is crucial for early diagnosis.

However, detection of the nodules is not always a straightforward task for radiologists because nodules are heterogeneous in different factors such as shape, size, location, margin, calcification, and texture. Typically, they are round or oval structures with dimensions of up to 30 mm in their greatest diameters. They are mostly located inside the lungs, either isolated or touching nearby pulmonary structures. Subject to their locations, nodules can be divided into three types: (i) isolated nodules which reside within the lungs without touching other lesions; (ii) juxta-pleural nodules which adhere to the parenchyma wall; and (iii) juxta-vascular nodules which attach to vessels. Furthermore, the margins of the pulmonary nodules are also another significant factor of nodule variety. In detail, the nodules can be categorized into six groups based on their margins. They comprise: (i) round nodules with smooth circular or oval-shaped margins; (ii) lobulated nodules with well-defined margins containing some large convexities along the margins; (iii) speculated nodules with irregular margins having multiple radiating fined stands; (iv) ragged nodules with irregular margins having small serrations; (v) polygonal nodules with polygonal or angular margins; and (vi) halo nodules with margins showing ground-glass opacity [5].

Similarly, calcification, an effect of calcium deposition inside the body, also produces different patterns of nodules. Based on calcification, nodules are divided into four types: (i) central dense, (ii) diffuse solid, (iii) laminate, and (iv) popcorn [6]. Another essential factor that dominates the variety of nodules is the texture. Texture determines the clarity of nodules on the radiographic scans; that is, some nodules are easily detectable, but some are not. There are two main types of nodule based on texture. They are (i) solid nodules that have high intensity and are easy to detect on the scan, and (ii) ground-glass (non-solid) nodules that contain obscure portions and are challenging to detect. Ground-glass nodules can be sub-divided into two types: part-solid nodules, which have a mixture of solid and ground-glass opacity, and pure ground-glass nodules, in which the entire nodule has only ground-glass opacity. Figure 10.1 summarizes the various types of pulmonary nodules depending on different characteristics. The CT slices of pulmonary nodules which are described throughout this chapter are freely accessible from The Cancer Imaging Archive [7].

In clinical practice, half of the patients who undergo chest screening usually present more than one nodule [8]. According to [9], a pulmonary nodule appears at least once in every 500 chest scans. However, every nodule discovered on the chest radiographic or CT scans is not malignant. The percentage of nodule malignancy varies depending on the characteristics mentioned above. The most important criterion that influences the malignancy of a nodule is the size. Generally, larger nodules are more likely to be malignant compared to smaller ones. A meta-analysis of nodules in [10] studied the malignancy percentage of nodules depending upon the

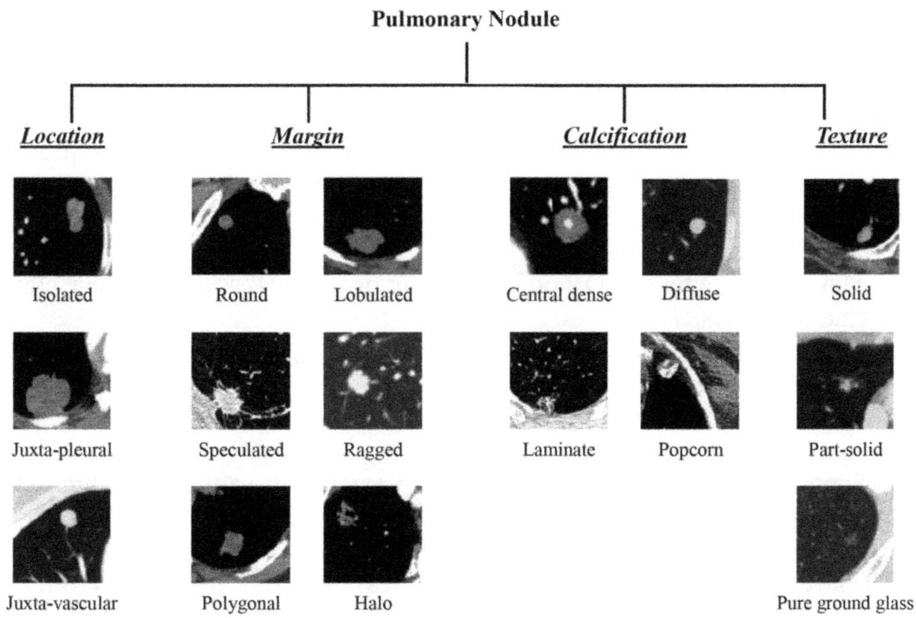

Figure 10.1. Types of nodules based on different characteristics.

sizes. They reported that the malignancy of nodules $\leqslant$5 mm was 0% to 1%, for nodules >5 mm and $\leqslant$10 mm it was 6%–28%, and for nodules $\geqslant$20 mm it was 64%–82%, respectively.

Additionally, the likelihood of malignancy also depends on the margins of the pulmonary nodules. Nodules with irregular margins often show a higher malignancy rate compared to the smooth or well-bordered ones. A study conducted by [11] proved that only 21% of smooth bordered nodules showed malignancy. In addition to margins, the calcification patterns of nodules can also help to determine the malignancy of nodules. In particular, diffuse, central, and laminated nodules are highly suggestive of being benign while other patterns are regarded as malignant [12]. Also, texture features are crucial for distinguishing malignant and benign nodules. The clinical experiments in [13] showed that nodules with a part-solid texture have a higher potential of malignancy compared to the pure ground-glass nodules.

With the increasing incidence of lung cancer day by day, radiologists are dealing with the difficulty of diagnosing multiple lung nodules. As the malignancy of lung cancer depends on several criteria, radiologists have to analyze the nodular characteristics precisely to differentiate between the benign and malignant. Incorrect or missed detection of malignant nodules is very serious because it may severely affect the patients' survival chances. Unfortunately, the manual way of nodule detection is effort-intensive and error-prone. In addition, the availability of skillful radiologists may also be a problem in some rural hospitals. For these reasons, computer-aided detection (CAD) for pulmonary nodule detection has been promoted to overcome these challenges. CAD for nodule detection has emerged in the last two decades, and now its performance has become better and better with the help of advanced technologies. However, the ground-glass opacity (GGO) nodules remain a diagnostic problem in both manual and computer-aided detection due to their indistinct appearance. Therefore, a more systematic approach which can accurately detect GGOs is still lacking in existing CADs [14].

The primary intention of this chapter is to study the GGO nodules, and their detection from CT scans using automated diagnosis methods. We aim to provide the reader with the following knowledge:

i. The definition of GGO nodules.
ii. The reasons why GGO nodules appear on the CT scan and their clinical characteristics.
iii. The importance of GGOs in lung cancer diagnosis and the correlation between malignancy and GGO nodules.
iv. The image characteristics of GGOs and the difficulties of GGO detection in computer-aided diagnosis systems.
v. Some examples of image processing and machine learning algorithms which emphasize the detection of GGOs.

We believe this chapter will provide a great deal of help to researchers to further improve the detection of GGO nodules in automatic diagnosis systems.

10.2 Ground-glass opacity (GGO) nodules

A GGO nodule is a radiological finding with a hazy morphologic description in chest scans. GGO nodules are usually small in size, ranging from 5–10 mm in greatest diameter and are troublesome to detect in the conventional chest x-ray scans [15]. However, recent breakthroughs and the widespread use of low-dose computed tomography (LCT) have produced a significant increase in the detection of pulmonary nodules with GGO nodules. GGOs are very important in lung cancer oncology because the incidence of cancer in GGO is up to 63% [16]. As we described in the introduction, GGO nodules can be further classified into two types: (i) part-solid nodules which show both ground-glass and solid consolidation; and (ii) pure ground-glass nodules in which the entire nodule possesses only ground-glass opacity. In the whole chapter, we will use the term 'GGOs' to represent both part-solid and pure ground-glass nodules.

As an illustration, representative CT slices containing the three types of pulmonary nodule can be seen in figure 10.2. Figure 10.2(a) represents a solid nodule, and it has a very sharp intensity on the CT scan while the other two GGO

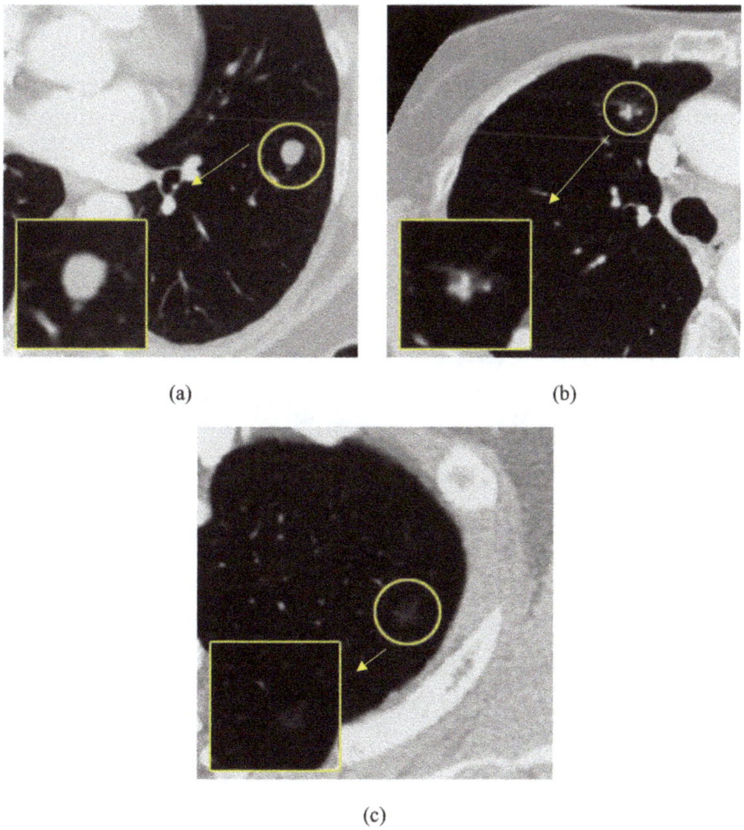

Figure 10.2. Three different types of pulmonary nodules based on texture: (a) solid, (b) part-solid (mix ground-glass), and (c) pure ground-glass.

nodules (figures 10.2(b) and (c)) possess lesser intensity compared to figure 10.2(a). Next, figure 10.2(b) is a part-solid nodule, and it shows a mixture of both solid and ground-glass intensities. The last one, figure 10.2(c), is a pure ground-glass nodule which presents only the ground-glass intensity. The circles in the figures denote the positions of the nodules, and the rectangles display the zoom-in views of the nodule regions.

10.2.1 Clinical and radiological characteristics of GGO nodules

According to [17], GGO nodules can be defined by two main radiological characteristics: (i) hazy and amorphous focal areas with increased lung densities; and (ii) areas with no observation of underlying vessels and bronchial walls. The density of the lungs is a proportion of the other pulmonary structures such as blood, vessels, extravascular water, and tissues. An increase in lung density usually occurs when the amount of air in the airspaces and lumens of the airways is reduced, and the spaces (reduced areas) are filled with cells or fluid. In addition, pulmonary hyperperfusion, an increased blood volume in lung capillaries, can also increase the lung density. These increases in density can cause diffuse or focal ground-glass opacities on chest scans. The occurrence of GGOs due to hyperperfusion is commonly minimal [17].

Once the alveolar wall is filled with fluid or cells, the alveolar interstitium becomes thick, as shown in figure 10.3. Pure GGOs are the growth of the alveolar wall with

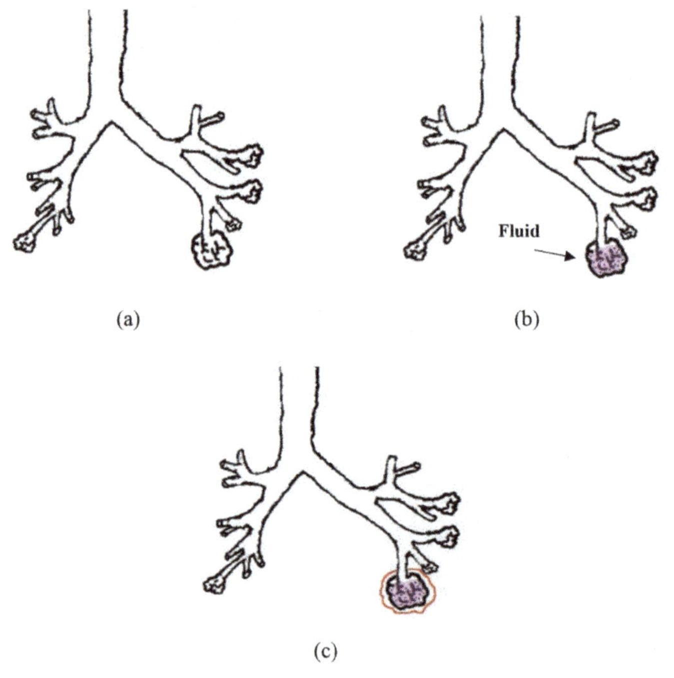

Figure 10.3. Increase in lung density: (a) normal alveoli, (b) alveoli filled with fluid or cells, and (c) the thickness of the alveoli interstitium.

no destruction of the alveolar structures. However, mixed GGOs are the effect of the partial filling of fluid or cells that makes it not possible for the complete consolidation of lung parenchyma to occur on CT scans [14]. Mixed GGOs or partly solid opacities can also result when pure GGOs increase in size and alveolar structure collapses, fibroblasts proliferate, and solid components increase [18].

GGO nodules can manifest in either benign or malignant conditions; however, the part-solid GGOs show a higher malignancy percentage compared to the solid ones. The experiments of the Early Lung Cancer Action Project (ELCAP) revealed that the malignancy rates in part-solid, pure ground-glass, and solid nodules were 63%, 18%, and 7%, respectively. The solid component of a part-solid GGOs is more critical than the ground-glass regions because they are the indicators of malignancy. Research conducted by the Fleischner society stated that a GGO nodule with a solid component >5 mm should be regarded as malignant [19].

Moreover, the presence of solid portions in GGOs is also an indicator of a historical invasion, for example, alveolar collapse, inflammation, fibrosis, and, occasionally, mucus, and so on [13]. A measurement known as the consolidation/tumour (*C*/*T*) ratio, which is the proportion of solid component to the whole tumour, is usually used to distinguish between invasive and non-invasive malignant nodules. Figure 10.4 demonstrates how to measure the *C*/*T* ratio in some representative part-solid GGO nodules. In the figures, *a* and *b* denote the greatest diameters of the entire tumor and consolidation part, respectively, and the *C*/*T* ratio is the ratio of *b* to *a*.

GGO nodules are difficult to manage because the solid components in some GGOs are gradually enlarged over time, but some remain unchanged for years. According to retrospective studies, nearly 20% of pure GGOs and 40% of part-solid

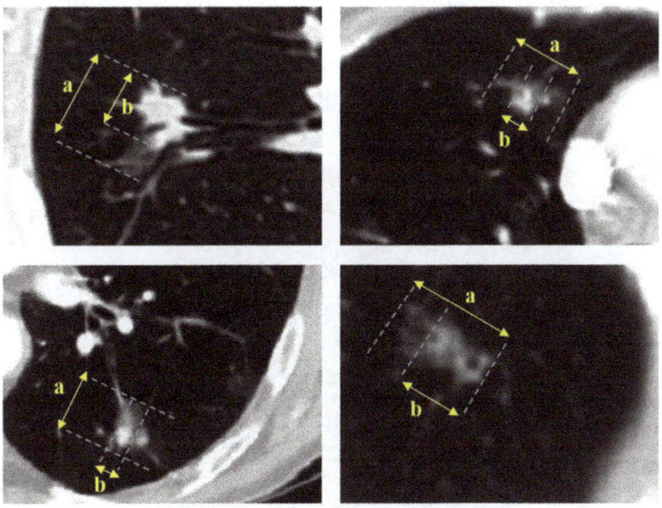

Figure 10.4. Measurements of the consolidation/tumour (*C*/*T* ratio) in representatives of part-solid GGO nodules in high-resolution computed tomography.

GGOs expand their solid regions [20]. Compared to the pure GGOs, part-solid ones grow faster in shorter volume doubling times. However, all GGOs do not increase in size. Some part-solid nodules are transient and disappear in follow-up studies, in particular when there are infectious or inflammatory conditions, lesion multiplicity, large solid partitions, ill-defined lesion borders, and blood eosinophilia. According to [13], persistent GGO nodules that grow very slowly or remain unchanged are associated with atypical adenomatous hyperplasias (AAH) and invasive adenocarcinomas.

10.2.2 The importance of GGO nodules: the correlation between malignancy and GGO nodules

Once a pulmonary nodule is malignant or cancerous, it can be clinically termed as an adenocarcinoma. GGOs may be either adenocarcinomas or their precursors, ranging from pre-invasive lesions to minimally invasive and invasive carcinomas. Adenomatous hyperplasia (AAH), which is a precursor lesion of adenocarcinoma, shows GGO on CT scans. AAH usually appears as focal regions with small ($\leqslant$5 mm), well-defined oval or round pure GGO on CT scans, as illustrated in figure 10.5.

Several pathological studies reported that the bronchioloalveolar carcinomas (BACs) could be observed as part-solid opacity on the CT, as can be seen in figures 10.6 and 10.7. BACs are also termed adenocarcinoma *in situ* (AIS), and they are small tumours arising in the bronchioles or alveoli. Generally, BACs are a non-invasive form of lung adenocarcinoma. Mostly, nonmucinous AISs under normal conditions show pure ground-glass opacity (figure 10.6), but nonmucinous AISs with focal collapsed alveoli appear as part-solid opacity (figure 10.7).

Another type, minimally invasive adenocarcinoma (MIA), which are lepidic and invasive lesions, are also revealed by GGO on the CT scans as illustrated in figures 10.8 and 10.9. MIA can represent either pure GGN (figure 10.8) or part-solid opacity, in particular the central solid component (figure 10.9). This solid consolidation of MIA occurs due to fibrosis, atelectasis, or invasive cancer.

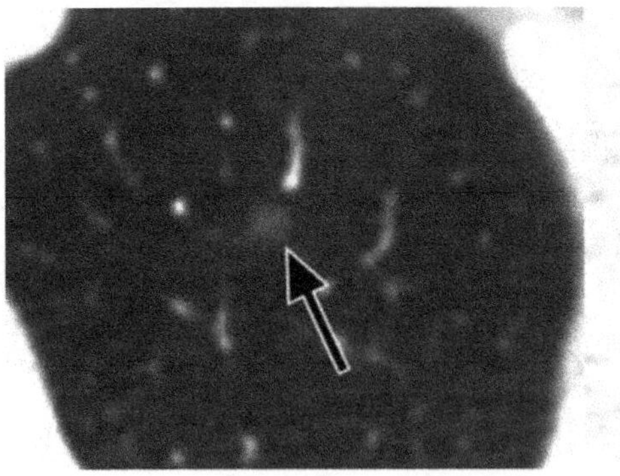

Figure 10.5. An AAH nodule (arrow) with smooth margins and pure ground-glass opacity. Reproduced from [21]. CC BY 4.0.

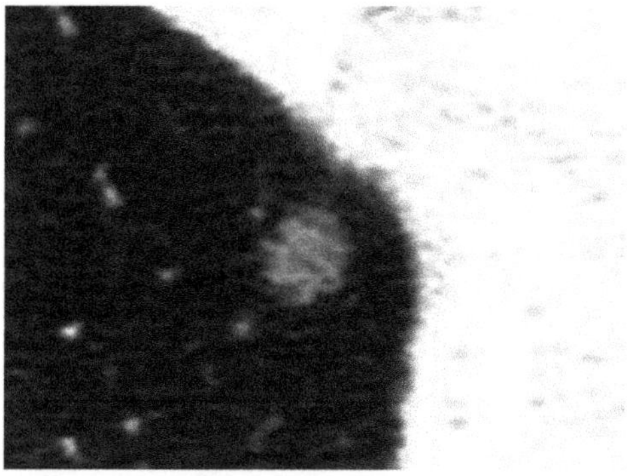

Figure 10.6. Adenocarcinoma *in situ* (AIS) with nonmucinous AIS with pure ground-glass opacity. Reprinted from [22], copyright 2019 with permission from Elsevier.

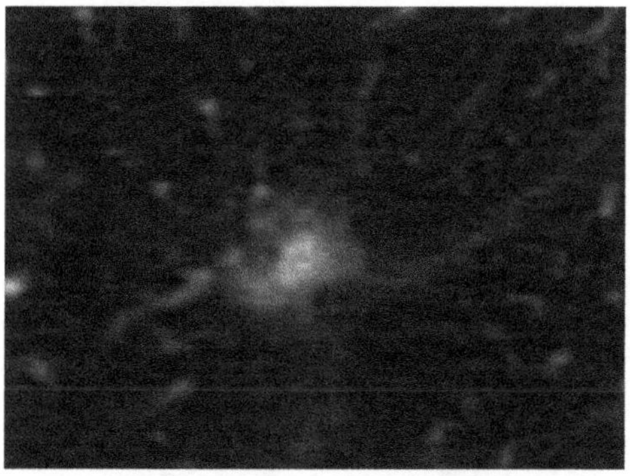

Figure 10.7. Adenocarcinoma *in situ* (AIS) with nonmucinous AIS with part-solid opacity. Reprinted from [22], copyright 2019 with permission from Elsevier.

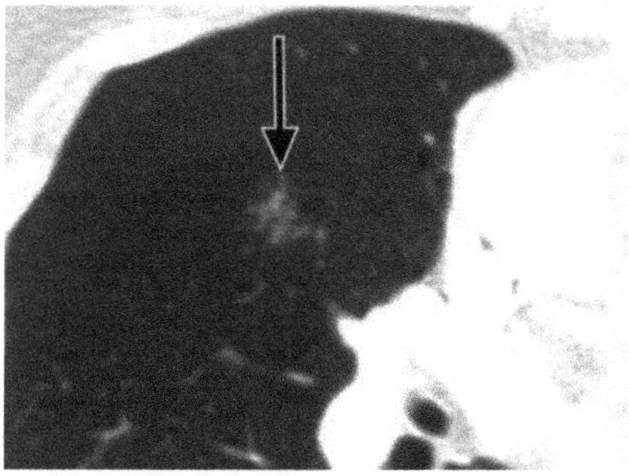

Figure 10.8. Minimally invasive adenocarcinoma (MIA) with pure ground-glass opacity. Reproduced from [21]. CC BY 4.0.

Next, mucinous BACs are another type of invasive adenocarcinoma, and their opacities can vary from solid to sub-solid GGOs. These types of nodules are generally multifocal and multi-lobar, as illustrated in figure 10.10.

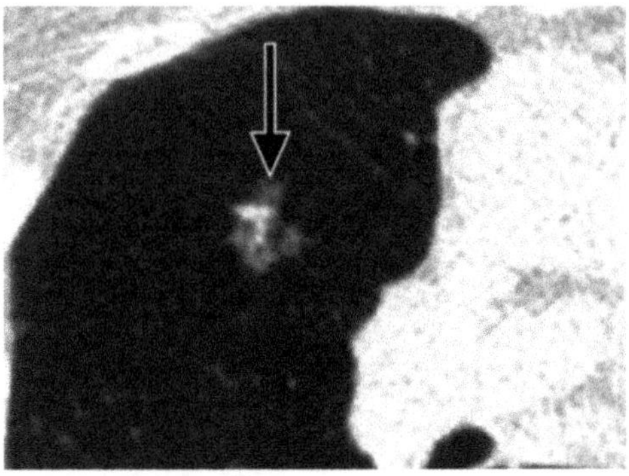

Figure 10.9. Minimally invasive adenocarcinoma (MIA) with part-solid opacity. Reproduced from [21]. CC BY 4.0.

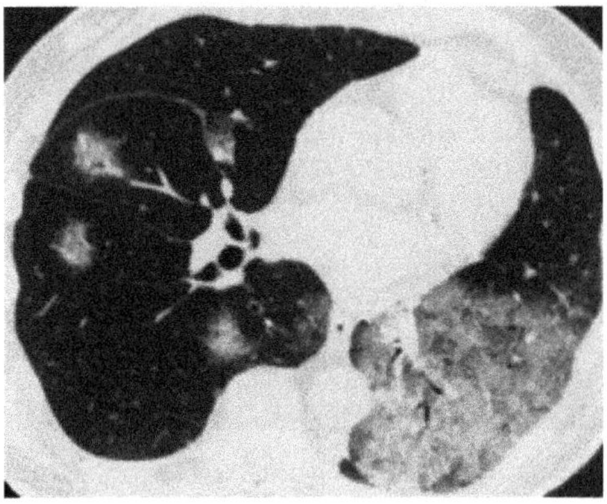

Figure 10.10. Mucinous BACs with multifocal and multi-lobar nodules. Reproduced from [21]. CC BY 4.0.

Table 10.1. Types of adenocarcinomas in GGO nodules.

Malignancy	Adenocarcinomas	CT findings
Precursors	Adenomatous hyperplasia (AAH)	Ground-glass
Pre-invasive	Adenocarcinoma *in situ* (AIS)	Ground-glass, part-solid
Minimally invasive	Minimally invasive adenocarcinoma (MIA)	Ground-glass, part-solid
Invasive	Mucinous BACs	Solid, part-solid

In table 10.1, we summarize the type of adenocarcinomas, their severity, and radiological findings on the CT scans to show the correlation between malignancy and GGO nodules.

10.2.3 Image analysis of GGO nodules from CT scans

The appearance of GGO nodules on CT scans is significantly different from solid nodules due to their increased density. A CT scan represents a particular constituent

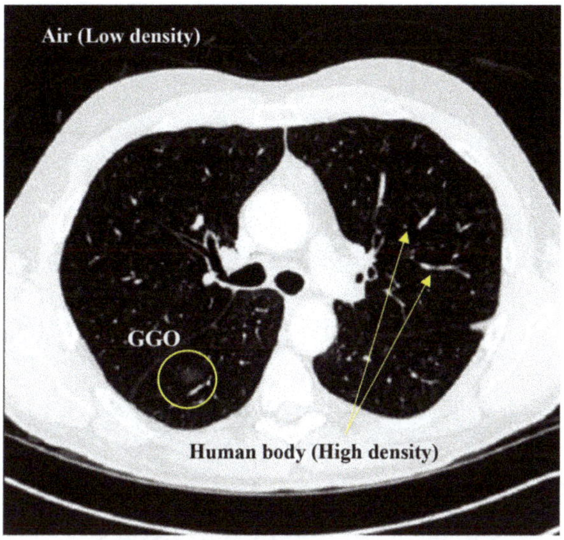

Figure 10.11. A chest CT slice containing a GGO nodule showing a different density between GGO and human body tissues.

of the human body with a range of radiological densities, which can be measured in Hounsfield units (HU). Lung CT comprises two primary constituents, namely the air region with a lower density (−1000 HU) and the human body region with a higher density (−400 HU to 1000 HU) as illustrated in figure 10.11. In image analysis, these HU values are translated as a particular range of the grey level, for instance, lower density air is translated as black pixels while the higher density human body is represented as various shades of grey. The human body region, similarly, is also a composition of other structures, such as parenchyma, fluid, fat, soft tissues, bones, and vessels, showing a variety of HU values, as listed in figure 10.12 [8].

The pulmonary nodules generally present soft tissue attenuation when they are in a pure solid-state. However, in most cases, the nodule attenuation is usually interfered with by adjacent parenchymal lesions such as the lung wall, vessels, and bronchi. As a negative consequence, the precise identification of HU intervals for pulmonary nodules is difficult.

Generally, nodules reveal a relatively higher intensity and contrast than other parenchymal lesions. As a demonstration, figure 10.13 describes the probability density distribution of solid nodule. Figure 10.13(a) is a representative CT slice containing a solid nodule, and its probability density distribution can be seen in (b). After that, in (c), we manually segment the solid nodule and study the probability of the density distribution of only the nodule area, as shown in (d). Similarly, figures 10.14 and 10.15 demonstrate the probability density distribution of part-solid and pure GGO nodules. From this observation, we can know that the nodules have a higher intensity (the middle peak of the histograms) than other structures, and that they show a uniform density distribution. Moreover, we analyse the

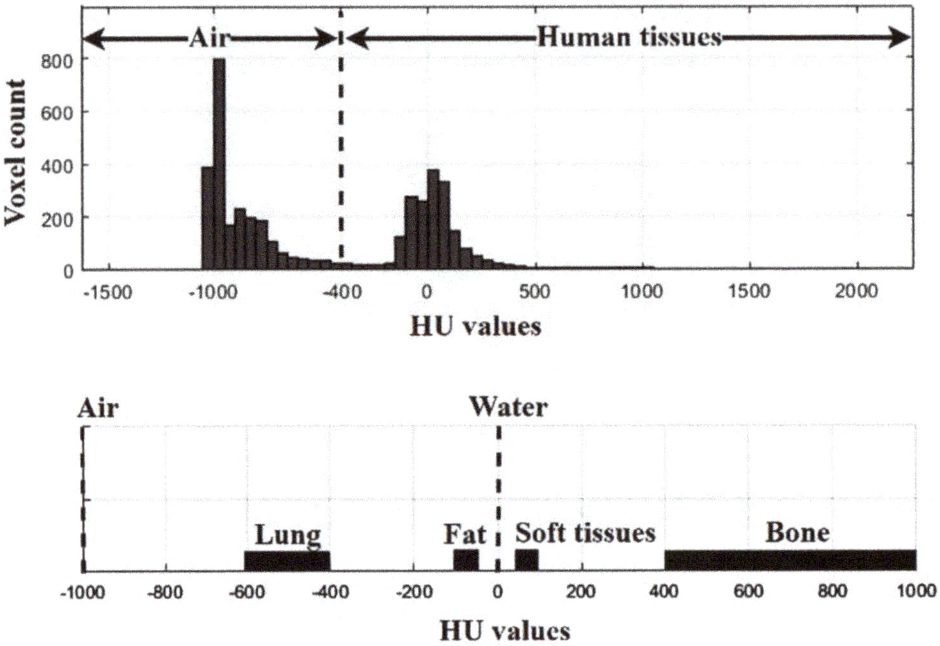

Figure 10.12. Range of radiological densities on a lung CT scan. Reproduced from [8]. CC BY 4.0.

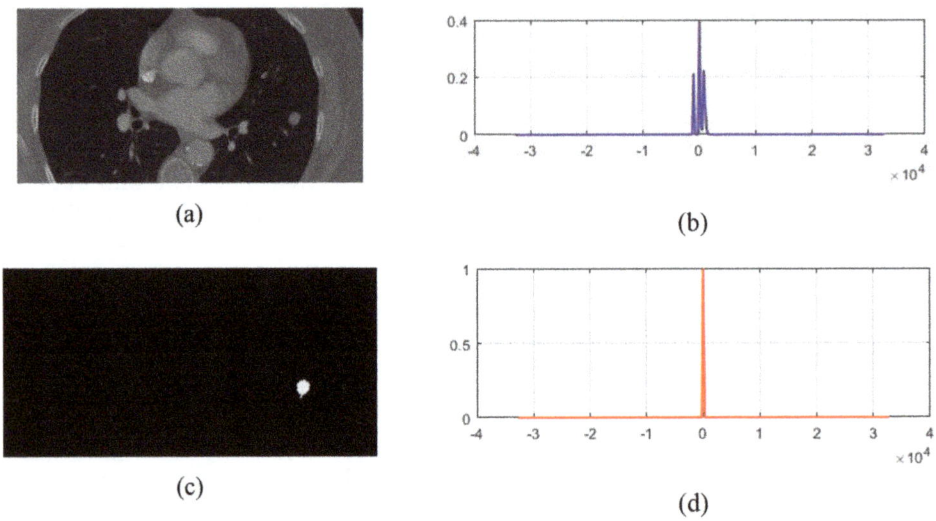

Figure 10.13. The probability density distribution of solid nodules.

intensity of each representative of the solid, part-solid, and pure ground-glass nodules. The mean intensity value of each nodule from figures 10.13, 10.14, and 10.15 is 29.9, 21.8, and 16.91, respectively. From these values, we found that the solid nodule has the highest intensity value, and the intensity of part-solid nodules is higher than that of the pure GGOs due to the intensity of solid consolidation.

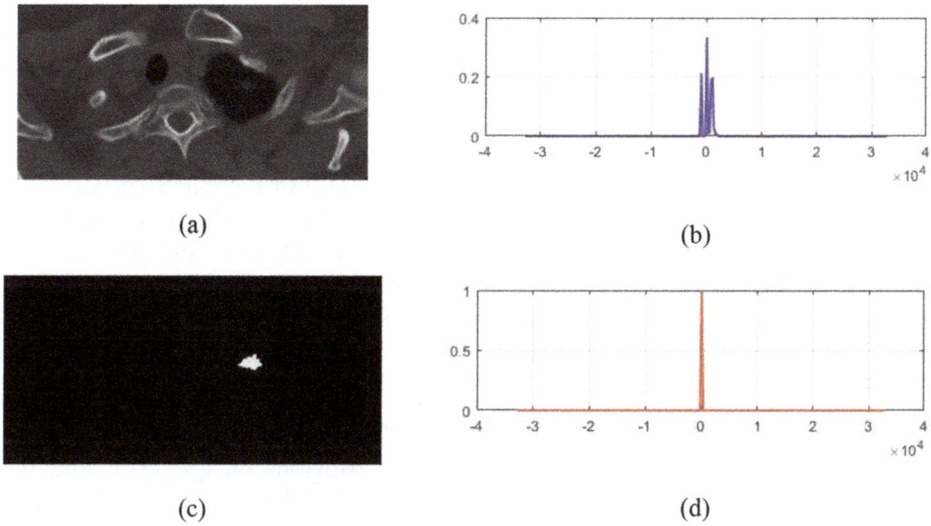

Figure 10.14. The probability density distribution of part-solid nodules.

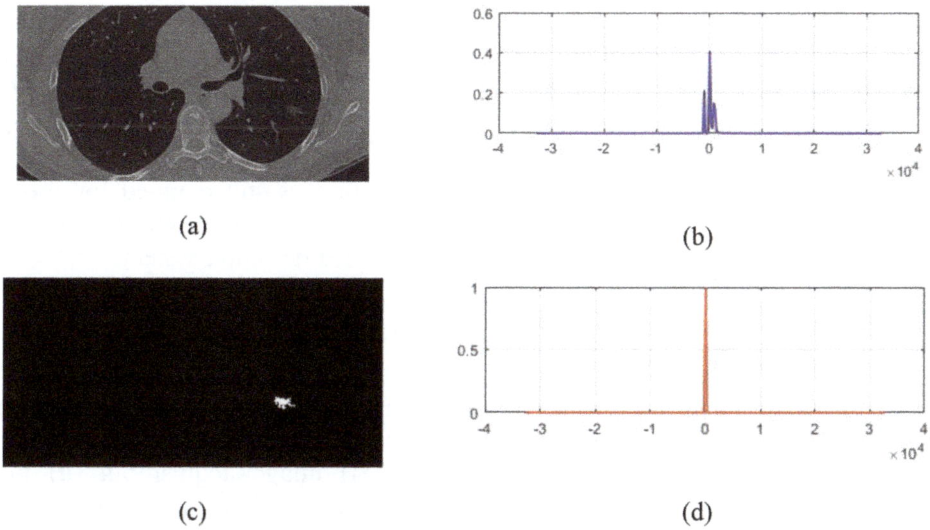

Figure 10.15. The probability density distribution of pure GGO nodules.

10.3 Computer-aided detection of GGO nodules

In practice, the detection of pulmonary nodules on CT scans is a challenging problem for radiologists because misdetection of potentially malignant nodules is hazardous and high-risk for the patient. To overcome this problem, the European CT screen studies proposed a double reading method. This method aims to reduce the false-negative rate by allowing two readers to analyze all CT scans independently. If there is any inconsistency between the two results, an additional reader will arbitrate to make a more precise decision [23]. Nonetheless, even double reading cannot promise accurate detection because it sometimes misses the early stage of cancer nodules. Research conducted by [24] compared the accuracy of the manual double reading method and computer-aided detection (CAD) using randomized trials of the NELSON nodules. They found that 22% of nodules were misdetected by double reading and, significantly, 3% of them were diagnosed as malignant the following year. Fortunately, the nodules misdetected by double reading can be identified by CAD. For these reasons, CADs are highly recommended and widely used as assistant tools for radiologists to provide accurate diagnosis results [25]. Typically, most CADs for automatic pulmonary nodule detection exclusively focus on the detection of solid nodules. As the appearance of GGO nodules varies highly from solid nodules, the CADs designated for solid nodule detection are very likely to predict incorrect diagnosis results when detecting GGOs.

10.3.1 Challenges of GGOs in automated detection

Due to their haziness characteristic, GGOs are not obvious on CT scans and their detection usually encounters difficulties in both manual and computer-aided detection (CAD). Even a CAD which emphasizes GGO nodules detection cannot ensure accurate predictions for both part-solid and pure GGOs. As we discussed in section 10.2.3, the intensity of pure ground-glass presents a constant character while that of part-solid nodules is significantly heterogeneous, as it is a combination of solid and ground-glass intensity. Moreover, the intensity of GGO nodules is sometimes interfered with by other lung lesions, in particular the parenchyma wall and vessels. In such situations, GGOs need to be detached from the interfering structures as well. However, clinical practice, a high-performing CAD which can detect any variant of nodules such as solid, part-solid, and pure GGOs regardless of shape, size, and location, is still required for precise diagnosis results. Therefore, in the next section, we will discuss some effective ways to handle the detection of GGO nodules in computer-aided detection systems.

10.4 Different ways to handle GGOs in automated detection

An automated nodule detection system is impossible to develop using a single algorithm. Instead, it is a combination of one or more image processing and machine learning algorithms. Commonly, most of the automated pulmonary nodule detection systems work in four fundamental steps: (i) image acquisition, (ii) pre-processing, (iii) segmentation of candidate lesions, and (iv) false-positive reduction. In image acquisition, the chest CT slices from the database are inputted into the detection system to initiate the process. Subsequently, pre-processing improves the quality of the input CT slices using suitable enhancement filters and noise removing algorithms. In this task, the unwanted objects from the slices, for example the background and outer contour of the lung regions, are also eliminated to reduce the extra effort and possible error. After that, the candidate lesions that are objects with a high likelihood of being ROIs are segmented, applying an appropriate segmentation algorithm. Finally, the real ROIs can be segregated by false-positive reduction using a prediction model. Currently, there are a diversity of existing works for lung nodules detection. Among them, this section will focus on some examples of segmentation algorithms specifically designed for the detection of GGO nodules.

10.4.1 Markov random field-based GGO segmentation

A Markov random field (MRF), a stochastic approach, is handy for image segmentation processes. The principal intention of any segmentation algorithm is to divide the image pixels into different regions where the pixels in each region possess homogeneity; that is, the neighbouring pixels show similar features such as texture, intensity, and colour. Suppose I is the input image, and then the algorithm segments I into the disjoint parts I_k such that each of them belongs to different objects in the input image [26]. Alternatively, the segmentation process can be assumed as a pixel labelling task where each pixel of I is assigned a label based on specific criteria, and the particular label represents a category of the input image.

For GGO segmentation, Y is assumed as an observation image with L categories of regions (numbers of class labels). On the CT scans, we can assume that there are four different regions (labels), namely background, normal opacities, ground-glass opacities, and high-intensity regions that contain consolidations and blood vessels [27]. As the labels of neighbouring pixels are dependent on each other, the MRF is suitable for handling such dependency. To perform the segmentation, MRF calculates a probability measure on the set of all possible labels and then select the most appropriate one. X is the labelling field, and X_S is a random variable (pixel) having values in a common set of labels $\Lambda = \{1, 2, \dots, L\}$. Then, the posterior distribution can be calculated by

$$P(x, y) = P(x|y)P(x),$$

where $P(x)$ is an MRF segmentation model which uses a Gibbs distribution. Then, $P(x|y)$ is the data model that is the conditional probability of a label for a given observed feature y using a Gaussian distribution. In [27], the MRF segmentation model was created, applying intensity-based statistical features from each category. These categories were manually extracted and assigned by field expert radiologists.

For the data model, they proposed an adaptive approach which can ensure heterogeneous intensities of GGOs by calculating the local Gaussian distribution in pixels of a given category:

$$P_{Y_s|X_s}(Y_s|X_s) = \frac{1}{\sqrt{2\pi\sigma_{X_s}^2}}\exp\left\{-\frac{(y_s - \mu_s)^2}{2\sigma_{X_s}^2}\right\},$$

where μ is the mean and σ is the standard deviation of the local image, and both μ and σ depend on the neighbourhood of pixel s. Then, the simulated annealing algorithm with a Gibbs sampler is applied to find optimal labelling for the best segmentation results. Figure 10.16 demonstrates the GGO detection using MRF based segmentation where an input CT slice containing a GGO is segmented into four different regions such as background, normal opacities, ground-glass opacities, and high-intensity regions.

10.4.2 Template matching based GGO segmentation

Template matching, which segments a region of interest (ROI) by creating templates or reference models, is also applicable for GGO nodule detection. The templates or

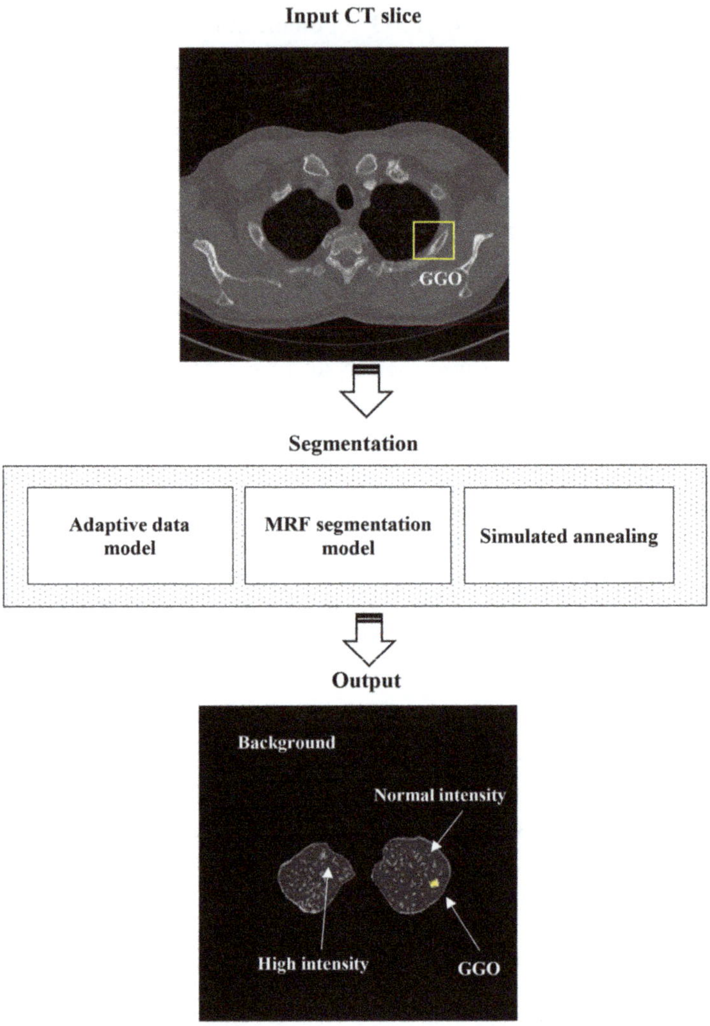

Figure 10.16. Markov random field-based GGO segmentation [27].

reference models simulate the ROI, and then they are matched with the small parts of the input image to detect the ROIs. A matching operation is usually required to measure the similarity between the template and the ROIs of the input image.

According to the investigation in [28], nodules are spherical, and their CT values tend to follow a Gaussian distribution. Based on this knowledge, a volumetric template model which represents the nodules (including both solid and GGOs) can be created using 3D Gaussian distributions:

$$V_{x,y,z} = m^* e^{-\frac{(x^2 + y^2 + k \cdot z^2)}{n}},$$

where $V_{x,y,z}$ is the voxel value at the coordinate (x, y, z), and m and n are the maximum and variance of the distribution, respectively; k is the parameter which controls the

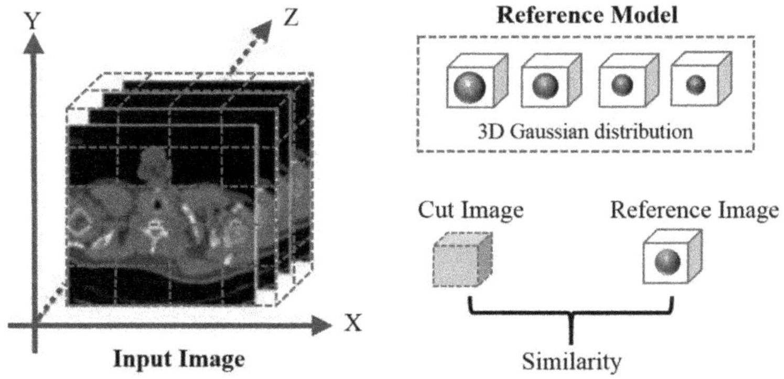

Figure 10.17. Template matching based GGO segmentation [28].

scaling in z [28]. After creating the reference images, the matching process is conducted by extracting small parts from the input image, as illustrated in figure 10.17. Each part has the same dimension as a reference image, and it can be termed as the 'cut image'. After that, the similarity between the 'cut image' and 'reference image' can be measured by the cross-correlation coefficient normalized covariance:

$$\text{Similarity}_{c,r} = \frac{\sum_i \sum_j (c_{ij} - m_c)(r_{ij} - m_r)}{\sqrt{\sum_i \sum_j (c_{ij} - m_c)^2} \sqrt{\sum_i \sum_j (r_{ij} - m_r)^2}},$$

where c_{ij} and r_{ij} are the intensity values, and m is the mean intensity value of cut image c and reference image r at the coordinate points i and j. The similarity value can vary from -1 to 1 and suspected GGO regions in the input image can be detected when $|\text{Similarity}_{c,r}|$ is greater than a predefined value. The potential effectiveness of the template-based segmentation method for GGO nodule detection is successfully proved in [29].

10.4.3 Multi-level learning-based GGO segmentation

The multi-level learning-based approach is proposed by [30] for the early detection of GGO nodules from lung CT scans. The primary concept of this approach is to seamlessly combine the segmentation and detection processes using two-level classification: voxel-level and object-level. The input of this method is a sub-volume of nodule candidate lesions. At the initial stage of the algorithm, each voxel from the input sub-volume is identified into two categories, 'ground-glass opacity' and 'non-ground-glass opacity', using the voxel-level classification. Subsequently, in object-level classification, the labelled voxels (outputs of voxel-level classification) are further classified to detect the appearance of GGOs.

As shown in figure 10.18, multi-level learning works in two steps: (i) segmentation using voxel-wise soft labelling and (ii) detection using object-scale image classification. The first step, segmentation, begins by extracting intensity–texture features from each volume candidate. Subsequently, the dimensions of the extracted features

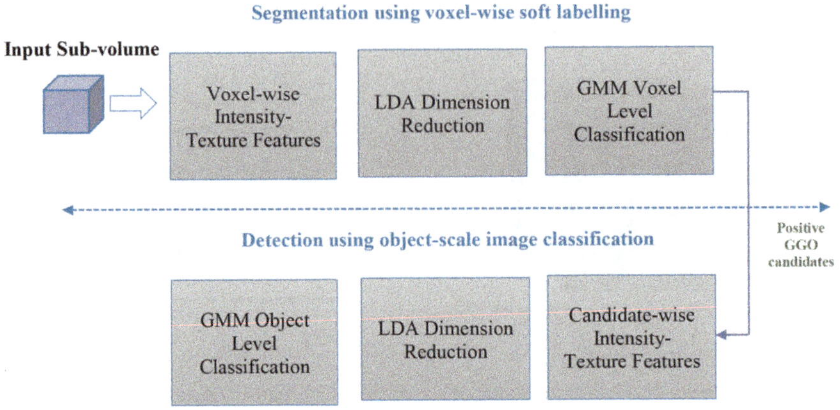

Figure 10.18. Multi-level learning-based GGO segmentation [30].

are reduced by linear discriminant analysis (LDA). The low dimensional feature subspace projected by LAD is then fed into Gaussian mixture models (GMM) to classify voxels into two classes (positive and negative). The output of this step is a class probability map which assigns each voxel with a certain label or weight values. The positive class label of GMM represents the voxels with ground-glass opacities, and the negative class represents non-ground-glass opacities.

On the lung CT scans, there are not only GGOs but also other lesions such as parenchyma, vessels, and airways, hence a single layer classifier for voxel-wise soft labelling is not sufficient to remove the vast number of false positives. For this reason, multiple-phase classification approaches are applied in the first step. The positive class voxels which are predicted from the single layer classifier are reused as the new input and repeat the classification. The next rounds of voxel-level classification are iterated using both original input and new input. The main advantage of multi-phase classification is that it can improve the overall performance as well as speed of the supervised enhancement by rejecting negative probability samples.

The second step, detection using object-scale image classification, aims to locate and extract GGO nodule candidates produced from the previous step, voxel-level classification. As nodules are spherical, multiscale blob enhancement filtering can help to capture GGO candidates. Otsu thresholding and connected component labelling methods are also applied to disconnect candidates from other attached lesions. Next, volume size and prior position information can be applied to reduce the number of candidates. After reducing, object-level classification is carried out in the same way as for the previous segmentation phase. Candidate-wise volumetric feature vectors including intensity–texture features, volume size, sphericity, and mean of positive GGN class probability maps are extracted and fed into LDA-GMM classification to identify the presence of GGNs within input CT sub-volume candidates.

10.4.4 Deep learning-based GGO segmentation

In recent years, deep learning in CAD systems has become very popular as a research topic. This involves very powerful learning algorithms and can give better

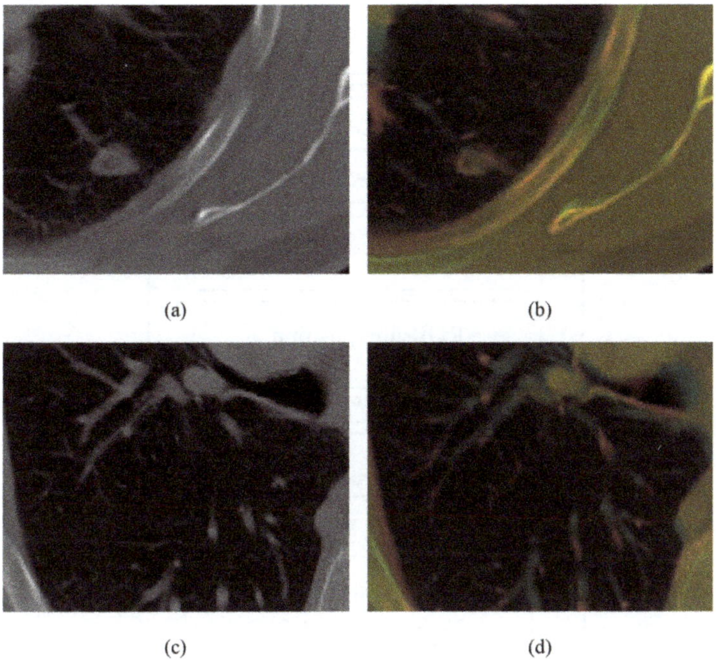

Figure 10.19. ROI superposition: (a) original CT image of a nodule, (b) pseudocolour image of a nodule (spheroidal structures), (c) original CT image of vessels, and (d) pseudocolour image of vessels (longitudinal stripes) [31].

performance compared to other traditional models. These systems work with multiple processing layers which can learn image features automatically from the input data. GGO detection using deep learning can also be found in [31]. Although deep learning can learn features directly from the input CT slices, [31] initially reduces the unnecessary areas outside the lung regions in order to minimize the processing effort and conceivable errors. Then threshold binarization and connected component labelling are applied to remove the external regions of the lungs. After that, the corrosion process is conducted to separate the touching lesions inside the lung regions. Subsequently, the ROIs from three continuous slices are cut out from the lung regions using 64×64 blocks by taking the centroid location as the centre.

Next, the superposition of ROIs is conducted to distinguish between the potential nodules and the normal tissues, in particular the blood vessels. In this purpose, the pseudocolour images are created by superimposing three channels (RGB) on each of three continuous slices of the ROI. In a pseudocolour format, nodules can be seen as spheroidal structures while the vessels appear as longitudinal stripes, as illustrated in figure 10.19. Finally, the deep learning models such as AlexNet, GoogleNet and RestNet50 are trained and tested using pseudocolor images, as shown in figure 10.20.

10.5 Conclusion

This chapter described the clinical and image features of ground-glass opacity (GGO) pulmonary nodules in automated detection systems. GGO nodules are

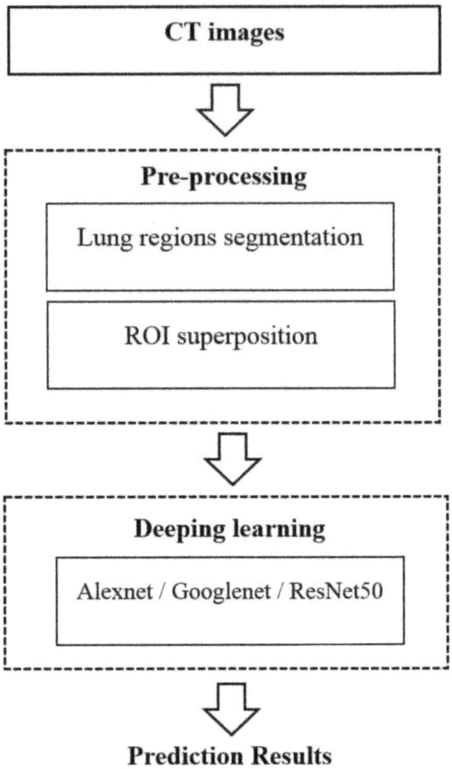

Figure 10.20. Deep learning-based GGO segmentation [31].

frequently detected on the computed tomography (CT) scans, and they are very dangerous as they possess a higher malignancy likelihood compared to solid nodules. Thus, precise detection of GGOs is crucial and beneficial in improving lung cancer prognosis. However, the hazy structures and faint intensities of GGOs cause difficulties in the detection process. For these reasons, this chapter mainly focused on GGO nodules and studied the following: (i) the clinical characteristics of GGO nodules, (ii) the correlation between GGOs and malignancy, (iii) analysis of GGO image features on the CT scans, (iv) the difficulties of GGO nodule detection in automated detections, and (v) some sample image processing and machine learning algorithms that are designated for the detection of GGO nodules. We believe that this chapter provides fundamental knowledge about GGO nodules for the reader and will assist in providing some advanced research ideas for GGO nodule detection.

References

[1] Bray F, Ferlay J, Soerjomataram I, Siegel R L, Torre L A and Jemal A 2018 Global cancer statistics 2018: GLOBOCAN estimates of incidence and mortality worldwide for 36 cancers in 185 countries *CA Cancer J. Clin.* **68** 394–424

[2] Siegel R L, Miller K D and Jemal A 2019 Cancer statistics, 2019 *CA Cancer J. Clin.* **69** 7–34

[3] Detterbeck F C, Mazzone P J, Naidich D P and Bach P B 2013 Screening for lung cancer *Chest* **143** e78S–92S
[4] Haidekker M A 2013 *Medical Imaging Technology* (New York: Springer)
[5] Paing M P and Choomchuay S 2073 Classification of margin characteristics from 3D pulmonary nodules *2017 10th Biomedical Engineering Int. Conf. (BMEiCON), Hokkaido* pp 1–5
[6] Khan A, Al-Jahdali H, Allen C, Irion K, Al Ghanem S and Koteyar S 2010 The calcified lung nodule: what does it mean? *Ann. Thorac. Med.* **5** 67
[7] Clark K *et al* 2013 The Cancer Imaging Archive (TCIA): maintaining and operating a public information repository *J. Digit. Imaging* **26** 1045–57
[8] Paing M P, Hamamoto K, Tungjitkusolmun S and Pintavirooj C 2019 Automatic detection and staging of lung tumors using locational features and double-staged classifications *Appl. Sci.* **9** 2329
[9] Barnett P G, Ananth L and Gould M K 2010 Cost and outcomes of patients with solitary pulmonary nodules managed with PET scans *Chest* **137** 53–9
[10] Wahidi M M, Govert J A, Goudar R K, Gould M K and McCrory D C 2007 Evidence for the treatment of patients with pulmonary nodules: when is it lung cancer? *Chest* **132** 94S–107S
[11] Brandman S and Ko J P 2011 Pulmonary nodule detection, characterization, and management with multidetector computed tomography *J. Thorac. Imaging* **26** 90–105
[12] Rivera M P, Mehta A C and Wahidi M M 2013 Establishing the diagnosis of lung cancer *Chest* **143** e142S–65S
[13] Kim H, Park C M, Koh J M, Lee S M and Goo J M 2014 Pulmonary subsolid nodules: what radiologists need to know about the imaging features and management strategy *Diagn. Interv. Radiol.* **20** 47–57
[14] Pedersen J H, Saghir Z, Wille M M W, Thomsen L H, Skov B G and Ashraf H 2016 Ground-glass opacity lung nodules in the era of lung cancer CT screening: radiology, pathology, and clinical management *Oncology* **30** 266–74
[15] Evangelista L, Panunzio A, Scagliori E and Sartori P 2018 Ground glass pulmonary nodules: their significance in oncology patients and the role of computer tomography and 18F–fluorodeoxyglucose positron emission tomography *Eur. J. Hybrid Imaging* **2** 2
[16] Migliore M *et al* 2018 Ground glass opacities management in the lung cancer screening era *Ann. Transl. Med.* **6** 90
[17] Yamaguchi T, Ashizawa K, Nagaoki K and Hayashi K 1998 High-resolution CT evaluation of ground-glass opacity in diffuse lung disease *Acta Med. Nagasakiensia* **43** 1–11
[18] Wang J, Ma H, Ni C-J, He J-K, Ma H-T and Ge J-F 2019 Clinical characteristics and prognosis of ground-glass opacity nodules in young patients *J. Thorac. Dis.* **11** 557–63
[19] Naidich D P *et al* 2013 Recommendations for the management of subsolid pulmonary nodules detected at CT: a statement from the Fleischner Society *Radiology* **266** 304–17
[20] Kobayashi Y, Ambrogio C and Mitsudomi T 2018 Ground-glass nodules of the lung in never-smokers and smokers: clinical and genetic insights *Transl. Lung Cancer Res.* **7** 487–97
[21] Seidelman J L, Myers J L and Quint L E 2013 Incidental, subsolid pulmonary nodules at CT: etiology and management *Cancer Imaging* **13** 365–73
[22] Ishida H *et al* 2019 Distinctive clinicopathological features of adenocarcinoma *in situ* and minimally invasive adenocarcinoma of the lung: a retrospective study *Lung Cancer* **129** 16–21

[23] Baldwin D R, Duffy S W, Wald N J, Page R, Hansell D M and Field J K 2011 UK Lung Screen (UKLS) nodule management protocol: modelling of a single screen randomised controlled trial of low-dose CT screening for lung cancer *Thorax* **66** 308–13

[24] Zhao Y *et al* 2012 Performance of computer-aided detection of pulmonary nodules in low-dose CT: comparison with double reading by nodule volume *Eur. Radiol.* **22** 2076–84

[25] Benzakoun J *et al* 2016 Computer-aided diagnosis (CAD) of subsolid nodules: evaluation of a commercial CAD system *Eur. J. Radiol.* **85** 1728–34

[26] Kato Z 2011 Markov random fields in image segmentation *Found. Trends Signal Process.* **5** 1–155

[27] Zhu Y, Tan Y, Hua Y, Zhang G and Zhang J 2012 Automatic segmentation of ground-glass opacities in lung CT images by using Markov random field-based algorithms *J. Digit. Imaging* **25** 409–22

[28] Lee Y, Hara T, Fujita H, Itoh S and Ishigaki T 2001 Automated detection of pulmonary nodules in helical CT images based on an improved template-matching technique *IEEE Trans. Med. Imaging* **20** 595–604

[29] Bastawrous H A, Nitta N and Tsudagawa M 2006 A new CAD system for detecting localized ground glass opacity nodules in lung CT images using cross and coronary section images *IEEE Int. Workshop on Medical Measurement and Applications, 2006. MeMea 2006. (Benevento, Italy)* pp 54–7

[30] Tao Y *et al* 2009 Multi-level ground glass nodule detection and segmentation in CT lung images *Medical Image Computing and Computer-Assisted Intervention—MICCAI 2009* vol 5762 ed G-Z YangG-Z, D Hawkes, D Rueckert, A Noble and C Taylor (Berlin: Springer), pp 715–23

[31] Ye W *et al* 2019 Detection of pulmonary ground-glass opacity based on deep learning computer artificial intelligence *Biomed. Eng. OnLine* **18** 6

Chapter 11

Electromagnetic imaging and lung ablation

Lulu Wang

11.1 Introduction

Lung cancer has been considered the number one public health problem and is associated with a low survival rate [1]. Approximately 80%–85% of lung cancers are non-small cell lung cancer (NSCLC) [2]. The 5-year survival rate of lung cancer remains low (about 15%) [3] due to most lung cancers being diagnosed at an advanced stage [4]. Early diagnosis and appropriate treatment play an important role in improving 5-year survival [5]. The commonly available lung imaging techniques include computed tomography (CT) [6], chest radiography (CRG) [7], and positron emission tomography (PET) [8]. CT is the current standard lung imaging tool, but it is expensive, and produces radiation and allergic reactions to the contrast dye [9]. Regular CT examinations increase the risk of cancers, in particular in children [10]. Although low-dose CT (LDCT) can reduce lung cancer mortality by about 20%, this method has very high false-positive rates [11]. Physicians have applied 18F-fluorodeoxyglucose PET/CT for oncological imaging but this is associated with inaccurate results [12, 13].

Biopsy is another commonly available clinical lung cancer detection method, which is relatively expensive and requires a trained physician [14]. Over the past two decades, biosensor and biomarker based techniques for lung tumor detection have received increasing attention [15, 16]. Proteomic biomarkers have been used within a panel of protein biomarkers, but they are not recommended for individual marker detection. Clinicians cannot obtain sufficient information on cancer cells from the individual marker. In this case, making a clinical decision is challenging. The disadvantages of biomarker based techniques also include their high cost, time-consuming nature, and low sensitivity for low marker concentrations. The disadvantages of biosensor based techniques include small target size, marker levels, and the possibility of high non-specific binding in real patient samples. The obtained experimental results have demonstrated that the available biosensor and biomarker based techniques are still immature for early lung cancer detection [9]. Thus,

doi:10.1088/978-0-7503-2540-0ch11

developing an inexpensive and highly sensitive method for early lung cancer detection is a critical task.

Electromagnetic (EM) imaging has been extensively studied for imaging of human organs such as the lung [17], breast [18], and head [19]. This noninvasive technique aims to image the EM properties (permeability, permittivity, and conductivity) of the target biological object without causing damage. In other words, the technique is highly dependent on the EM properties' contrast between the abnormal tissue and healthy tissue at radio frequencies (RF) [20]. Existing EM imaging approaches can be classified into three groups: electrical impedance tomography (EIT), magnetic induction tomography (MIT), and microwave imaging (MI). EIT aims to map the conductivity distribution of the object, while MIT and MI aim to map the dielectric property distribution of the object. EIT has received much attention over the past few years because it can monitor lung ventilation and perfusion continuously at the bedside [21]. MIT has been considered as an additional or alternative tool to CT for accessing lung diseases due to its advantages of low cost and being less complicated than other medical imaging methods [22]. The recently published clinical studies on microwave breast imaging have proved that MI has the potential to become an alternative or additional imaging tool to mammography for breast cancer detection [23, 24]. Some researchers have recently studied the feasibility of the use of MI for lung cancer detection [25].

Chemotherapy is the primary care method used for lung patients with small cell lung carcinoma (SCLS) [26, 27], and surgical treatments are generally applied for patients with NSCLS [28, 29]. RF ablation and microwave ablation have been applied as tumor control treatments by heating tissues with EM waves [30]. The frequency spectrum of 300 MHz–300 GHz results in a large zone of active heating [31]. Coagulation necrosis occurs when the temperature of 65 °C–160 °C is used in ablation [32]. Microwave ablation is an alternative therapeutic method used for NSCLC patients with high surgery risk [33]. Several clinical studies on microwave ablation and the combination of microwave ablation with chemotherapy have been carried out for the treatment of lung tumors [34–36].

This chapter reviews the recently developed EM-based techniques for the diagnosis and treatment of pulmonary diseases. EM imaging approaches, include EIT, MIT, and MI, are discussed with a particular focus on the diagnosis of pulmonary diseases. Recent developments in RF ablation and microwave ablation for lung tumor treatment are also addressed. Both the advantages and disadvantages as well as future research directions of the EM-based approaches for biomedical applications are discussed in this chapter.

11.2 Electrical impedance tomography

To date, EIT based techniques have been applied to monitor head injuries and diseases [37], lung disease [38], heart disease [39], liver disease [40], and some other diseases.

11.2.1 Working principle

EIT aims to reconstruct the impedance of a target biological object from the measured boundary voltages by injecting a constant voltage or current signals using a voltage source or current source using the sensors. Previous studies have shown that 2D or 3D images of the impedance of the object can be reconstructed using an EIT system with the frequency range of 100 Hz–1 MHz [41, 42]. In an EIT system, an array of sensors (silver chloride electrodes [42] or square metallic patches [43]) are placed on the surface of the object with each sensor inducing eddy currents and recording boundary voltages. Some EIT systems induce voltages and measure current signals [44]. The image quality of EIT is determined mainly by the conductivity of the object and the geometry of the measurement system. EIT based techniques have some advantages, including non-invasiveness, no harmful radiation, low cost, and real-time functional images. Some disadvantages include skin allergies caused by electrodes and low image resolution. Most EIT devices are related to external devices and power amplifiers to produce high-power signals with less noise.

11.2.2 Imaging methods

Imaging reconstruction algorithms of EIT are usually related to solving Maxwell's equations [45, 46]. EIT includes solving forward and inverse problems. Several imaging methods, such as the boundary-element method (BEM), finite-element method (FEM), hybrid FEM BEM, and the Gauss–Newton method, have been developed to solve the forward problem [46].

Various imaging reconstruction methods have been developed for EIT applications [47, 48], including the linearized imaging algorithms and iterative imaging algorithms. However, it seems inadequate to achieve robust time domain EIT images with regularization in the spatial domain [49, 50]. More accurate results could be obtained by applying prior probability in EIT [51]. EIT imaging reconstruction is a nonlinear problem. A generalized inverse operator is usually ill-posed and ill-conditioned. Therefore, the solutions for EIT are not unique and are highly sensitive to measurement noise [52].

Artificial intelligence (AI) has been recently applied in EIT to solve inverse problems to improve image quality [53, 54]. Moreover, noise and modeling errors are non-negligible in clinical measurements. Martin *et al* proposed a new method based on AI and linear approximations to solve the 3D EIT inverse problem [55]. This method combined the benefits of linear and nonlinear approximations. Compared with other inverse problem solvers such as the linear approach, nonlinear iterative, and AI-based inverse solver, the proposed method has the potential to produce high quality, stable, and nonlinear EIT images.

Interoperating the EIT image is a challenging task due to the region above and below the electrodes. This difficulty may be compensated by volumetric EIT images with two or more electrodes. The Graz consensus reconstruction EIT (GREIT) algorithm is a popular reconstruction method used in lung EIT. However, this algorithm produces a 2D image only, which cannot produce accurate results. To solve this limitation, Grychtol *et al* proposed a 3D EIT algorithm based on the

GREIT method and developed an open-source tool to demonstrate that the proposed 3D GREIT algorithm is a function for stimulation and measurement patterns [56]. The proposed algorithm offered significantly more uniform sensitivity profiles through the chest region.

In 2016, Constantin *et al* developed a new EIT method to reliably assess extravascular lung water [57]. In this study, thirty domestic pigs were randomly divided into three categories: no lung injury, acute lung injury, and vascular lung injury. A noninvasive technique using changes in thoracic electrical impedance with lateral body rotation was applied to measure the lung water ratio, which reflected total extravascular lung water. There was a significant correlation between extravascular lung water measured by postmortem gravimetric analysis and EIT. Results have shown that extravascular lung water could be identified by measuring characteristic changes observed by EIT during lateral body rotation. The lung water ratio provided the potential to become a noninvasive method to monitor pulmonary edema at the bedside.

11.2.3 Measurement system

Figure 11.1 shows a schematic design of a typical EIT system that consists of a wave generator, current source, differential amplifier, synchronous voltmeter, two multiplexers, and a control and data storage block. There are 16 electrodes attached to the skin of the subject's body.

The wave generator not only generates a synchronous signal used by the demodulator but also serves as a reference signal of the sinusoidal current source. There are two major types of solutions, which are the analog solution and digital solution. The digital solution has been commonly applied in the newly developed EIT systems. These solutions provide stored samples for digital-to-analog converters. Spectral purity and its signal-to-noise ratio measure the performance of the unit. The current source is driven by a wave generator signal, which is converted into current and injected into the human body through electrodes. The single-ended and floating sources are commonly used in current sources. The single-ended source is an excellent choice for systems with multiple sources, while the floating source is commonly used for systems with a single source. The measurement of resistivity and permittivity values or the resistivity value are necessary to reconstruct the EIT image. Multiplexers are applied to select channels for injecting current and

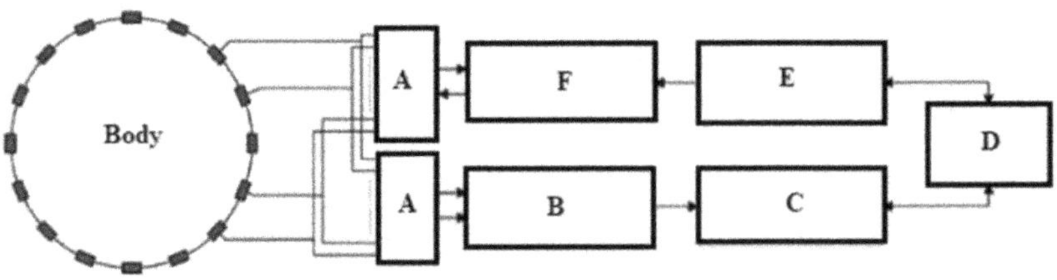

Figure 11.1. A typical EIT system. A: multiplexer; B: differential amplifier; C: synchronous demodulation; D: control and data storage; E: signal and generation; and F: current source.

measuring voltage. Control is necessary to synchronize all other blocks, store the measured data, and transmit it to the computer to display the reconstructed image [58]. Various newly developed EIT systems including IMPETOM, Shield system, open access, 128 element system, and active electrodes have been studied, compared, and reported in [58].

11.2.4 Clinical trails

The clinical application of EIT requires consensus examination, nomenclature, data analysis, and interpretation schemes. In 2014, Van *et al* compared cross-sectional and whole lung volume changes using EIT and respiratory inductive plethysmography (RIP) [59]. EIT and RIP continuously and simultaneously measured the cross-sectional and whole lung volume changes during a stepwise recruitment procedure. Twenty-three infants were involved in this study. Results have demonstrated that the cross-sectional lung volume changes measured by EIT are representative for the whole lung and that this concept also applies to newborn infants.

Krause *et al* conducted a study to determine the value of EIT as an additional monitoring tool to assess regional lung ventilation after pediatric cardiac surgery for congenital heart disease in infants and children [60]. EIT was performed for 30 patients who were mechanically ventilated after cardiac surgery. It has been found that 96.67% of patients could be monitored for regional lung ventilation using EIT.

In 2015, Reinius *et al* conducted a clinical study on the online physiological effects of lung ventilation/capnothorax using EIT [61]. In this study, five piglets were involved. The obtained results confirmed that EIT could detect dynamic changes in real-time during pulmonary ventilation and perfusion distributions.

In 2017, Vogt *et al* applied EIT to evaluate regional lung function in healthy children before and after an exercise challenge [62]. One hundred children between the ages of 74–195 months were involved in this study. The authors compared the results of the studied children with three cystic fibrosis (CF) children. EIT detected the distinctly higher ventilation heterogeneity in the CF children. Research findings have demonstrated that exercise does not affect the global and regional lung functions of healthy children, and exercise does not increase ventilation inhomogeneity.

In 2017, Zhou *et al* developed a monotonicity-based spatiotemporal conductivity imaging for continuous lung monitoring by EIT during inhalation and exhalation [63]. The feasibility of the proposed method for monitoring lung disease has been validated through various simulations, phantom experiments, and human experiments. The proposed method allowed lung EIT to visualize the monotonically varying conductivity distribution during inhalation and exhalation.

The TREND study group conducted a study on how EIT can be used as a powerful tool in clinical decision and therapy planning [64]. The research findings confirmed that EIT has the potential for monitoring patients with chronic lung diseases. Conventional techniques, terminology, coordination, and consensus on EIT application with large multicenter clinical trials are needed to promote the clinical use.

In 2018, Santos *et al* conducted an animal study on whether multi-frequency EIT can provide diagnosis, monitor, and differentiate between pathologies associated with acute respiratory distress syndrome (ARDS) [65]. Seven pigs with ARDS and five healthy pigs were involved in this study. The animals were monitored with multi-frequency EIT. It has been found that the proposed multi-frequency EIT could diagnose lung edema, differentiate this from atelectasis, and monitor their progress over time in terms of global and regional differences.

11.3 Magnetic induction tomography

11.3.1 Working principle

MIT is a relatively new tomographic imaging method that can map all EM properties of a target object. Typical MIT usually aims to map the conductivity of the object, which can be obtained by modeling eddy currents in the forward model and identifying the conductivity in the inverse model. Over the past two decades, various low-conductivity MIT methods have been developed for medical imaging applications [66–69], and several high-conductivity MIT methods have been proposed for industrial applications [70, 71]. Unlike EIT, MIT is a contactless method which does not suffer from poor electrode contact, and it can look better through insulating tissues. Various MIT approaches and systems have been developed for biomedical applications with a particular focus on the diagnosis of diseases, including lung disease [66], brain stroke [67], heart disease [68], and liver disease [69].

11.3.2 Measurement system

A typical MIT system normally consists of several excitation coils and detection coils, interface electronics, and a computer with a matched imaging program. The MIT system applies a magnetic field from an excitation coil to induce eddy currents in the target object which changes the excitation magnetic field distribution, and the backscattered magnetic field from the object is then measured by each detection coil. During imaging data acquisition, each excitation coil induces a primary field in the conductive medium, and the induction of eddy currents accompanies the interaction in the object as the primary field propagates and penetrates the object [9]. The eddy current is changed immediately once the conductivity of the tissue is changed due to the disease, which means the MIT can be applied for biomedical applications with a particular focus on the diagnosis of disease.

Griffiths *et al* developed a single-channel MIT system consisting of one excitation coil and one detection coil with the working frequency of 10 MHz [72]. This MIT system induces eddy currents to the object causing perturbations in the sensed magnetic field, and the detection coil measures the scattering field. This design was improved by applying the back-projection algorithm [73]. However, a long image data collection time was required due to only one channel being available. Therefore, several multi-channel MIT systems have been developed and validated both numerically and experimentally to overcome the limitation of single-channel MIT systems [74, 75].

Watson *et al* developed a 16 channel MIT system to investigate low-conductivity (<10 s m^{-1}) objects at the frequency of 10 MHz [76]. Heterodyne was employed in this system to reduce the received signals to 10 kHz. This 16 channel MIT system was experimentally validated on pipeline phantom and human legs. The proposed system could reconstruct the low-conductivity object. Another multi-channel MIT system was developed using the down-conversion method with a capability of simultaneous parallel readouts [77]. However, noise appeared in the MIT images.

Gürsoy *et al* studied the feasibility of lung imaging using the MIT approach [78]. Various MRI images of a thorax model were applied to reconstruct the lung image using different datasets (static, temporal, and spectral). Results have shown that MIT has the potential for lung imaging. However, the improvement of the design is required before the system can be used in hospitals. Watson *et al* proposed MIT with a phase-stable amplifier for biomedical applications [79]. Using more coils could improve the image quality but increases the cost, complexity, and image data collection time.

Recently, Wang *et al* proposed a single frequency holographic electromagnetic induction (HEI) algorithm for biomedical imaging applications [22]. The proposed method was numerically validated on various realistic thorax models. Small lung tumors with correct size and location information could be successfully obtained in the reconstructed images. The proposed method provided crucial priority information that can be exploited to improve the capabilities of MIT diagnostics methods.

Scharfetter *et al* developed a rotational MIT system which offers better field penetration depth information on the object [80]. The measurement results can easily be affected by the capacitance coupling between coils. Therefore, eliminating capacitive coupling is necessary to provide more accurate results. Although various MIT devices have been proposed, developed, and validated for biomedical imaging applications, they have not been widely used in hospitals and clinics due to limited image resolution and not meeting commercial standards.

11.3.3 HMI imaging algorithm

This section presents the development of the HMI algorithm for imaging of the thorax model [22].

11.3.3.1 Imaging algorithm

As shown in figure 11.2, the HEI system includes a cylindrical tank, a 3D thorax model, an EM source generator, 16 excitation coils, 16 detection coils, and a host computer with the HEI program. All excitation and detection coils are equally placed in circle excitation and detection coil array planes, respectively. The excitation coil array is positioned at the bottom of the tank, and the detection coil array is mounted on the wall of the tank and is designed to be moveable in the *Z*-direction. The chamber is filled with a matching solution medium that helps to measure the scattering field accurately.

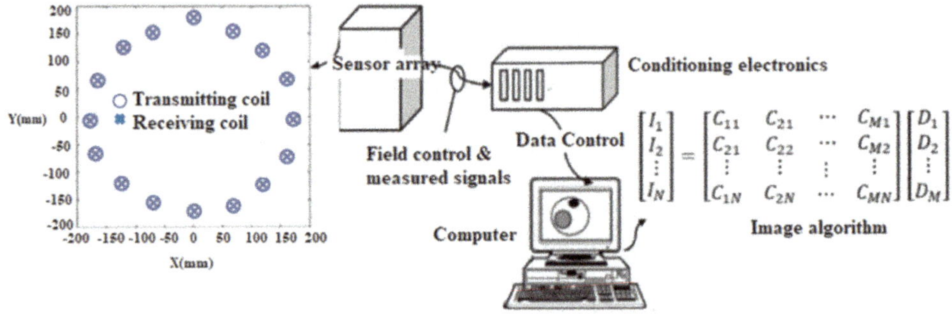

Figure 11.2. HEI system. © [2017] IEEE. Reprinted, with permission, from [22].

As shown in figure 11.3(a), any pair of detection coils measure reflections from the target point P within the thorax model to compute the visibility data that can be applied to reconstruct an image of the thorax model:

$$\vec{M}_{vi}(\vec{r}_i, \vec{r}_j) = \left\langle \vec{M}_{\text{scat}}(\vec{r}_i) \cdot \vec{M}^*_{\text{scat}}(\vec{r}_j) \right\rangle, \tag{11.1}$$

where $\vec{M}_{\text{scat}}(\vec{r}_i)$ and $\vec{M}^*_{\text{scat}}(\vec{r}_j)$ are the scattering magnetic field and the conjugate complex of the scattering magnetic field recorded by coils located at $\vec{r}_i$ and at $\vec{r}_j$, respectively, $\langle\rangle$ means the time average.

Let us define the density distribution of the thorax model:

$$I(\vec{s}) = \left(\frac{j\omega\mu_0}{4\pi}\right)^2 |\sigma(s) + j\omega\varepsilon_0\varepsilon_r - \sigma_{\text{bg}}|^2 \vec{M}_{\text{scat}}(\vec{s}) \cdot \vec{M}^*_{\text{scat}}(\vec{s}), \tag{11.2}$$

where σ_{bg} denotes the background medium conductivity.

The visibility data over the thorax model becomes

$$\begin{aligned} \vec{M}_{vi}(\vec{r}_i, \vec{r}_j) = \left(\frac{j\omega\mu_0}{4\pi}\right)^2 \iiint_V |\sigma(s) + j\omega\varepsilon_0\varepsilon_r - \sigma_{\text{bg}}|^2 \\ \times \vec{M}_{\text{scat}}(\vec{s}) \cdot \vec{M}^*_{\text{scat}}(\vec{s}) \frac{e^{-jk_0(\vec{r}_i - \vec{r}_j)\cdot \hat{s}}}{s^2} dV. \end{aligned} \tag{11.3}$$

Equation (11.1) can be simplified with the combination of equations (11.2) and (11.3):

$$\vec{M}_{vi}(\vec{D}_{ij}) = \iiint_V I(\vec{s}) \frac{e^{-j2\pi\vec{D}_{ij}\cdot\hat{s}}}{s^2} dV, \tag{11.4}$$

where $\vec{D}_{ij} = (\vec{r}_j - \vec{r}_i)/\lambda_b$, λ_b is the background wavelength, $\hat{s} = \sin\theta\cos\phi\hat{\underline{x}} + \sin\theta\sin\phi\hat{\underline{y}} + \cos\theta\hat{\underline{z}}$, $dV = s^2\sin\theta\, d\theta\, d\phi\, ds$. Change Cartesian coordinates to spherical coordinates, and define variables $p = \sin\theta\cos\phi$, $q = \sin\theta\sin\phi$, $n = \cos\theta = \sqrt{1 - p^2 - q^2}$. Then, the element dV can be represented as

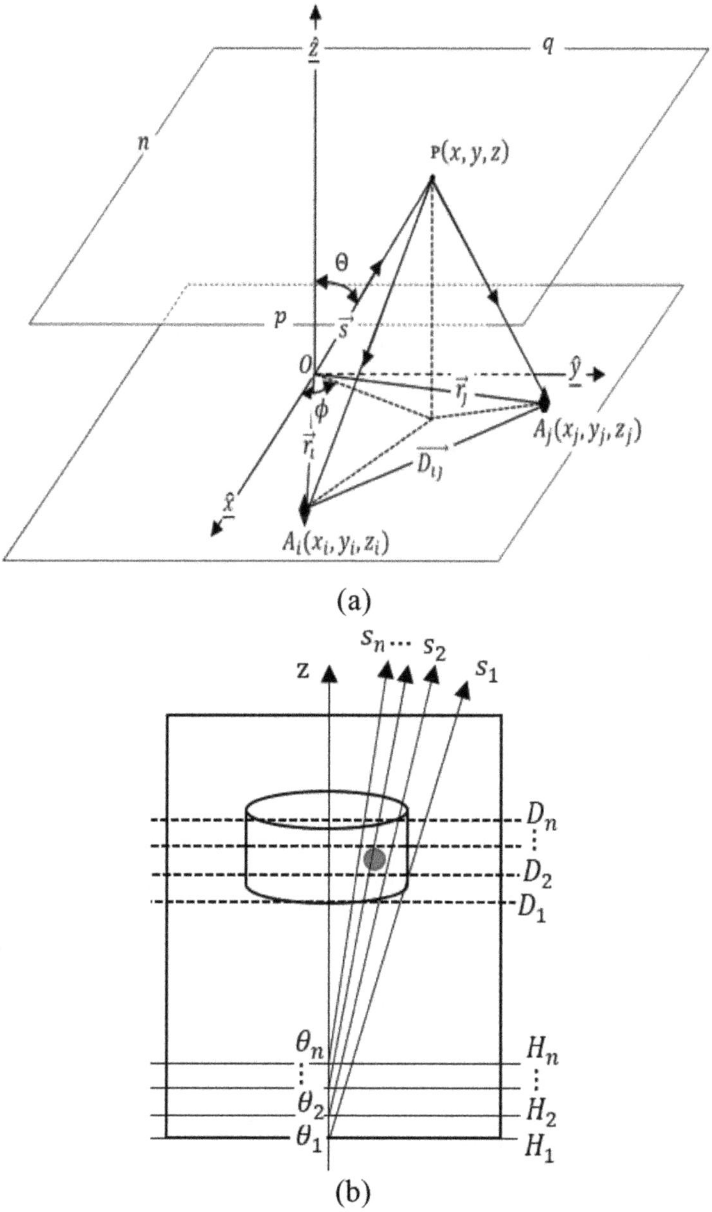

Figure 11.3. (a) A set-up of a pair of HEI detection coils. (b) Side view of coil array plane.

$$dV = s^2\ dp\ dq\ ds/n. \tag{11.5}$$

The visibility function can be simplified as

$$\vec{M}_{vi}(\vec{D}_{ij}) = \iiint_V I(\vec{s})\frac{e^{-j2\pi\vec{D}_{ij}\cdot\hat{s}}}{n}dp\ dq\ ds, \tag{11.6}$$

where $\vec{D}_{ij}$ can be represented by $u_{ij} = (\vec{x}_j - \vec{x}_i)/\lambda_b$, $v_{ij} = (\vec{y}_j - \vec{y}_i)/\lambda_b$, and $w_{ij} = (\vec{z}_j - \vec{z}_i)/\lambda_b$. If the coil array is positioned at a target vertical location, the visibility function can be expressed by the following equation:

$$\vec{M}_{vi}(u_{ij}, v_{ij}, w_{ij}) = \int_p \int_q \int_n \frac{I(s, p, q)}{\sqrt{1 - p^2 - q^2}} e^{(-j2\pi\Phi_{ij})} dp\, dq\, ds, \tag{11.7}$$

where

$$\Phi_{ij} = u_{ij}p + v_{ij}q + w_{ij}n.$$

As all receiving sensors located on a planar plane ($w_{ij} = 0$), the line integral can be obtained:

$$\tilde{I}(p, q) = \int_s \frac{I(s, p, q)}{\sqrt{1 - p^2 - q^2}} ds. \tag{11.8}$$

The visibility function changes to

$$\vec{M}_{vi}(u_{ij}, v_{ij}) = \iint \tilde{I}(p, q) e^{-j2\pi(u_{ij}p + v_{ij}q)} dp\, dq. \tag{11.9}$$

A 2D lung image can be removed by applying the inverse Fourier transform of equation (11.9):

$$\tilde{I}(p, q) = \iint \vec{M}_{vi}(u_{ij}, v_{ij}) e^{j2\pi(u_{ij}p + v_{ij}q)} du\, dv. \tag{11.10}$$

The detection coil array is then repositioned at a new vertical location, and the 2D image data measurement process is repeated until the target object has been fully scanned. Therefore, a 3D lung image can be reconstructed by combining a set of 2D images.

As shown in figure 11.3(b), the information on the depth of lung is obtained:

$$D_n = s_n \cos(\theta_n), \tag{11.11}$$

where θ_n denotes the coil detection angle. Then:

$$dD = \frac{dz}{\cos(\theta_n)} = \frac{dz}{\sqrt{1 - p^2 - q^2}}. \tag{11.12}$$

With the combination of all measured 2D images, when the coil array placed at different vertical positions we can produce a 3D image:

$$dI(\vec{V}_{vi} = z_n, p, q) = \frac{d\tilde{I}(p, q) \cdot \sqrt{1 - p^2 - q^2}}{dz}. \tag{11.13}$$

Equation (11.13) can be rewritten as

$$\frac{d\tilde{I}}{dz} = \frac{\tilde{I}_{z_n} + \tilde{I}_{z_{n-1}}}{z_n + z_{n-1}}. \tag{11.14}$$

It can be seen that the 3D image of the lung can be represented by combining formulas (11.13) and (11.14).

11.3.3.2 Forward model

The time-harmonic vector wave equation was applied in the forward model to solve the electric field:

$$\nabla \times \left(\mu_r^{-1} \nabla \times \vec{E}\right) - k_0^2 \varepsilon_r \vec{E} = -j\omega\mu_0 \vec{J}_s, \tag{11.15}$$

where ∇ denotes the divergence operator, $\mu_r = \mu/\mu_0$, $\varepsilon_r = \frac{\varepsilon}{\varepsilon_0} + \frac{j\sigma}{\varepsilon_0\omega} = \varepsilon' + j\varepsilon''$ with μ_0 and ε_0 are free-space permeability and free-space permittivity and σ the conductivity, $\omega = 2\pi f$, $k_0 = \omega\sqrt{\mu_0\varepsilon_0}$, $\vec{E}$ denotes the electric field, $\vec{E} = \vec{E}_{\text{inc}} + \vec{E}_{\text{scat}}$ with $\vec{E}_{\text{inc}}$ and $\vec{E}_{\text{scat}}$ are the induced and recorded electric field in each coil, $j = \sqrt{-1}$, and $\vec{J}_s$ is the excitation current density in the excitation coil.

The magnetic field strength can be computed as

$$\vec{M} = j(\omega\mu_0\mu_r)^{-1} \cdot (\nabla \times \vec{E}), \tag{11.16}$$

where $\vec{M} = \vec{M}_{\text{inc}} + \vec{M}_{\text{scat}}$ with $\vec{M}_{\text{inc}}$ the magnetic field induced by each excitation coil and $\vec{M}_{\text{scat}}$ the magnetic field recorded by each detection coil.

11.3.3.3 Backward model

The excitation coil array is fixed at the vertical selection location, and each detection coil measures the scattering magnetic field from the object which can be modeled as [22]

$$\vec{M}_{\text{scat}}(\vec{r}_0) = \frac{-j}{4\pi\omega\mu_0} \int_V \left[(\vec{J}_m \cdot \nabla) \times \nabla + k_0^2 \vec{J}_m + j\omega\mu_0 \vec{J}_s \nabla\right] G(\vec{r}, \vec{r}_0) dV, \tag{11.17}$$

where $\vec{r}_0$ and $\vec{r}$ are the vector position from the origin to the point source and the vector position from the detection coil to the point source, respectively, and G means Green's function. We can calculate the induced electric and magnetic current signals as

$$\begin{aligned} \vec{J}_s &= j\omega\varepsilon_0(\varepsilon_r - 1)\vec{E} \\ \vec{J}_m &= j\omega\mu_0(\mu_r - 1)\vec{M}. \end{aligned} \tag{11.18}$$

Formula (11.17) is represented as

$$\vec{M}_{\text{scat}}(\vec{r}_0) = \frac{k_0^2}{4\pi} \int_V [(a\vec{M} + b(\vec{M} \cdot \underline{\hat{r}})\underline{\hat{r}})] G(\vec{r}, \vec{r}_0) dV \tag{11.19}$$

where $\underline{\hat{r}}$ denotes the unit vector, $a = \mu_r\varepsilon_r - \frac{j(\mu_r - 1)}{k_0R}(1 - \frac{j}{k_0R})$, $b = (\mu_r - 1)(-1 + \frac{3j}{k_0R} + \frac{3}{(k_0R)^2})$, R means the distance from the source to the target point. Hence $k_0^2 a \cong -(\mu_r - 1)/R^2$ and $k_0^2 b \cong 3(\mu_r - 1)/R^2$.

The scattering magnetic field can be rewritten as

$$\vec{M}_{\text{scat}}(\vec{r}_0) \cong \frac{1}{4\pi}\int_V \left[\frac{\mu_r - 1}{R^2}(-\vec{M} + 3(\vec{M}\cdot\underline{\hat{r}})\underline{\hat{r}})\right]G(\vec{r}, \vec{r}_0)dV. \tag{11.20}$$

The Born approximation has been used in equation (11.20) when performing a predictive forward model [81].

11.3.3.4 Experiment

Various numerical simulations have been carried out using MATLAB software to validate the proposed HEI method on various realistic thorax models. Two multi-layer thorax models were developed using the published studies of tissues at RF frequencies [82]. The first model is made of seven tissues and a spherical lesion. Model II includes several small lung tumors with arbitrary shapes, sizes, and locations developed using human CT datasets [83]. The working frequency of the HEI system was 10 MHz.

Figure 11.4 shows the thorax model I and its reconstructed images. It can be seen that the internal structure of the model I and target lesion (10 mm in diameter, black square) could be displayed in the reconstructed images.

Figure 11.5 displays thorax model II and its reconstructed images. The internal structure of thorax model II and the lesions could be fully detected in the reconstructed images. Color bars in the thorax models demonstrate the dielectric properties of the model, while in reconstructed images they present scale energy density.

11.4 Microwave imaging

Since the first study on the use of a microwave detector for monitoring pulmonary activity of the dog in 1978 [84], scientists worldwide have extensively studied MI techniques for the diagnosis of diseases such as stroke [85], breast cancer [86–88], and lung cancer [89].

11.4.1 Imaging methods

Existing MI techniques can be classified into three groups: the passive MI, hybrid MI, and active MI approaches. The passive MI techniques identify malignant tumors by relying on the temperature difference between malignant tumors and healthy tissues. The hybrid MI approaches apply microwave waves to illuminate the organ, such as the breast, and measure pressure waves caused by the expansion of heated tumors by ultrasound transducers. The active MI techniques to detect malignant tumors based on the electrical properties contrast between malignant tumors and healthy tissues at microwave frequencies. Three types of active MI

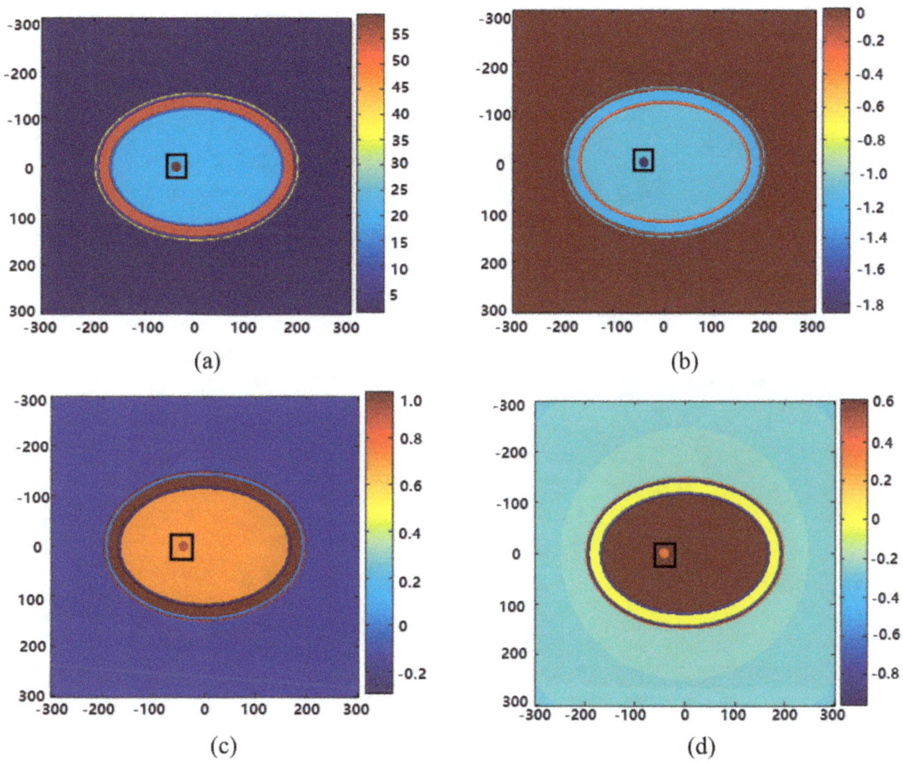

Figure 11.4. Thorax model I: (a) permittivity distributions and (b) conductivity distributions. Reconstructed image of thorax model I: (c) real part and (d) imaginary part.

approaches, including microwave tomography (MT), ultra-wideband (UWB) MI, and holographic MI, have obtained promising results for biomedical applications.

The MT-based techniques seek to reconstruct the electrical properties of the target organ from the measured data by using near-field tomographic imaging methods. The UWB microwave imaging techniques aims to identify the presence and location of significant backscatters such as tumors. One major challenge of MI techniques is to develop a robust reconstruction algorithm that offers high image quality and fewer artifacts. During the past few decades, many imaging algorithms, including the delay-and-sum algorithm [90], microwave imaging via space–time [91], generalized likelihood ratio test [92], finite-difference time-domain (FDTD) [93], time-reversal [94], multistatic adaptive microwave imaging [95], and delay-multiply-and-sum [96], have been developed and validated for MI approaches.

11.4.2 Measurement systems

In 2005, Camacho *et al* proposed an MI method using the FDTD to demonstrate the feasibility of the proposed method for lung cancer detection [97]. They numerically validated the proposed method on the torso model using different frequencies.

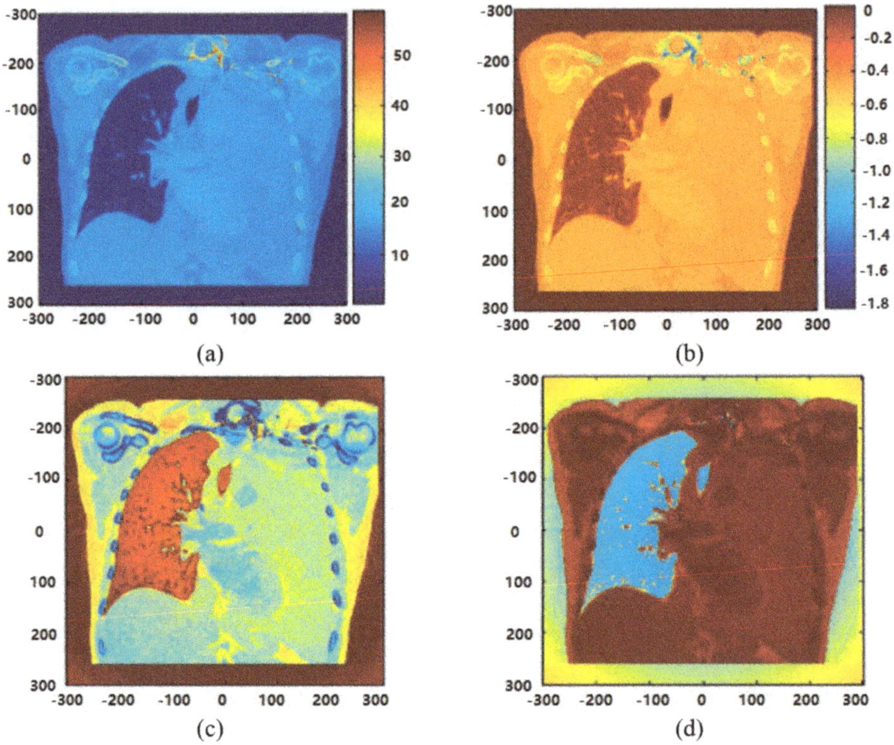

Figure 11.5. Thorax model III: (a) permittivity distributions and (b) conductivity distributions. Reconstructed image of thorax model III: (c) real part and (d) imaginary part. © [2017] IEEE. Reprinted, with permission, from [22].

The proposed MI approach offers promise for the diagnosis of lung cancer, and better results could be achieved at 3 GHz.

In 2015, Zamani *et al* developed a frequency-domain MI for imaging of a torso phantom [89]. An array of 12 slot antennas with fixed locations was placed around the phantom. During image data collection, the phantom was rotated every 30 degrees, each antenna transmitted EM waves to the phantom and recorded the backscattered waves from the phantom in the frequency range 1.5–3 GHz. The authors applied the Bessel function to analyze and reconstruct the image using measured data. The phantom experimental results have confirmed that the frequency-domain MI has the potential for lung cancer detection in the future.

In 2016, Babarinde *et al* studied the feasibility of the use of the confocal MI device with the delay-and-sum imaging method for lung tumor detection in a frequency range of 3–5 GHz [98]. Phantom experimental results have proved that the proposed MI approach has the ability to detect lung tumors. However, more investigations, including developing an improved imaging algorithm to reduce image noise and evaluate the proposed technique on a more realistic phantom, are required in the future.

11.5 Lung ablation

Approximately 33% of patients with NSCLC are unresectable. Thus, it is necessary to develop an ablation technique for the treatment of primary lung cancer [99]. The thermal ablation technique has been widely applied in the treatment of lung cancer with primary and secondary thoracic malignancies. RF ablation and microwave ablation are the commonly available ablation techniques for tissue heating, and have been applied to treat disease, including in the lung [100], kidney [101], liver [102], and bone [103]. RF ablation is the predominant ablation method. During RF ablation, electrodes and grounding pads are placed on the patients' legs, and a sinusoidal current of frequency 400–500 kHz is passed through the tissue. It is well known that coagulation and cell death are induced when the temperature is 50 °C–60 °C, and protein denaturation occurs when the temperature is higher than 60 °C. Microwave ablation utilizes the frequency range of 915 MHz to 2.45 GHz for tissue heating, which is much higher than that of RF ablation.

Compared with RF ablation, microwave ablation offers several advantages include enlarged ablation zones, shorter ablation times, and fewer heat-sink effects [104]. Microwave ablation may lead to some significant complications. Therefore, some researchers have studied the risks for major complications after microwave ablation [105, 106]. The research group from Shandong University has performed microwave lung ablation on 253 lesions during 2011–13 [107]. Research outcomes have proved that microwave lung ablation could induce severe complications. Clinicians should pay more attention to patients with emphysema, subpleural, or large target tumor.

In 2015, Wei *et al* reported their clinical studies on whether the combination of microwave ablation with chemotherapy can improve treatment outcomes for thirty-nine patients with advanced NSCLC [108]. The clinical results have shown that there is no correlation between microwave ablation and chemotherapy. For chemotherapy, 28.2% of patients achieved a partial response, 46.2% of them showed stable disease, and 25.6% of patients had progressive disease. 56.4% of patients had complications, and 7.9% of patients had grade 3 adverse events.

Clinical studies have demonstrated that thermal ablation obtains similar results with sublobar resection, and ablation has an advantage in unfit patients [109]. RF ablation offered a 5-year control rate of 58%–68% compared to 83.0%–89.5% with stereotactic ablative therapy [110]. Stereotactic ablative therapy produced better overall survival (38%–84.7%) and cancer-specific survival (64%–88%) with 3-year overall survival [110]. However, the overall survival of RF ablation was 47%–74% [110]. Furthermore, the post-procedural morbidity was higher for RF ablation at 33%–100%, mainly owing to the incidence of pneumothorax. Hiraki *et al* reported a similar research conclusion with RF ablation in NSCLC [111]. RF ablation might be the right choice for patients with early-stage NSCLC who are unfit for surgery or sublobar lung resection.

11.6 Current trends and future perspectives

The available EM imaging techniques offer the potential for lung cancer detection. MIT has been recommended as an additional or alternative method to CT for lung disease detection, but it has some challenges such as high computational cost, leak of realistic phantoms, complicated clinical application devices, and limited image resolution. Therefore, developing a high dynamic MIT device is urgently needed. The image quality of MIT could be improved using more coils, but this also produces more coupling noises between coils. In addition, using more coils also increases the total computational cost, scanning time, and device complexities. Recent studies have proved that optimization of coil arrays may overcome some limitations of the current MIT approaches, and a suitable coil array configuration provides benefits in terms of high image resolution, inexpensive systems, and short data collection times. Moreover, the complexity of the device may be improved by applying the multiple in a multiple out technique. In the future, scientists and engineers should pay more attention to developing a robust image algorithm and clinically applicable device as well as experimental validations of the proposed theory and device on more realistic thorax phantoms and human subjects. The risks for significant complications after EM imaging approaches should be another research direction.

11.7 Conclusion

This chapter reviewed the up-to-date status of research in EM modalities for lung disease diagnosis and therapy. Recent developments in biomedical imaging techniques, including CT, PET, EIT, MIT, and MI based approaches, were discussed with particular focus on the diagnosis of lung disease. Clinical trials of EIT and MIT for the diagnosis of lung diseases have proved that EM imaging technique have the potential to become a cost-effective and low-risk tool for lung disease detection. EM imaging techniques show a high potential to improve the diagnosis of lung disease. Some RF lung ablation and microwave lung ablation techniques were also reviewed. RF and microwave ablation techniques may offer excellent treatment opportunities for patients with early-stage NSCLC who are unfit for surgery or sublobar lung resection.

To data, EM techniques still face some challenges and disadvantages that need to be solved before they can be introduced into wide-scale utilization in clinics. Integrating more than one EM technique has shown the potential to resolve some of these limitations. In the future, researchers should pay more attention to several areas, including robust imaging algorithms, compact and clinical applicable devices, realistic phantoms, and experimental clinical validation studies, to improve the EM imaging-based techniques.

Acknowledgments

The author gratefully acknowledges the financial support from the National Natural Science Foundation of China (grant No. 61701159).

References

[1] Tammemägi M C 2015 Application of risk prediction models to lung cancer screening a review *J. Thorac. Imaging* **30** 88–100

[2] Lee C B, Stinchcombe T E, Rosenman J G and Socinski M A 2007 Therapeutic advances in local-regional therapy for stage II non-small-cell lung cancer: evolving role of dose-escalated conformal (3-dimensional) radiation therapy *Clin. Lung Cancer* **8** 195–202

[3] Jemal A *et al* 2005 Cancer statistics *CA Cancer J. Clin.* **55** 10–30

[4] Ruiz M and Ramirez R A 2015 Lung cancer in HIV-infected patients and the role of targeted therapy *J. Community Support. Oncol.* **13** 282

[5] Ryo M and Junji Y 2011 Lung cancer—CT screening for lung cancer dramatically improved survival after surgical resection *Gan to Kagaku Ryoho (Cancer Chemother.)* **38** 197–201

[6] Li X, Dong X, Lian J, Zhang Y and Yu J 2019 Knockoff filter-based feature selection for discrimination of non-small cell lung cancer in CT image *IET Image Process.* **13** 543–8

[7] Moore W, Riptonsnyder J, Wu G and Hendler C 2011 Sensitivity and specificity of a CAD solution for lung nodule detection on chest radiograph with CTA correlation *J. Digit. Imaging* **24** 405–10

[8] Chien C R, Liang J A, Wang H N, Lin C C and Kao C H 2011 Diagnostic performance of selective positron emission tomography for lung cancer computed tomography screening: a meta-analysis *Eur. J. Cancer* **47** S211

[9] Wang L 2017 Screening and biosensor-based approaches for lung cancer detection *Sensors* **17** 2420

[10] Journy N, Rehel J L, Pointe H D L, Lee C, Brisse H, Chateil J F, Caer-Lorho S, Laurier D and Bernier M O 2015 Are the studies on cancer risk from CT scans biased by indication? Elements of answer from a large-scale cohort study in France *Br. J. Cancer* **112** 1841–2

[11] Church T R *et al* 2013 Results of initial low-dose computed tomographic screening for lung cancer *N. Engl. J. Med.* **368** 1980–91

[12] Chicklore S, Goh V, Siddique M, Roy A, Marsden P K and Cook G J R 2013 Quantifying tumour heterogeneity in F-18-FDG PET/CT imaging by texture analysis *Eur. J. Nucl. Med. Mol. Imaging* **40** 133–40

[13] Ippolito D, Capraro C, Guerra L, De Ponti E, Messa C and Sironi S 2013 Feasibility of perfusion CT technique integrated into conventional (18) FDG/PET-CT studies in lung cancer patients: clinical staging and functional information in a single study *Eur. J. Nucl. Med. Mol. Imaging* **40** 156–65

[14] Cheng B Y 2016 Development of a chemiluminescent immunoassay for cancer antigen 15-3 *Labeled Immunoassay Clin. Med.* **23** 1348–51

[15] Lizuka S, Taniguchi N and Makita A 1984 Enzyme-linked immunosorbent assay for human manganese-containing superoxide dismutase and its content in lung cancer *J. Natl. Cancer Inst.* **72** 1043–9

[16] Eftekhari-Sis B, Aliabad M A and Karimi F 2016 Graphene oxide based nano-biosensor for the detection of deletion mutation in exon 19 of EGFR gene, leading to lung cancer *Mater. Lett.* **183** 441–3

[17] Gex G, Pralong J A, Combescure C, Seijo L, Rochat T and Soccal P M 2014 Diagnostic yield and safety of electromagnetic navigation bronchoscopy for lung nodules: a systematic review and meta-analysis *Respiration* **87** 165

[18] Poplack S P *et al* 2007 Electromagnetic breast imaging: results of a pilot study in women with abnormal mammograms *Radiology* **243** 350–9

[19] Acar Z A and Makeig S 2010 Neuroelectromagnetic forward head modeling toolbox *J. Neurosci. Methods* **190** 258–70

[20] Hassan A M and El-Shenawee M 2011 Review of electromagnetic techniques for breast cancer detection *IEEE Rev. Biomed. Eng.* **4** 103–18

[21] Richard J C, Pouzot C, Gros A, Tourevieille C, Lebars D and Lavenne F 2009 Electrical impedance tomography compared to positron emission tomography for the measurement of regional lung ventilation: an experimental study *Crit. Care* **13** R82

[22] Wang L and Aljumaily A M 2017 Imaging of lung structure using holographic electromagnetic induction *IEEE Access* **5** 20313–8

[23] Meaney P M *et al* 2017 Initial clinical experience with microwave breast imaging in women with normal mammography *Acad. Radiol.* **14** 207–18

[24] O'Loughlin D, O'Halloran M J, Moloney B M, Glavin M, Jones E and Elahi M A 2018 Microwave breast imaging: clinical advances and remaining challenges *IEEE Trans. Biomed. Eng.* **65** 2580–90

[25] Babarinde O J, Jamlos M F and Ramli N B 2014 UWB microwave imaging of the lungs: a review *IEEE Int. Symp. on Telecommunication Technologies* pp 188–93

[26] Hara N, Ichinose Y, Motohiro A, Noge S, Miyake J, Ohta M and Hata K 1986 Combination chemotherapy and radiation therapy for small cell carcinoma of the lung *Gan Kagaku Ryoho Cancer Chemother.* **13** 80–5

[27] George S, Schell M J, Detterbeck F C and Socinski M A 1998 Adjuvant chemotherapy for resected non-small cell carcinoma of the lung: why we still don't know *Oncologist* **3** 35–44

[28] Stamatis G, Eberhard W and Pöttgen C 2004 Surgery after multimodality treatment for non-small-cell lung cancer *Lung Cancer* **45** S107–12

[29] Abdel-Rahman O 2018 Outcomes of surgery as part of the management of metastatic non-small-cell lung cancer: a surveillance, epidemiology and end results database analysis *Cancer Invest.* **36** 238–45

[30] Healey T T, March B T, Baird G and Dupuy D E 2017 Microwave ablation for lung neoplasms: a retrospective analysis of long-term results *J. Vasc. Interv. Radiol.* **28** 206–11

[31] Lee W K, Lau E W F, Chin K, Sedlaczek O and Steinke K 2013 Modern diagnostic and therapeutic interventional radiology in lung cancer *J. Thorac. Dis.* **5** S511–23

[32] Goldberg S N, Stein M C, Gazelle G S, Sheiman R G, Kruskal J B and Clouse M E 1999 Percutaneous radiofrequency tissue ablation: optimization of pulsed-radiofrequency technique to increase coagulation necrosis *J. Vasc. Interv. Radiol.* **10** 907–16

[33] Dupuy D *et al* 2013 Radiofrequency ablation of stage 1A NSCLC in medically inoperable patients: results from ACOSOG Z4033 (Alliance), an NCI funded multicenter trial *Chest* **144** 86A

[34] Yang X *et al* 2018 Microwave ablation for lung cancer patients with a single lung: clinical evaluation of 11 cases *Thorac. Cancer* **9** 548–54

[35] Wei Z *et al* 2015 Microwave ablation in combination with chemotherapy for the treatment of advanced non-small cell lung cancer *Cardiovasc. Interv. Radiol.* **38** 135–42

[36] Sun Y H *et al* 2015 Effects of microwave ablation or its combination with whole-body chemotherapy on serum vascular endothelial growth factor levels in patients with stage IIIB/IV NSCLC *Genet. Mol. Res.* **14** 10015–25

[37] Hopfer M, Planas R, Hamidipour A, Henriksson T and Semenov S 2017 Electromagnetic tomography for detection, differentiation, and monitoring of brain stroke: a virtual data and human head phantom study *IEEE Antennas Propag. Magn.* **59** 86–97

[38] Makris D *et al* 2007 Electromagnetic navigation diagnostic bronchoscopy for small peripheral lung lesions *Eur. Respir. J.* **29** 1187–92

[39] Fred G 2001 Cardiac electromagnetic imaging as an inverse problem *Electromagnetics* **21** 559–77

[40] Banovac F, Wilson E, Zhang H and Cleary K 2006 Needle biopsy of anatomically unfavorable liver lesions with an electromagnetic navigation assist device in a computed tomography environment *J. Vasc. Interv. Radiol.* **17** 1671–5

[41] Kalager M, Zelen M, Langmark F and Adami H O 2010 Effect of screening mammography on breast-cancer mortality in Norway *N. Engl. J. Med.* **363** 1203–10

[42] Kerner T E, Paulsen K D, Hartov A, Soho S K and Poplack S P 2002 Electrical impedance spectroscopy of the breast: clinical imaging results in 26 subjects *IEEE Trans. Med. Imaging* **21** 638–45

[43] Boverman G, Kao T J, Kulkarni R, Kim B S, Isaacson D, Saulnier G J and Newell J C 2008 Robust linearized image reconstruction for multifrequency EIT of the breast *IEEE Trans. Med. Imaging* **27** 1439–48

[44] Boverman G, Isaacson D, Saulnier G J and Newell J C 2009 Methods for compensating for variable electrode contact in EIT *IEEE Trans. Biomed. Eng.* **56** 2762–72

[45] Luís A M M, Sturler E D, Paulino G H and Emílio C N S 2010 Recycling Krylov subspaces for efficient large-scale electrical impedance tomography *Comput. Method Appl. Mech. Eng.* **199** 3101–10

[46] Lionheart W R 2004 EIT reconstruction algorithms: pitfalls, challenges and recent developments *Physiol. Meas.* **25** 125–42

[47] Kang S I, Khambampati A K, Kim B S and Kim K Y 2017 EIT image reconstruction for two-phase flow monitoring using a sub-domain based regularization method *Flow Meas. Instrum.* **53** 28–38

[48] Kang S I, Khambampati A K, Kim B S and Kim K Y 2016 A sub-domain based regularization method with prior information for human thorax imaging using electrical impedance tomography *Meas. Sci. Technol.* **27** 025703

[49] Gong B, Schullcke B, Krueger-Ziolek S, Zhang F, Mueller-Lisse U and Moeller K 2018 Higher order total variation regularization for EIT reconstruction *Med. Biol. Eng. Comput.* **5** 1–12

[50] Goharian M, Bruwer M J, Jegatheesan A, Moran G R and Macgregor J F 2007 A novel approach for EIT regularization via spatial and spectral principal component analysis *Physiol. Meas.* **28** 1001–16

[51] Dunlop M M and Stuart A M 2016 The Bayesian formulation of EIT: analysis and algorithms *Inverse Probl. Imaging* **10** 1007–36

[52] Oh S, Tang T and Sadleir R 2007 Quantitative analysis of shape change in electrical impedance tomography (EIT) *13th Int. Conf. on Electrical Bioimpedance and the 8th Conf. on Electrical Impedance Tomography* **vol 17** 424–7

[53] Nan G F 2004 Neural network models for electrical impedance tomography *Pattern Recogn. Artif. Intell.* **17** 94–7

[54] Sébastien M and Choi C T M 2017 A novel post-processing scheme for two-dimensional electrical impedance tomography based on artificial neural networks *PLoS One* **12** e0188993

[55] Martin S and Choi C T M 2017 A new divide-and-conquer method for 3-D electrical impedance tomography *IEEE Trans. Magn.* **54** 17596167

[56] Grychtol B, Müller B and Adler A 2016 3D EIT image reconstruction with GREIT *Physiol. Meas.* **37** 785–800

[57] Constantin J C T, Charles R P, Josep S, Andy A, Sebastian A, Michael R, Stephan H B and Daniel A R 2016 Electrical impedance tomography (EIT) for quantification of pulmonary edema in acute lung injury *Crit. Care* **20** 18

[58] Santos E and Simini F 2012 Electrical impedance tomography for pulmonary oedema extent monitoring: review and updated design *J. Phys. Conf. Ser.* **407** 012024

[59] Van D B P S, Miedema M, De Jongh F H, Frerichs I and Van Kaam A H 2014 Cross-sectional changes in lung volume measured by electrical impedance tomography are representative for the whole lung in ventilated preterm infants *Crit. Care Med.* **42** 1524–30

[60] Krause U, Becker K, Günter H, Dittmar J, Ruschewski W and Paul T 2014 Monitoring of regional lung ventilation using electrical impedance tomography after cardiac surgery in infants and children *Pediatr. Cardiol.* **35** 990–7

[61] Reinius H *et al* 2015 Real-time ventilation and perfusion distributions by electrical impedance tomography during one-lung ventilation with capnothorax *Acta Anaesthesiol. Scand.* **59** 354–68

[62] Vogt B *et al* 2017 Regional lung function testing in children using electrical impedance tomography *Pediatr. Pulmonol.* **53** 293–301

[63] Zhou L, Harrach B and Seo J K 2018 Monotonicity-based electrical impedance tomography for lung imaging *Inverse Prob.* **34** 045005

[64] Frerichs I *et al* 2017 Chest electrical impedance tomography examination, data analysis, terminology, clinical use and recommendations: consensus statement of the translational EIT development study group *Thorax* **72** 83–93

[65] Santos S A, Czaplik M, Orschulik J, Hochhausen N and Leonhardt S 2018 Lung pathologies analyzed with multi-frequency electrical impedance tomography: pilot animal study *Respir. Physiol. Neurobiol.* **254** 1–9

[66] Gürsoy D and Scharfetter H 2010 Anisotropic conductivity tensor imaging using magnetic induction tomography *Physiol. Meas.* **31** S135–45

[67] Liu R, Li Y, Fu F, You F, Shi X and Dong X 2014 Time-difference imaging of magnetic induction tomography in a three-layer brain physical phantom *Meas. Sci. Technol.* **25** 065402

[68] Marmugi L and Renzoni F 2016 Optical magnetic induction tomography of the heart *Sci. Rep.* **6** 23962

[69] Hu G, Cressman E and He B 2011 Magnetoacoustic imaging of human liver tumor with magnetic induction *Appl. Phys. Lett.* **98** 023703

[70] Watson S *et al* 2007 Developments in magnetic induction tomography for oil-industry applications *Mater. Sci. Technol.* **47** 22–7

[71] Zakaria Z *et al* 2013 Magnetic induction tomography: a review on the potential application in agricultural industry of Malaysia *J. Agric. Sci.* **5** 78–82

[72] Griffiths H, Stewart W R and Gough W 1999 Magnetic induction tomography: a measuring system for biological tissues *Ann. NY Acad. Sci.* **873** 335–45

[73] Ke L, Lin X and Du Q 2013 An improved back-projection algorithm for magnetic induction tomography image reconstruction *Adv. Mater. Res.* **647** 630–5

[74] Xu Z, Luo H, He W, He C, Song X and Zahng Z 2009 A multi-channel magnetic induction tomography measurement system for human brain model imaging *Physiol. Meas.* **30** S175–86

[75] Ran P, Xiao X, He W and Li Z 2015 Biological impedance cross evaluation and imaging from composite measurements of magnetic and electrical methods *Bio-Med. Mater. Eng.* **26** S1695

[76] Watson S, Williams R J, Gough W and Griffiths H 2008 A magnetic induction tomography system for samples with conductivities below 10 Sm^{-1} *Meas. Sci. Technol.* **19** 45501
[77] Hamsch M, Igney C H and Vauhkonen M 2007 16 channel magnetic induction tomography system featuring parallel readout *13th Int. Conf. on Electrical Bioimpedance and the 8th Conf. on Electrical Impedance Tomography* (Berlin: Springer)
[78] Gürsoy D and Scharfetter H 2009 Feasibility of lung imaging using magnetic induction tomography *World Congress on Medical Physics and Biomedical Engineering* (Berlin: Springer)
[79] Watson S, Wee H C, Griffiths H and Williams R J 2011 A highly phase-stable differential detector amplifier for magnetic induction tomography *Physiol. Meas.* **32** 917–26
[80] Scharfetter H, Merwa R and Pilz K 2005 A new type of gradiometer for the receiving circuit of magnetic induction tomography (MIT) *Physiol. Meas.* **26** S307–18
[81] Born M, Wolf E and Hecht E 1975 *Principles of Optics: Electromagnetic Theory of Propagation, Interference and Diffraction of Light* (New York: Pergamon)
[82] Italian National Research Council 2019 *An Internet Resource for the Calculation of the Dielectric Properties of Body Tissues in the Frequency Range 10 Hz–100 GHz* http://niremf.ifac.cnr.it/tissprop (Accessed: 1 August 2019)
[83] ELCAP Public Lung Image Database 2019 http://via.cornell.edu/lungdb.html (Accessed: 1 August 2019)
[84] Pedersen P C, Johnson C C, Durney C H and Bragg D G 1978 Microwave reflection and transmission measurements for pulmonary diagnosis and monitoring *IEEE Trans. Bio-med. Eng.* **25** 40–8
[85] Bialkowski K, Ireland D and Abbosh A 2013 Microwave imaging for brain stroke detection using born iterative method *IET Microwaves Antennas Propag.* **7** 909–15
[86] Kwon S, Son S and Lee K 2018 Experimental demonstration of in CC lace calibration for time domain microwave imaging system *Radio Sci.* **53** 429–39
[87] Zarnaghi Naghsh N, Ghorbani A and Amindavar H 2018 Compressive sensing for microwave breast cancer imaging *IET Signal Proc.* **12** 242–6
[88] Santis V D, Sill J M, Bourqui J and Fear E C 2012 Safety assessment of ultra-wideband antennas for microwave breast imaging *Bioelectromagnetics* **33** 215–25
[89] Zamani A, Rezaeieh S A and Abbosh A M 2015 Lung cancer detection using frequency-domain microwave imaging *Electron. Lett.* **51** 740–41
[90] Lim H B, Nhung N T, Li E P and Thang N D 2008 Confocal microwave imaging for breast cancer detection: delay-multiply-and-sum image reconstruction algorithm *IEEE Trans. Biomed. Eng.* **55** 1697–704
[91] Davis S K *et al* 2003 Microwave imaging via space–time beamforming for early detection of breast cancer: beamformer design in the frequency domain *J. Electromagn. Waves Appl.* **17** 357–81
[92] Davis S K, Tandradinata H, Hagness S C and Van Veen B D 2005 Ultrawideband microwave breast cancer detection: a detection-theoretic approach using the generalized likelihood ratio test *IEEE Trans. Biomed. Eng.* **52** 1237–50
[93] Bardak C and Saed M 2014 Microwave imaging with a time-reversed finite-difference time-domain technique *J. Electromagn. Waves Appl.* **28** 1455–67
[94] Hossain M D, Mohan A S and Abedin M J 2013 Beamspace time-reversal microwave imaging for breast cancer detection *IEEE Antennas Wirel. Propag. Lett.* **12** 241–4

[95] Xie Y *et al* 2006 Novel multistatic adaptive microwave imaging methods for early breast cancer detection *EURASIP J. Appl. Signal Process.* **2006** 091961
[96] Elahi M A *et al* 2017 Adaptive artifact removal for selective multistatic microwave breast imaging signals *Biomed. Signal Process. Control* **34** 93–100
[97] Camacho L M and Tjuatja S 2005 FDTD simulation of microwave scattering from a lung tumor *IEEE Antennas and Propagation Society Int. Symp.*
[98] Babarinde O J, Jamlos M F, Soh P J, Schreurs D M M P and Beyer A 2016 Microwave imaging technique for lung tumour detection *IEEE Microwave Conf.*
[99] Smith S L and Jennings P E 2015 Lung radiofrequency and microwave ablation: a review of indications, techniques and post-procedural imaging appearances *Br. J. Radiol.* **88** 20140598
[100] Rakovich G, Carignan S, Caty V and Bujold A 2018 Thoracoscopic ultrasound-guided radiofrequency ablation for lung cancer *Canadian J. Respir. Crit. Care Sleep Med.* **2** 84–6
[101] Kelly E F and Leveillee R J 2018 Image guided radiofrequency ablation for small renal masses *Int. J. Surg.* **36** 525–32
[102] Cirimbei C, Rotaru V, Chitoran E, Pavaleanu O and Cirimbei S E 2017 Immediate and long-term results of radiofrequency ablation for colorectal liver metastases *Anticancer Res.* **37** 6489–94
[103] Dierselhuis E F, Jutte P C, Eerden P J M V D, Suurmeijer A J H and Bulstra S K 2010 Hip fracture after radiofrequency ablation therapy for bone tumors: two case reports *Skeletal Radiol.* **39** 1139–43
[104] Huang S J, Yu J and Liang P 2014 Percutaneous microwave ablation for liver tumors adjacent to large vessels *Microwave Ablation Treatment of Solid Tumors* 79–87
[105] Splatt A M and Steinke K 2015 Major complications of high-energy microwave ablation for percutaneous CT-guided treatment of lung malignancies: single-centre experience after 4 years *J. Med. Imaging Radiat. Oncol.* **59** 609–16
[106] Carrafiello G *et al* 2012 Complications of microwave and radiofrequency lung ablation: personal experience and review of the literature *Radiol. Med.* **117** 201–13
[107] Zheng A *et al* 2014 Major complications after lung microwave ablation: a single-center experience on 204 sessions *Ann. Thorac. Surg.* **98** 243–8
[108] Wei Z, Ye X, Yang X, Zheng A, Huang G, Li W, Ni X, Wang J and Han X 2015 Microwave ablation in combination with chemotherapy for the treatment of advanced non-small cell lung cancer *Cardiovasc. Intervent. Radiol.* **38** 135–42
[109] Kwan S W, Mortell K E, Talenfeld A D and Brunner M C 2014 Thermal ablation matches sublobar resection outcomes in older patients with early-stage non-small cell lung cancer *J. Vasc. Interv. Radiol.* **25** 1–9.e1
[110] Renaud S, Falcoz P E, Olland A and Massard G 2013 Is radiofrequency ablation or stereotactic ablative radiotherapy the best treatment for radically treatable primary lung cancer unfit for surgery? *Interact. Cardiovasc. Thorac. Surg.* **16** 68–73
[111] Hiraki T *et al* 2006 Risk factors for local progression after percutaneous radiofrequency ablation of lung tumors: evaluation based on a preliminary review of 342 tumors *Cancer* **107** 2873–80

Lightning Source UK Ltd.
Milton Keynes UK
UKHW051303020220
358013UK00003B/38

9 780750 325387